AF512719

A Complete Guide to
HOMEOPATHY

"Alan Schmukler has gifted us with a survival kit packed full of vital and usable information, helpful tips, delightful tidbits, and, best of all, hope and empowerment. With this work, homeopathy has indeed become medicine for the people's liberation."

—Lucille Balukian
President, Citizen's Alliance for
Progressive Health Awareness (CAPHA)
Editor, Progressive Health

"Alan Schmukler has an amazing ability to bring homeopathy to life in a clear and precise way. This book is valuable to the novice as well as the most experienced homeopath. I feel it is the best overview of homeopathy I have seen and will recommend it to all my patients!"

—Beth Rotondo, HCE
Homeopathic consultant and educator
Fourth-generation homeopath and mother of five

A Complete Guide to
HOMEOPATHY

Alan V. Schmukler

New Age Books

ISBN: 978-81-7822-302-5

First Indian Edition: Delhi, 2007

Reprinted from 'Homeopathy: An A to Z Home Handbook'
Published by Llewellyn Publications Woodbury, MN 55125 USA
www.llewellyn.com

© 2006 by Alan V. Schmukler

All rights reserved. No part of this publication may be reproduced or transmitted in any form or by any means, electronic or mechanical, including photocopying, recording, or by any information storage and retrieval system, without permission in writing from the publishers.

Published by
NEW AGE BOOKS
A-44 Naraina Industrial Area, Phase-I
New Delhi 110 028
INDIA
Email: nab@vsnl.in
Website: www.newagebooksindia.com

Printed in India
at Shri Jainendra Press
A-45 Naraina Phase-I
New Delhi 110 028
INDIA

Contents

Acknowledgments

I want to thank all those people who inspired, assisted, taught, and healed me over the years. Deep appreciation to Dr. Henry Williams, Beth Rotondo, Dr. Lance Wright, Dr. Luelle Hamilton, Dr. William Block, Dr. Bernardo Merizalde, Dr. Bonnie Bennett, Bernie Havilland, Lucille Balukian, Richard Salloum, Richard Levey, Judy Mendelsohn-Mackey, Marie Ruxton, Alice Schwartz, Ronald Gonski, Elaine Lewis, Janice Zalewski, Michael and Penny Zalewski, Shelley Epstein VMD, Deva Khalsa VMD, Dorothy Montgomery, Gorby Montgomery, and Rose Schmukler, my mother.

This book has been prepared using a wide variety of sources. Due to the nature of these sources and in the interest of preserving the text's readability, I have opted not to annotate individual citations. Instead, I would like to direct readers to the bibliography, which includes all materials used for my research.

The information in this book is based on the teachings of homeopathic physicians over the last two hundred years. It is for educational purposes and is not intended to replace services of health care professionals. It does not constitute medical advice or medical opinion.

Introduction

About sixteen years ago I developed an abscess in the root of a tooth. Both a dentist and a doctor insisted on antibiotics, in spite of the fact that I do badly on them. A friend suggested I try a homeopath. The homeopath was not alarmed and handed me some little pills made from oyster shells. In a couple of hours the pain was gone, and in a few days the infection disappeared.

Millions of people are suffering needlessly because they don't know about homeopathy, don't believe in it, or because it isn't covered by their health insurance.

Every day people die from falls, auto accidents, allergic reactions, heart attacks, or shock. Many of those lives could have been be saved for eight cents' worth of homeopathic remedy, administered by someone who has read this book.

I've taught homeopathy to hundreds of people, most of whom had no medical training. They can now ease pain and suffering in many instances, without rushing to a doctor.

My mother is ninety years old. About ten years ago, I bought her a kit of remedies. For the first couple months, she would call and ask what remedy to use. Now she calls to tell me what she took and how great it worked.

Laypeople can use homeopathy for treating injuries and acute ailments, and for preventing illness. By following a few basic rules, anyone can use homeopathy safely. (See "Rules for Using Remedies" in chapter 2.) Selecting the remedies for injuries is incredibly easy. Each type of injury has one or two remedies that are specific for it. You just look it up. A dose of Arnica after a bruising blow, Hypericum after a spine injury, or Ledum after a puncture wound can mean the difference between quick recovery and long-term suffering, or even death.

Using homeopathy for minor ailments doesn't require any medical training or a brilliant mind. Each remedy is associated with a particular set of symptoms. If the patient has those symptoms, the remedy can cure. It doesn't matter what the name of the disease is. You don't need perfect knowledge for good results.

This book takes the reader one step further, by including remedies for serious diseases such as cholera and anthrax. It also describes how you can use homeopathic remedies to prevent illness during an epidemic.

One wouldn't ordinarily suggest that laypeople attempt such a feat, but these are not ordinary times. In the next ten years we may find ourselves in survival situations, either as a community or as individuals. This book was written to provide laypeople a means to treat injuries and acute ailments where conventional care is either not available or not effective. It is for situations involving pain, threats to life, or problems that might become serious if not treated. It is not meant as a substitute for professional medical care, when that care is available.

There is also a section specifically dealing with preventing illnesses, such as in epidemics. Homeopathy has a long history of successes in that area.

I don't mean to imply that this book will make you an expert in cholera or anthrax, nor are most doctors experts in those exotic ailments. But with the information in this book you will be able to act, even if imperfectly. In a critical situation, that makes all the difference.

Note: *All the remedies described in this book also apply to animals.* So don't deprive your pets of this effective healing tool. My dog's life has been saved a number of times by homeopathic remedies. There are veterinarians who specialize in homeopathy. A call to the National Center for Homeopathy can elicit the nearest homeopathic vet.

If you have a chronic health problem, such as diabetes, arthritis, cancer, chronic fatigue syndrome, ulcerative colitis, or functional heart disease, then you need to see a professional homeopath. These conditions are treatable, but require considerable experience. However, this book will offer remedies for the acute phases of some chronic ailments (e.g., asthma, arthritis).

I call this a handbook for survival, because in the coming years we may find ourselves in survival situations for the following reasons:

1. **Natural disasters:** Weather cycles, disrupted by global warming, are becoming increasingly extreme. Natural disasters, such as droughts, severe floods, snowstorms, and heat waves, could easily disrupt everyday medical service.
2. **Terrorism:** We live in an age of increasing unrest, where terrorism always looms as a possibility. A large-scale attack in a crowded urban area could temporarily overwhelm the medical system.
3. **Antibiotic-resistant infections**: For the last several decades, antibiotics have been overused. This has given rise to infections that are more virulent and transmissible, while being resistant to all or most antibiotics. Pharmaceutical companies will not be able to keep up with this rapid escalation in antibiotic resistance. Bacteria can produce a new generation every twenty minutes. The world's leading experts in antibiotic-resistant microbes have predicted that it is just a matter of time before killer strains develop for which there will be no cure.

   At the 1994 annual meeting of the American Association for the Advancement of Science, Dr. Alexander Tomasz, a leading authority on antibiotic-resistant bacteria, stated, "In the postantibiotic world, the simplest infections could quickly escalate into fatal illnesses. It would be nothing short of a medical disaster."

The medical system could easily be overwhelmed by thousands of cases of untreatable infections. For example:

- **Staphylococcus aureus** is the leading cause of infection in hospitals. It can be fatal in up to 40% of the cases. Recently the Center for Disease Control (CDC) found strains that were resistant to all antibiotics. This is so serious that the CDC has a task force developing contingency plans for an outbreak.
- **Enterococcus:** In 1996, the federal government reported that 14% of all hospital-acquired enterococcus infections were resistant to all antibiotics.
- **Pneumococcus:** Many strains of it are resistant to all antibiotics except vancomycin. It's just a matter of time.
- **Tuberculosis:** There are now strains that resist all known treatment.
- **Plague:** There are now strains that resist all known treatment.
- **Group A streptococcus** (toxic shock syndrome and necrotizing fasciitis, popularly known as flesh-eating infection): In 1993, 5% of cases were resistant to erythromycin. Two years later, 30% of cases were resistant to erythromycin.

4. **Exotic diseases**, such as Ebola and hantavirus, can be expected to occur more often due to destruction of rainforests, overpopulation, increased trade between nations, and global temperature changes. Global warming allows vector insects carrying these diseases to travel farther north.
5. **Chemical or drug sensitivity:** More and more people have become allergic to conventional drugs. When that happens, the side effects of the drug can be more dangerous than the disease itself. If you are allergic to the drugs you need, the doctor may have nothing more to offer you. Homeopathic remedies are effective for most conditions now treated conventionally and are without any side effects.

6. **Genetic engineering:** The biotechnology industry has been playing mix-and-match with the basic units of life. Genes from animals have been inserted into plants and genes from humans have been placed into animals. Genetically engineered foods are on supermarket shelves, often without any long-term testing for safety. People and animals may develop new diseases for which there is no conventional treatment. Homeopathic remedies are ideal for such a situation. To choose a remedy, all you need are the symptoms.
7. **No medical insurance:** 45.8 million Americans have no medical insurance. If you can't afford medical care for acute ailments, homeopathy may help you avoid needless suffering.

1

The What, How, and Why of Homeopathy

What Is Homeopathy?

Homeopathy is a medical science that uses natural substances to mimic illness and stimulate healing. It is based on the idea of "like cures like." Any substance that can produce symptoms in a healthy person can cure those same symptoms in a sick person.

Here are several examples of this principle:

a. An onion is a substance that makes your eyes water and your nose burn. So if you are having an attack of hay fever with watering eyes and a burning nose, a few doses of homeopathic onion can relieve it.

b. Poison ivy causes redness, small blisters, intense itching, and stiff muscles. Homeopathically it has been used for everything from herpes and burns to eczema and arthritis.

c. Coffee can overstimulate the mind and trigger insomnia. Homeopathic coffee can help restore sleep disturbed by an overactive mind.

d. When you are stung by a bee you feel a burning, stinging pain, and the tissues surrounding the area swell up. Some relief is obtained from applying cold to the area. If you had swollen tonsils with burning and stinging pain relieved by cold, homeopathic bee sting could cure.

Over two thousand substances are now used as remedies to treat everything from colds and cough to arthritis and cancer.

Why Turn to Homeopathy?

1. **When antibiotics fail, homeopathic remedies will still work. Germs can never develop a resistance to homeopathic remedies.** The remedies do not kill the germs directly, but rather, they stimulate the immune system to do the healing. For the last two hundred years, homeopaths have cured meningitis, endocarditis, pneumonia, nephritis, tuberculosis, plague, and venereal diseases using homeopathic remedies alone.

   Homeopathic remedies are effective against viruses, but antibiotics are not. In 1918, the worldwide influenza epidemic killed over twenty million people, and over five hundred thousand in the United States. At a time when survival rates were 70% with conventional medicine, they were 98% with homeopathy.

   Some other viral diseases are Ebola, hantavirus, viral pneumonia, viral hepatitis, yellow fever, polio, rabies, viral meningitis, viral encephalitis, dengue fever, mumps, chickenpox, measles, herpes simplex and zoster, and mononucleosis.

2. **Homeopathy is affordable—homeopathic remedies cost about eight cents per dose.** Thousands of people could be treated during an emergency for just a few dollars. The antibiotic used to treat sepsis infections costs $4,000 for one day's treatment. The equivalent homeopathic remedies cost 8¢ per dose.

3. **You can begin prescribing without a diagnosis.** Homeopathic remedies are prescribed based on the person's symptoms. You don't have to know the name of the disease. This is especially important when new or exotic diseases arise.
4. **Homeopathic remedies are extremely safe and free of chemical side effects.** By following a few simple rules, any intelligent person can use the remedies without danger. Prescription drugs, on the other hand, are not safe for amateurs. In fact, they are quite dangerous even when used by doctors. A recent study published in the *Journal of the American Medical Association* (April 15, 1998) concluded that prescription drugs, properly prescribed and properly taken, are between the fourth and sixth leading cause of death in the United States (after heart attack, stroke, and cancer). The study found that prescription drugs kill over one hundred thousand Americans a year.
5. **Homeopathic remedies can be used prophylactically, much like vaccines.** Thousands of people could be inoculated quickly and cheaply if an epidemic threatened. A remedy made from the chick pea (Lathyrus) has been used with great success during polio epidemics.
6. **People who are allergic to antibiotics and other drugs can still use homeopathic remedies.** Homeopathic remedies can substitute for almost all conventional drugs.
7. **You can heal faster.** Conventional drugs can relieve pain or reduce inflammation, but they don't speed healing. All homeopathic remedies, when properly selected, speed the healing process.
8. **You can sometimes avoid surgery.** Polyps, tonsillitis, hemorrhoids, ulcers, abscesses, gall bladder problems, and more, often yield to homeopathic treatment. Surgery is always an option, but when possible, why not try a less invasive method first?
9. **Homeopathic remedies remove toxins from the body.** Conventional drugs increase the toxic load.

What You Can Accomplish with Homeopathy

If conventional medical care were not available, what could the average person hope to accomplish with homeopathy? You wouldn't be an expert, but you could still prevent illness, relieve pain, and save lives.

First Aid

Just as a person can learn conventional first aid, so one can learn homeopathic first aid. This includes treating anything from cuts and sprains to concussions and broken bones. For first aid injuries, you simply look up the type of injury. The book will list the appropriate remedy. For example, bruises require Arnica and burns need Cantharis. It's quite straightforward. **You can look up the remedies for first aid in chapter 3, "Ailments A to Z."**

Acute Care

This involves anything from colds and coughs to influenza, infected wounds, and pneumonia. If you know the name of the ailment, you can look it up in this book. It involves more decisions than treating first aid problems, because you'll have more remedies to choose from. Match the remedy to the patient's symptoms. Just do your best! You don't have to get it right the first time, or even the second or third time. Trained homeopaths often try several remedies before they get the right one. **You can look up the remedies for acute health problems in chapter 3, "Ailments A to Z."**

Preventing Illness

Homeopathic remedies can also help prevent illness. If there were an epidemic and you had no vaccines available, you could use remedies to help prevent the disease or reduce its severity. This is similar to vaccination, but without the side effects. **You can read more about this and look up the remedies in chapter 7, "Preventing Illness."**

Homeopathy's Track Record

You may be wondering what kind of track record homeopathy has for treating serious diseases. A look at the past will establish that homeopathy has proven itself reliable and is often much more effective than conventional treatment. It has also saved countless lives when used preventively.

- The worldwide influenza epidemic of 1918 killed over twenty million people and more than five hundred thousand in the United States. At a time when when survival rates were 70% with conventional medicine, they were 98% with homeopathy. Most of the homeopathic remedies that were used are the same ones you will have in your kit (e.g., Gelsemium, Arsenicum, and Bryonia).
- During the cholera and typhus epidemics in Europe from the 1860s to early 1900s, people using homeopathy had survival rates 50% or greater than those treated by conventional medicine.
- In an epidemic of typhus in Leipzig in 1813, Dr. Samuel Hahnemann treated 180 cases of typhus, losing only two patients. Mortality rates for conventional treatment were over 30%.
- During the cholera epidemic of 1849 in Cincinnati, with survival rates between 40%–52%, those treated by homeopathy had a 97% survival rate. These results were published in the local newspapers.
- During the 1831–32 cholera epidemic in Europe, the mortality rate was between 40%–80%. The mortality rate in the ten homeopathic hospitals was 7%–10%. Homeopathy was so effective that the law forbidding the practice of homeopathy in Austria was repealed.
- In 1878, the mortality rate for yellow fever in New Orleans was 50% for conventional care, but only 5.6% with homeopathic care.
- Records from Broome County, New York (1862–64), show diphtheria mortality at 83.6%, but only 16.4% for those treated homeopathically.

Prevention

In the 1957 polio epidemic in Buenos Aires, the remedy Lathyrus was given to thousands of people. Not one case of polio was reported in these individuals.

In a 1974 epidemic of meningicoccal meningitis in Brazil, 18,640 children were given a homeopathic remedy for prevention. Only four cases of meningitis occurred in these children.

In the smallpox epidemic of 1902 in Iowa, the homeopathic remedy Variolinum was given as prophylaxis to 2,806 patients of fifteen doctors. The protection rate was 97%.

See chapter 7, "Preventing Illness," for a more detailed discussion.

How Homeopathy Got Started

Homeopathy was developed by Dr. Samuel Hahnemann (1755–1843), a German physician, in the period from 1790 until his death in 1843. In addition to being a physician, he was a pharmacist, and wrote seventy original works on chemistry and medicine. He was also a translator, fluent in seven languages. With his theoretical and practical discoveries in homeopathy, he developed an entire system of medicine.

Hahnemann was ahead of his time in many respects, being one of the first people to promote compassionate treatment for the mentally ill. He used homeopathy to cure many individuals so afflicted. He grasped the principles of contagion long before the germ theory, and wrote about the need for public sanitation.

There is a monument to Hahnemann in Washington, D.C., at Scott Circle, at the junction of Massachusetts Avenue and Sixteenth Street. Hahnemann is buried in Père-Lachaise Cemetery in France, along with other renowned individuals such as Molière, Sarah Bernhardt, Edith Piaf, Marcel Proust, Balzac, Oscar Wilde, and Modigliani. He is honored in countries throughout the world.

Homeopathy is based on the idea of "like cures like," a principle that was understood by Aristotle, Hippocrates, and Paracelsus, and mentioned in ancient Hindu manuscripts. It was Hahnemann, however, who turned it into a science of healing.

Hahnemann wondered why cinchona bark, from which quinine is derived, was effective in treating malaria. As an experiment he consumed some cinchona bark and soon developed the symptoms of malaria. From this experience, he reasoned that a substance can cure an ailment if it is able to produce the symptoms of that ailment. He concluded that a true medicine is something that can produce the symptoms it is trying to cure. He thus hypothesized the principle of "like cures like." This principle is also called the "law of similars."

To prove this hypothesis he experimented on himself, his family, and friends. Initially, he used tinctures or concentrated doses. Later, in an effort to prevent side effects, he began diluting his medicines. At each stage of dilution, he would firmly tap the bottle of liquid. To his amazement, this process of diluting and tapping, called "potentizing," increased the healing power of the remedies. The more he diluted and tapped them, the deeper and longer-acting the remedies became. From those experiments, he confirmed two important principles of homeopathy:

Like cures like: A substance that causes symptoms of illness can cure those same symptoms.

Minimum dose: To cure without harm, use the least amount of medicine necessary.

Hahnemann experimented with other substances, learning what symptoms they would produce and, therefore, what symptoms they could cure. He taught others his new method of healing, and soon homeopathy spread from Germany to the rest of the continent. By 1829, Hahnemann was famous throughout Europe. He produced amazing cures in some of the worst epidemics of the time. During a typhus epidemic in 1813, Hahnemann cured 179 of 180 cases. Survival rates in homeopathic hospitals during epidemics were usually 50%–75% greater than in conventional hospitals. Because of its success in healing the most serious diseases without harm to the patient, homeopathy was soon practiced all over the world.

How Homeopathic Remedies Are Made

The first step in making a homeopathic remedy is to dissolve a substance in water or grain alcohol. It then goes through a process of successive dilutions, either one part to one hundred or one part to ten. At each stage of dilution, the container of liquid is tapped firmly fifty to one hundred times (called *succussion*). The process of dilution and succussion may be carried out anywhere from three to one hundred thousand times. This whole operation is called *potentization*. It removes the original substance, but leaves its energy pattern.

The more dilutions and succussions, the stronger, deeper, and longer-acting the remedy is. The healing effect of a remedy that has been diluted fifty thousand times and succussed five million times can easily last a year.

The more diluted, the stronger it is? This may seem paradoxical. In fact, for years no one was sure how the remedies worked. But recent research has helped explain it. When something is dissolved in water and then potentized, the water molecules form clusters.The character of the clusters is specific for each substance. Further, these clusters can carry complex information and communicate it to other water molecules. The energy pattern of the original substance affects the water, and this effect is transmitted through each dilution.

Homeopathic remedies cure by presenting the body with an energy pattern that mimics the energy pattern of the disease. This triggers exactly the correct healing response.

The remedy does not add any chemicals to your body. Rather, it contains information about how to heal. It is similar to a floppy disc in your computer. People who are not knowledgeable about homeopathy often try to disparage it, saying there is nothing in the remedy. Well, there is no "thing" or chemical in the remedy, but rather, information. It would be as foolish to say there is nothing in a floppy disc. The remedy gives your body instructions for healing, in the same way the floppy disc instructs the hard drive.

How Does Homeopathy Work? Why Should an Energy Pattern Heal Disease?

Homeopathy has some basic assumptions about disease and healing.

1. *Living beings are alive because they have energy flowing through them.* Hahnemann called this energy the "Vital Force." In India it is referred to as *prana*, and in China it is known as *chi*. Wilhelm Reich named it the *orgone*. Whatever it is called, this energy is the spark that animates us. Without it, all plant and animal life would be a pile of inert chemicals.
2. *Disease is a disturbance in the body's energy.* Those things normally thought of as disease, such as fevers, inflammations, blocked vessels, and growths, are the result of disturbed energy flow. They are the symptoms, signs, and results of disease, but not the disease itself. The disease is the disrupted energy.
3. *To cure disease you have to restore the body's energy flow.*
4. *Since disease is a disturbance of energy, you need an energy medicine to correct it.*

Homeopathic remedies are essentially energy patterns.

How Does a Particular Remedy Help Heal a Particular Disease?

The famous physicist Louis de Broglie demonstrated that all matter (living or inert) has wavelength and frequency. That is to say, everything is vibrating. That includes people, animals, rocks, and homeopathic remedies.

When we are healthy, we are vibrating in a particular way. This changes during illness. A homeopathic remedy that matches the sickness vibration will mimic your disease. This stimulates and guides the healing process. The symptoms disappear because the remedy corrected the underlying energy problem.

Each remedy represents a different vibration. Since we can't see these vibrations, what we actually match are the symptoms of the remedy and the symptoms of the patient.

The idea that disease is due to an energy imbalance is very different from the conventional view. The conventional view is that disease is caused by a chemical imbalance and needs to be fixed with chemicals. Rather than a sign of healing, symptoms are seen as the disease itself and are suppressed with strong chemicals, called drugs. The suppression of symptoms is basic to that view.

Treating disease this way has serious drawbacks. Since it doesn't address the underlying problem, symptoms frequently return. This requires ever-stronger drugs, often with dangerous side effects. The ineffectiveness of this approach is quite apparent in chronic disease. Most people with chronic ailments have to take drugs the rest of their lives. It is clear that the problem hasn't been fixed.

Further, suppressing symptoms can make one sicker. When your body needs to rid itself of toxins, you might get a runny nose, watery eyes, vomiting, diarrhea, perspiration, or a fever. These are signs that your body is trying to heal itself. When a drug stops this from happening, where do the toxins go? The body's natural expression has been thwarted.

According to homeopathy, suppressing symptoms over time can create a deeper and more serious illness. For example, homeopaths have observed that minor skin ailments suppressed with drugs give rise to asthma. What's more, if the asthma is then treated suppressively, it can give rise to colitis, arthritis, heart disease, etc. The proof of this is that the process reverses itself under homeopathic treatment. As the colitis is cured, symptoms of asthma briefly return. When the symptoms of asthma disappear, a skin rash erupts for a day or two. The process is complete.

Occasionally, symptoms themselves can become life-threatening, such as an allergic reaction to a bee sting. In such cases, it makes sense to suppress. For the most part, however, symptoms represent a healing process.

The Minimum Dose

By using potentized remedies, homeopaths are able to adhere to a second principle, the minimum dose. This principle states that the homeopath should use the least amount of medicine (or energy) needed to trigger healing. Thus, the remedies stimulate the body to make changes, rather than forcing it to do so. Because they are so dilute, they produce no chemical side effects. This is a very different approach from conventional medicine, which uses toxic doses of chemicals that kill over one hundred thousand Americans a year.

The potentization process allows homeopaths to make perfectly safe remedies from substances that were toxic in their crude form. In fact, the more toxic something is, the better a remedy it makes. That's because whatever symptoms a substance can cause, it can cure. Arsenic produces many serious symptoms, and therefore has a wide range of healing properties when used homeopathically.

There are currently about two thousand homeopathic remedies. Most are made from plants, minerals, or elements. A handful of remedies are made from animal substances such as bee sting toxin and snake venom. There are also some remedies made from diseased tissue, such as tuberculosis or diphtheria. Those remedies are called *nosodes*. You can't catch any disease from them, because they contain nothing but an energy pattern. In fact, nosodes are often used to prevent those diseases during epidemics.

Examples of Substances Used to Make Remedies

Plants: Mountain daisy, sundew, St. Ignatius bean, wild rosemary.

Minerals: Calcium sulfate, potassium carbonate, sodium chloride, sodium sulfate.

Elements: Phosphorus, sulphur, gold, silver, copper.

Animal substances: Bee sting toxin, snake venom, cuttle fish ink.

Disease substances: Tuberculosis, diphtheria, influenza.

Once they have been potentized, they become quite safe and are able to stimulate healing. In this form, they act very differently from the crude substances.

Provings

How Homeopaths Discovered Which Substances Would Cure Specific Symptoms

Over the last two hundred years, various plants, minerals, animal substances, and disease extracts were tested on healthy volunteers to see what symptoms they would produce. This determined what symptoms those substances could cure.

This testing process is called a *proving*, from the German *Pruefung*, meaning test. The volunteers are called *provers*. They were usually given a homeopathic dose of something, over and over, until their bodies and minds reacted. They reported any changes they experienced to the homeopath, who also recorded his or her observations.

Provers experienced both physical and mental symptoms and changes. To date, these recorded symptoms number in the thousands and cover about every symptom known to man. Some examples of physical symptoms are headache, sore throat, aching bones, stomach ache, difficulty breathing, irregular menstruation, painful urination, and vision and hearing problems. Also observed were emotional symptoms such as anxiety, anger, fear, shame, depression, and jealousy. The provers sometimes experienced positive changes in personality, such as going from being aloof to being intensely sympathetic.

Each substance also produced specific feelings of "better or worse from." For example, a prover might have had a headache that was made better or worse from warmth, sleep, motion, eating, time of day, lying down, fresh air, pressure, bright light, or company. These conditions of "better or worse" are called *modalities*.

Some modalities of common remedies are:

- **Lachesis:** worse after sleep.
- **Hepar sulph:** worse from cold.
- **Pulsatilla:** worse in a closed room and better from fresh air.

- **Bryonia:** worse from any movement.
- **Rhus tox:** better from movement.
- **Natrum sulph:** worse from dampness.
- **Phosphorus:** better from company.
- **Arsenicum:** worse from midnight to 3 a.m.
- **Lycopodium:** worse from eating oysters.

Many of the substances produced very characteristic emotional and mental states. These turned out to be some of the best guides in choosing the right remedy.

Here are some of the mental states produced by specific substances:

Arsenicum (Arsenic trioxide): Great anxiety, especially when alone, fear of death, restlessness, tendency to be critical, conscientious about trifles, despair of recovery. Fear of cancer, robbers, poverty, and ghosts.

Aurum (Gold): Exaggerated sense of duty and the delusion that one has failed, accompanied by strong feelings of guilt, severe depression, fits of anger, desire for death, or suicidal intention.

Lachesis (Bushmaster snake venom): Extremely talkative, sarcastic, passionate, intense, jealous, and vindictive. Great clarity of mind or confusion. Fear of snakes, of evil, of going to sleep. Aversion to anything tight around the neck.

Lycopodium (Club moss): Extreme lack of confidence, anticipatory anxiety, fear of being alone, claustrophobia, feelings of helplessness, fear of strangers, becoming easily offended, weeping when thanked, dictatorial.

Sepia (Ink of the cuttlefish): Anger when contradicted, irritability, aversion to family, aversion to company yet fear of being alone, annoyed by consolation, fear of insanity, hysteria, overwhelming apathy.

Who Makes These Remedies and Where Do I Get Them?

Homeopathic remedies are made by homeopathic pharmacies around the world. They adhere to very strict guidelines laid down by organizations like the Homeopathic Pharmacopia of the United States. In the U.S., the remedies are all FDA approved.

Some homeopathic pharmacies sell directly to the public. Remedies are also available at health food stores, some pharmacies, and health food sections of supermarkets. The majority of remedies do not require any prescription. The exceptions are the nosodes, remedies made from diseased tissue. Some homeopathic pharmaceutical companies require a prescription for the nosodes, others do not. Another option is to find a friendly holistic doctor, dentist, or other health professional who can write a prescription for the nosode.

Homeopathic Kits

I highly recommend purchasing a kit. First, they are a real bargain. You can get a modest one for $85 to $200 that will contain between fifty and one hundred remedies. If you bought the remedies individually they would cost a third more. Secondly, the manufacturer has carefully chosen the remedies you will most often need. They will be effective for a wide range of ailments. If the need arises for other remedies, those can be ordered from a health food store or homeopathic pharmacy. I suggest buying a kit with remedies in the "30c" potency. See chapter 12, "Remedies for Your Home Kit," for a list of recommended remedies.

2

Finding and Using the Right Remedy

Rules for Using Remedies

To use remedies safely and effectively, follow these few rules.

1. **The most important rule is, as the patient improves, give the remedy less often. When the symptoms are much better, stop.** With homeopathy, less is more! The remedy triggers the healing and that process continues by itself. To continue taking the remedy after your symptoms are gone can be counterproductive.
2. **Tap three to five pellets (or eight to ten tiny granules) of the remedy into the cap of the bottle and toss them directly onto or under your tongue.** Let the remedy dissolve in your mouth. Remedies are not swallowed whole like regular pills. Try to avoid touching the remedy, since soaps, perfumes, or oils on your hands may interfere with its action.

   For infants, dissolve the remedy in a couple teaspoons of water and place a few drops on the tongue. **For animals**, crush the remedy between two spoons and tap the powder onto the gums or tongue. **For an unconscious patient**, place the remedy between the lip and teeth. This is to prevent it from being inhaled.

3. **Don't eat or drink anything for ten minutes**. Remedies are best taken ten minutes before or half an hour after eating or drinking, except water. The remedy works best if there are no food residues in your mouth. However, in an emergency, don't worry about this rule, just give the remedy!
4. **Certain substances can antidote the healing effect of the remedy.** These include mint (e.g., toothpaste, mint candies), coffee, camphor, and strong perfumes or essential oils. Try to avoid these when taking a remedy.

Note: If you ever want to stop a remedy from working, you could eat some strong mint, take a whiff of essential oils, or drink some coffee. If your body ever overreacted to a remedy, either because you repeated it too often or because you are one of those rare individuals who are oversensitive to remedies, you could intentionally antidote the effect with mint, coffee, etc.

Dosage

In a life-threatening situation such as heart attack, repeat the remedy as often as every fifteen minutes. For less serious problems such as sore throat, repeat every three to four hours. In both cases, as the patient improves, give it less often. When the symptoms are much better, just stop. The remedy keeps working by itself. If symptoms come back, repeat the remedy again. If you get no effect after three doses, then it's probably the wrong remedy. Try another one.

Potency

The strength of the remedy is called its *potency.* It is a function of how many times the substance has been diluted and succussed. The more dilutions and succussions, the stronger the remedy. By stronger, I mean it is deeper and longer-acting. This may seem paradoxical, but the effects have been demonstrated for over two hundred years.

Remedies come in different potencies, which are indicated by the number and letter on the tube or bottle. The number represents the number of dilutions. The higher the number, the deeper and longer-acting it is. *A 30c is stronger than a 12c.* Remedies marked "c" have been diluted 1:100 and are about twice as strong as the ones marked "x," which are diluted 1:10. *A 30c is about twice as strong as a 30x.*

As a beginner, it is best to use 30c for minor problems and 30c or 200c for emergencies. In a life-threatening situation such as heart attack, use the highest potency you have and repeat it as necessary. It's more important to get the right remedy than the right potency, so give whatever you have. There are potencies available that are thousands of times higher than what I have suggested here. Unless you are a professional homeopath, avoid them.

How Do You Select the Correct Remedy?

This book lists ailments alphabetically, in chapter 3, "Ailments A to Z." Look up the ailment and you will see a choice of remedies. Pick the one that best matches the patient's physical symptoms and mental state. It is not necessary for the person to have all the symptoms listed for that remedy. If he or she has the core symptoms, the remedy will probably cure.

If after two doses there is no effect, try the next closest remedy. The remedies with an asterisk (*) have been proven effective most often. They should be tried first, unless there is a clear indication for another.

What if You Take the Wrong Remedy?

Usually nothing happens. If the remedy is not tuned to your symptoms, then your body won't receive it. Your body is like a radio. There are lots of stations, but the radio only receives the one it's tuned to. If the remedy is close to being correct, it may cure some of the symptoms.

Store remedies away from light, heat, radiation (computer, TV, microwave oven), and they can last for decades, regardless of the date on the label.

The label on the bottle usually states that the remedy is good for only one condition, such as sore throat. Ignore that. Most remedies have scores of uses, but the manufacturer can't list them all on that tiny label.

Taking the Case

When you look up a typical ailment, there may be anywhere from three to fifteen remedies to chose from. The choice depends on the patient's symptoms. To select the correct remedy, you need to be aware of those symptoms. It is a good idea to take notes so you can remember what the patient said and what he or she looked like.

When you are with the patient, the most important things to look and listen for are:

1. **What makes the person feel better or worse?**
2. **Strange or unusual symptoms.**
3. **Possible causes of the ailment.**
4. **Changes in mental state.**
5. **Sensations.**

1. What makes the person feel better or worse? The person may feel better or worse from any number of conditions (modalities), including heat, cold, light, noise, company, certain times of day, lying or siting up, keeping still or moving, lying on the right or left side, from hot or cold drinks, after eating, after sleeping, etc.

Here are examples of remedies and some of their modalities:

Arsenicum: Better from heat, company, and small sips of water. Worse from cold, between midnight and 3 a.m., or when alone.

Belladonna: Better from rest, quiet, or being in a dark room. Worse from noise, light, being jarred, and drafts.

Bryonia: Better being still, or lying on the painful side. Worse from any motion, from exertion, or from warmth.

Lachesis: Better after discharges, from fresh air. Worse after sleep, from warmth, from tight clothing, from light touch, on the left side (left-sided symptoms).

Lycopodium: Better from moving around, cool air, and hot food or drink. Worse between 4 and 8 p.m., eating oysters, eating sweets, on the right side (right-sided symptoms).

Mercurius: Better at room temperature. Worse after sweating, from the warmth of the bed, at night.

Nux vomica: Better from a nap, moving the bowels, resting, damp weather. Worse in the morning, from mental exertion, spices, or stimulants.

Phosphorus: Better from company, short naps. Worse lying on the left side, during thunderstorms, being alone, from loud noises, and bright lights.

Pulsatilla: Better from company, sympathy, and fresh air. Worse from heat, being in a warm room, being alone, eating fats.

Rhus tox: Better from moving about, stretching, warmth, dry weather. Worse after resting, from dampness, cold, in the evening.

2. Strange or unusual symptoms. Other things to look for in your patient are unusual symptoms. These can help distinguish among several remedies. Here's a list of unusual symptoms and a sample of remedies associated with them:

Aversion to the smell of food (Arsenicum, Sepia, Ipecac, Colchicum)
Aversion to anything tight around the neck (Lachesis)
Burning pains, which are better from heat (Arsenicum)
Badly injured but says he's okay and refuses to be touched (Arnica)
Craves ice-cold drinks (Phosphorus)
Craves peanut butter (Pulsatilla)
Deep aching in bones (Eupatorium)
Excess salivation (even drooling) with great thirst (Mercurius)
Every stool is a different color (Pulsatilla)
Fever without thirst (Apis, Pulsatilla)

Flabby tongue with the imprint of teeth (Mercurius)
Hunger after diarrhea (Lycopodium)
High fever with slow pulse (Pyrogenium)
Itching without any eruption (Alumina, Mezereum, Arsenicum)
Left-sided symptoms (Lachesis)
Nausea not relieved by vomiting (Ipecacuanha)
Pain from the slightest touch, cold, or draft (Hepar)
Pain makes him double over (Colocynth)
Pain is worse after rest and better from continued motion (Rhus tox)
Painless diarrhea (Cinchona)
Right-sided complaints (Lycopodium)
Rolling from side to side with pain (Tarentula)
Symptoms keep changing in quality and location (Pulsatilla)
Sensitivity to noise with sounds felt in the teeth (Theridon)
Unendurable pain coupled with anger (Chamomilla)
Worse after sweating (Mercurius)
Worse after sleep (Lachesis)
Worse from the slightest movement (Bryonia)

3. Cause of illness. If you know what caused the illness, it can help you select the correct remedy. Some remedies are associated with specific causes. For example, Colocynth is effective for internal spasms caused by anger. Natrum sulphuricum is effective for symptoms caused by head injuries. Ignatia works well for ailments caused by grief.

The remedy may be effective days, months, or even years after the "cause." Natrum sulphuricum has healed symptoms from head injuries years after the injury. Here are some examples of causes and a sample of remedies that work for them.

Ailments Caused by:

Anger: Staphysagria, Colocynth, Nux vomica.

Antibiotics, overuse of: Nitric acid, Lycopodium, Cinchona.

Anticipation: Argentum nitricum, Gelsemium, Lycopodium.

Bad news: Gelsemium, Ignatia.

Breast, injury to: Conium, Bellis perennis.

Catheters: Aconite, Staphysagria, Calendula.

Cold wind: Aconite.

Constipation: Nux vomica, Bryonia, Aloe.

Dampness: Dulcamara, Natrum sulph, Rhus tox.

Dehydration: Cinchona, Carbo vegetabilis.

Drug abuse: Nux vomica, Gelsemium.

Foods, fatty: Pulsatilla.

Food, spoiled: Arsenicum, Cinchona, Carbo vegetabilis, Pyrogenium.

Fright: Aconite, Gelsemium, Ignatia, Stramonium.

Grief or loss: Ignatia, Natrum mur, Causticum.

Head injury: Arnica, Hypericum, Natrum sulphuricum.

Humiliation: Staphysagria, Ignatia, Lycopodium.

Injuries (bruising injuries, blows, trauma to the body): Arnica.

Influenza, weakness after: Gelsemium, Phosphoric acid, Cinchona.

Loss of fluids: Cinchona, Carbo vegetabilis.

Muscle injuries: Arnica, Rhus tox, Bryonia.

Nerve injury: Hypericum.

Poison ivy: Rhus tox, Anacardium.

Puncture wounds: Ledum, Hypericum.

Radiation, exposure to: Cadmium sulphuricum.

Rape or abuse: Staphysagria, Aconite, Ignatia.

Sexual abstinence: Conium.

Sharp object, cuts from: Staphysagria.

Shellfish: Urtica urens, Lycopodium.

Sleep, loss of: Cocculus.

Spine injuries: Hypericum.

Sun: Belladonna, Glonoine, Natrum carbonicum.

Teething: Chamomilla, Belladonna, Aconite.

Vaccination: Thuja, Silica.

Worms: Cina, Cicuta, Hyoscyamus.

4. Changes in mental state. When a person becomes ill, his or her mental state often changes. The change may be dramatic or quite subtle, and it can help you find the correct remedy. How has this person changed emotionally since getting sick? Has he gone from cheerful to depressed, from relaxed to anxious, from outgoing to withdrawn, or from friendly to uncivil? Does he suddenly desire sympathy or company, or does he want to be alone? Is he now anxious or fearful? Are there specific fears such as a fear of darkness, being alone, or dogs? Is he unusually restless, talkative, impatient, weepy, or lethargic? Is he unexpectedly jealous or full of rage?

5. Sensations. Try to find out what specific sensations the patient is experiencing. If there is pain, is it dull, sharp, aching, or burning? Does he experience tingling, itching, soreness, coldness, or pressure?

Finding the Remedy When You Don't Know the Name of the Ailment

There are several ways to solve this problem. Remember, we're dealing with a situation where there is no professional medical help available.

1. Look up whatever ailment this condition looks or feels like. Does it look like chickenpox, arthritis, food poisoning, flu? Look up that ailment and pick the remedy that best fits your patient. Why should this work? *Homeopathic remedies work because they match the patient's symptoms, not the name of the patient's disease.*

Suppose it looks like the flu. It might really be the beginnings of malaria, yellow fever, plague, anthrax, or hantavirus. Nevertheless, *if the remedy fits the symptoms, it will work*. Some of the same remedies used for flu are also used for those diseases. At that stage of the ailment, the person has flu-like symptoms and the flu remedies will often work.

The remedies have a lock-and-key relationship with specific clusters of symptoms, not with names of diseases. *Each remedy has certain symptoms associated with it. If a patient has those symptoms, the remedy can cure, regardless of the name of the ailment.* This is a basic axiom of homeopathy.

> **Example:** The remedy Belladonna is associated with redness, pain, heat, throbbing, spasms, and delirium. The patient is made worse from bright lights, noise, or being jarred. Belladonna may cure any ailment with that cluster of symptoms. Belladonna has cured cases of sore throat, headache, sunstroke, scarlet fever, abscess, ear infections, hydrophobia, meningitis, pneumonia, and more. But it will only cure when the Belladonna symptoms are present.

> **Example:** The remedy Arsenicum album is associated with anxiety, chills, restlessness, exhaustion, extreme thirst for small frequent sips, diarrhea, and burning pains that are better from heat (for instance, a burning throat that is better from hot tea). The patient is better from company and warmth. He's worse from midnight to 3 a.m. Arsenicum may cure any ailment with those symptoms. Arsenicum album has cured diarrhea, influenza, asthma, food poisoning, gangrene, blood poisoning, shingles, peritonitis, cholera, and more. But it only works when those Arsenicum symptoms are present.

2. If this ailment doesn't even look like anything you know, there are three approaches.

a. Read chapter 5, "Remedy Descriptions," and see if one of those remedies fits your patient. One of those descriptions may just pop out at you as being a good match.

b. See chapter 4, "Organ Remedies." It describes some top remedies for the heart, lungs, liver, and kidneys. In serious illnesses, one of these organs is usually affected.

c. Record your patient's symptoms and look them up in a *repertory.* A repertory is a book that lists thousands of symptoms and the remedies associated with them. You look up your patient's symptoms and see which remedy covers most or all of them. There's a sample repertory in this book at the end of chapter 11, "How to Use a Repertory."

3

Ailments A to Z

Select the remedy that best fits the patient's symptoms. The patient doesn't have to exhibit all the symptoms that are listed. If there is no effect after two doses, try the next-closest remedy. They are listed in the order of how closely they match the most common symptoms. Occasionally, part of a remedy description will be italicized as a *keynote*—this is used to emphasize the most important symptoms or modalities to observe. *The remedies most likely to work are marked with an asterisk (*) and listed first. Try these initially, unless another remedy is clearly indicated.*

> **Note:** The correctly chosen remedy will sometimes produce a temporary aggravation of the symptoms. This is a good sign and means that the healing process has begun. The aggravation usually lasts anywhere from a few minutes to several hours.

A remedy that is almost correct will sometimes give partial relief. If you don't have the exact remedy, give the closest remedy that you have.

> **Potency:** Unless otherwise indicated, use 30c. If the symptoms are either very intense, as in a toothache, or life threatening, as in heart attack, give 200c. If you don't have the recommended potency, give whatever you have.

Abscess

An abscess is a local infection with pus. When it forms at the base of a hair follicle it is called a furuncle. If it spreads to more hair follicles it is called a carbuncle. Squeezing an abscess can spread the infection. The following remedies can help the body find an opening for drainage. Hot salt water soaks or just hot water will also assist the process.

***Belladonna:** Red, hot, and throbbing—just starting. Sensitive to touch. Comes on quite rapidly.

***Hepar sulph** (6x to 6c)**:** Pus-filled wound. Hepar brings it to a head so it will drain. The abscess is very sensitive to touch, cold, or any draft.

***Myristica seb** (3c)**:** If Hepar fails. Helps bring inflammation to a head.

***Mercurius viv (or Merc sol):** Develops more slowly than Belladonna. The area is hard, and there is a sense of pressure from within. If the abscess is open, there may be thin, blood-streaked pus. Mercurius is especially useful for patients who perspire or have moist skin.

***Silica:** If it's taking a long time to heal and just keeps draining. Silica will help expel the pus. Also useful when every little injury goes to pus.

Arsenicum: Burning pain relieved by warmth. Bloody pus with foul odor. Restless, anxious.

Tarentula cubensis: Hard swelling with burning, stinging pain, and purple discoloration. Anxious and very restless.

Arnica: Abscess after an injury. Crops of small boils. Easy bruising. Hot, hard, shiny swelling. Worse from touch, cold.

Nitric acid: Abscess, especially at the outlets of the body such as the mouth, throat, and anus. Sticking pains as if from splinters, tendency to bleeding. Irritable.

Sulphur: Crops of boils. Every injury goes to pus. Itching followed by burning when scratched. Especially affects people who like a cool environment and can't stand heat.

Abscesses That Threaten to Become Blood Poisoning

If the bacteria from the abscess enter the bloodstream, blood poisoning (septicemia) can result. Symptoms include fever and chills, rapid respiration and heart rate, and great anxiety. This can progress further into septic shock, with pale face, cold clammy skin, weak rapid pulse, and shallow rapid breathing.

Lachesis: The inflamed area has a purplish color and foul-smelling pus, and the skin is highly sensitive to light touch. The person always feels worse after sleeping.

Anthracinum: May have started with a succession of boils, or black or blue blisters. Terrible burning pain with great weakness, high fever, restlessness, and foul secretions.

Pyrogenium: Horrible-smelling pus. Patient is better from warmth. His body feels bruised all over. High fever with low pulse rate, or low fever with high pulse rate.

Arsenicum: Intense burning pain relieved by warmth. Bloody pus with foul odor. Restless, anxious, weak, and thirsty for small frequent sips. Worse after midnight.

Agoraphobia: See "Fears"

Allergic Reaction: See "Anaphylaxis"

Amputations, Pain from

***Hypericum:** First choice for unbearable pain.

***Arnica:** 200c or higher.

***Calendula:** 30–200c.

If the Above Remedies Don't Give Full Relief, Go to

Staphysagria: Pain with anger, indignation.

Phosphorus: Burning pain, afraid to be alone, great thirst for cold drinks, tendency to hemorrhages of bright red blood.

Aconite: Unbearable pain accompanied by fear of death, unquenchable thirst.

Allium cepa: Pain like a fine thread. Patient is better in a cool room.

Coffea: Unbearable pain. Mentally hyper-alert and worse from noise and odors.

Anaphylaxis: Allergic Reaction

(See also "Hives—Allergic")

This is an extreme allergic reaction to such things as medicines, foods, and insect stings. It can be life threatening. The first symptoms include flushed face, itching, and palpitation. It then progresses to violent coughing, difficulty breathing, blue face, sudden drop in blood pressure, involuntary urination, convulsions, and shock. A frequent problem is suffocation from spasm or swelling of the airway. You must act quickly.

> **Note:** If the patient is unconscious, place the remedy between the lips and teeth to prevent it from being inhaled.

***Apis** (200c)**:** First choice. Burning, stinging pain in throat, etc. Throat swollen, difficulty breathing, can't pull air in. Suffocation imminent. Face may become swollen. Worse from warmth.

Urtica urens: With hives. Specific for shellfish reaction.

Arsenicum alb: Throat swollen, airway constricted, burning sensation in the throat, can't swallow, difficulty breathing. Very anxious and can't lie down for fear of suffocation. Restless, frightened, chilly, better from company.

Rhus tox: Skin red, raised, itching. Chest feels heavy. Sticking pains. Restless, anxious. Very thirsty prior to most severe symptoms. Better from warmth (opposite Apis). Joint pain.

Histaminum: If other remedies fail.

Anesthesia—Side Effects of Anesthetic Gases

(See also "Surgery")

Side effects of anesthetic gases include nausea and vomiting, headache, dry mouth, temporary loss of memory, and tiredness.

> **Caution:** If the patient is not fully conscious, dissolve the remedy in a tablespoon of spring water and place just a few drops of this on his tongue.

***Phosphorus:** First choice. Antidotes the effects of modern anesthetics as well as chloroform and ether.

***Acetic acid:** Antidotes all anesthetic gases. One dose should be sufficient.

Antimonium tart: Antidotes the effects of ether. Thick mucus in chest that can't be expelled by coughing.

Hepar sulph: Weakness from ether. Sensitive to the least draft or to cold.

Chloroformum: Liver problems after chloroform.

Angina

(See also "Heart Problems")

Angina is a type of chest pain caused by insufficient blood flow through the coronary vessels. The symptoms resemble a heart attack, except it only lasts between one and fifteen minutes, and does not produce permanent damage to the heart. If the attack is angina, it will usually be relieved by nitroglycerine tablets. Angina is most often due to atherosclerosis. Symptoms include severe pain or pressure near the heart, or pain radiating to the left shoulder and arm (also to the neck or back). The face is pale or blue, and there is much perspiration. There may be difficulty breathing and often fear of death. The attack may be triggered by exertion or stress. Chelation therapy may be the long term solution if blocked vessels are the cause.

***Aconite:** For the first attack. Intense fear of death, restlessness. It doesn't have the weakness of Arsenicum.

***Cactus grand:** *Feels like an iron band* around the chest being drawn tighter. Pulse fast but feeble. Worse lying on the left side.

***Arsenicum:** Tightness in the chest with a *burning sensation*. Very chilly and better from warmth and covers. Fear of death and being left alone. Restless, weak, thirsty for small sips. Face pale.

***Latrodectus mactans:** *Pain extends down the left arm to the fingers,* with numbness. Screams with pain. Gasps for breath. Skin cold. Constriction in the chest.

Iodum: *Feels like a tight band around the heart itself,* as opposed to the whole chest. Face flushed, worse from heat. Restless and anxious. Patient is usually very thin.

Spongia: *Heart feels as if it is getting bigger and bigger,* too large for the chest, and as if it might burst out. Worse lying down. Chilly and worse from any draft. Numbness in the arm or hand.

Animal Bite

If bleeding is not severe, bathe the wound with soap and running water for several minutes. If bleeding is a problem, apply direct pressure with a clean, dry cloth until it subsides.

***Ledum:** An excellent remedy for any puncture wound. Ledum and Hypericum are often used by homeopaths to prevent tetanus.

***Hypericum:** If there is much pain, and especially if the pain travels up the limb.

Hydrophobinum: If bitten by a rabid animal or if there is a high probability of rabies. A dose of hydrophobinum 30c should be repeated three times a day for a week and then Belladonna 3c twice a day for six months (see "Rabies"). Note: If the offending animal does not develop symptoms within ten days, it probably doesn't have rabies.

If Pus or Other Signs of Infection Appear

Pyrogenium 6c every 6 hours, or

Hepar sulph 6x or 6c, three or four times a day if pyrogenium is not available.

Anthrax

Anthrax is a serious infectious bacterial disease. One can get the disease from a scratch, eating infected food, or breathing the spores. There are three forms of anthrax, depending on whether it is contracted through the skin, the gastrointestinal tract, or the lungs. In the event of a terrorist attack using anthrax, the respiratory form would be the most likely. Antibiotics can prevent the disease in people who have been exposed. Treatment of the respiratory variety must begin as soon as suspected, because it runs its course rather quickly.

1. **The skin variety** forms as a reddish-brown elevation or boil. The skin becomes hardened, ulcerated, and black. Lymph nodes become enlarged. Exhaustion, muscle ache, fever, nausea, and vomiting follow.
2. **The gastrointestinal variety** may come from contaminated meat. It results in acute inflammation of the intestinal tract. Nausea, loss of appetite, vomiting, and fever are followed by abdominal pain, vomiting of blood, and severe diarrhea.
3. **The respiratory form**, called inhalation anthrax, initially looks like a cold or the flu. There is fatigue, aching muscles, cough, and fever. After a couple days the person may feel better, but this is the lull before the storm. Next comes difficulty breathing, chest pain, bloody foamy mucus, and finally respiratory failure.

Prevention

***Anthracinum** (nosode 30c): First choice.

***Lachesis.**

Remedies for Anthrax

***Arsenicum:** The boil is burning like fire, with purple spots that darken. The skin is cold and dry as parchment. It peels off. The patient is anxious, exhausted, restless, and thirsty for small sips. Wants company. Burning pains, which feel better from heat.

***Anthracinum:** Burning pain. Red lines running from the boil. Swelling of the tissue, foul-smelling pus. Hardening of tissue. Black, thick discharge. When Arsenicum fails. May also be effective as a preventive.

***Lachesis:** Dark, bloody pus, and burning pain better from cold application. Symptoms worse at night, after sleep, and on the left side. Patient is very talkative.

Secale: Skin feels cold to the touch, but there is burning pain internally. The patient is averse to heat and wants to be uncovered. Burning pains, which are relieved by cold. Worse from heat or warmth.

Belladonna: Heat, redness, throbbing pain, delirium. Worse from light, noise, or being jarred.

Rhus tox: Itching and burning at the site. Vertigo, restlessness, thirst. Bloody, foamy diarrhea. Better from warmth.

Carbo vegetabilis: Cough with burning in chest. Extremities cold. Cold breath. Craves fresh air and wants to be fanned. Hemorrhage from lungs. Constant belching. Face blue.

Phosphorus: Burning pain in chest. Feeling of tightness or a weight on the chest. Coughs up bloody sputum. Craves ice-cold drinks. Fear of being alone and wants company. Hypersensitive to odors, lights, and sounds. Tendency to bleeding.

Pyrogenium: Foul-smelling discharges of breath, stool, sweat, or vomit. The patient feels exhausted but extremely restless. Feels bruised all over. High fever with slow pulse or vice versa. Aware of his heart beating. Better from moving about, warmth. Worse from becoming cold.

Appendicitis

This sudden inflammation of the appendix often begins with pain near the bellybutton, nausea, and vomiting. After three to four hours, the pain shifts to the lower right abdomen. The pain may be dull and steady or very severe. The pain often feels worse from moving, coughing, or sneezing. Often the patient will draw up the right leg, which gives some relief.

Note: Because of the nature of the infection, the patient may seem better after a remedy, but then easily relapse. Try to get professional help, as this can quickly become a problem requiring surgery.

***Belladonna:** *Worse from touch,* area very sensitive, *patient can't stand light or noise. He feels better lying on back with knees drawn up.* Throbbing headache. Face may be red, hot. Pupils dilated. Worse from bending over or tight clothes. May be irritable, angry, or delirious.

***Bryonia:** *Worse from the slightest motion, better from lying on the right side,* lies still with legs drawn up, thirsty for large cold drinks, *better from pressure.* Burning pains. May be irritable, delirious. Worse in a warm room.

Lachesis: *Whole abdomen sensitive, pain goes down to thighs,* patient is hot and won't be covered. *Better lying on the back with the knees drawn up. Worse after sleep* and from the slightest touch.

Rhus tox: swelling over the right side of the abdomen, *extreme restlessness, worse after lying still.* Great thirst.

Ignatia: *Hysteria along with the physical symptoms.* Hyper-alert, fears an operation. The body is hot and rigid. Knees drawn up. Better changing position. Can't bear cigarette smoke.

Mercurius: *Much perspiration, breath foul.* Abdomen is hard, hot, and feels bruised. Great thirst in spite of excess salivation (the patient may even drool). Worse lying on the right side, from a warm room, and after perspiring. Stool green or blood-streaked. Tongue coated. Sometimes there is a metallic taste in the mouth.

Dioscorea: *Better bending backward, hyperextending.* Pain is constant and may radiate to surrounding areas. Worse lying down or doubling up (opposite Colocynth).

Colocynth: *Better doubling up.* Better from pressure, warmth. Bitter taste in the mouth. Irritable or angry.

Iris tenax: If available, begin with this remedy. Worse from touch, area very sensitive. Deathly sensation in the pit of the stomach. Green vomit. Exhaustion. Gloomy, weepy.

Pyrogenium: If patient keeps relapsing.

Appendicitis Complicated by Blood Poisoning

One or more of the following remedies may be needed if the infection in the appendix spreads to the bloodstream. The whole abdomen becomes painful again and vomiting continues.

***Pyrogenium:** High fever but low pulse, or vice versa. The bed feels too hard. Foul-smelling discharges and breath. Restless, anxious. Hot sweat.

***Arsenicum album:** Sudden exhaustion, diarrhea, restlessness, fear of death, thirst for small frequent sips of water, chills, burning pains that are better from warmth. Wants company.

***Lachesis:** Extremely sensitive to light touch, even the pressure of clothes, but oddly okay with firmer touch. Talkative. Can't stick out her tongue because it trembles. Worse from warmth. Feeling of suffocation when falling asleep.

***Echinacea:** Chilly, nauseous, limbs aching. Note: Only use *after* the appendix ruptures, never before. Use in tincture form (not potentized), 40 drops repeated. Can be used alone or with other remedies.

Belladonna: Worse from being jarred, from noise and light. Abdomen swollen and hard. Pupils dilated. Face may be red.

Bryonia: Intense thirst for large drinks, body is hot, worse from the slightest motion. Pain with each breath. Breathing is shallow and rapid.

Veratrum album: Extreme coldness, cold sweat, vomiting, diarrhea, weak rapid pulse, short labored breathing, restlessness, anxiety, and thirst.

Mercurius: A lot of perspiration, excess saliva but great thirst, foul breath, very chilly, bloody stools, tongue is flabby and shows the imprint of teeth. Chill alternates with feeling hot.

Arsenic Poisoning

Arsenic poisoning is characterized by agonizing, burning pain in the pit of the stomach, a metallic taste, cramping pain, vomiting, diarrhea that looks like rice water, bloody discharges, dry mouth and throat with intense thirst, tightness in the throat, and muscle cramps. The skin, especially on the hands and feet, is damp and blue. The pulse is fast and weak. The breath smells like garlic. There is sighing when breathing. Convulsions and coma follow. Standard treatment recommends administering an emetic such as ipecac, along with warm water to induce vomiting. This should remove some of the gross quantities of poison.

***Arsenicum:** Burning pain, extreme anxiety, great thirst for frequent small sips. Restless, chilly, weak, pale, exhausted by the least effort, and worse after midnight.

***Hepar sulph:** Chilly and can't get warm. Can't bear the slightest draft and worse from uncovering. Skin hypersensitive to touch. Faints from pain. Burning in the stomach, vomits all food. Profuse, foul-smelling sweat.

Carbo veg: Burning in the esophagus and stomach, short of breath and craves air, wants to be fanned, feels freezing cold. Lots of belching.

Ferrum metallicum: Face may be bright red or pale white and puffy. Spits up food by the mouthful. Can't bear the slightest noise. Chilly but with red hot face. Thirsty. Pain, vomiting, worse after midnight.

Ipecacuanha: Intense, continuous nausea not relieved by vomiting. Persistent vomiting. Clean tongue, profuse salivation, tendency to bright red hemorrhage. Thirstless. Better from open air, rest, pressure, and closing the eyes. Worse from the slightest motion and from warmth, especially damp warmth.

Mercurius: Profuse sweating, especially during sleep, after which the patient feels worse. Foul odor from the mouth. Excess saliva with drooling. Flabby tongue with the imprint of teeth. Great thirst for cold drinks. Creeping chilliness but worse from the warmth of the bed. Sensation as if hot vapors were rising into the throat. Trembling of the hands and tongue.

Phosphorus: Burning in the stomach. The patient throws up food by the mouthful, vomits water after it warms in the stomach, craves cold drinks. Afraid to be alone, desires company and reassurance. Hypersensitive to odors, sounds, and lights. Easily startled. Worse lying on the left side. Tendency to hemorrhage of bright red blood. Bloody urine or urinates pure blood.

Veratrum album: Freezing cold with profuse cold sweat on the face and forehead, etc. Skin pale or blue. Extreme weakness. Sudden, violent onset of symptoms. Wants to be covered. Craves cold drinks but vomits them immediately. Vomiting is worse from the least motion. Copious watery diarrhea, which exhausts. Delirium.

Arthritis Pain

Arthritis involves inflammation of one or more joints. There are over one hundred different kinds of arthritis, and multiple causes. Symptoms vary, but in general they include joint pain, joint swelling, stiffness in the morning, warmth around a joint, redness of the skin in the area, reduced mobility of the joint, and weakness that occurs with joint pain.

One of the first two remedies—Bryonia or Rhus tox—will bring relief in a majority of cases.

***Bryonia:** Worse from the slightest motion, exertion, or heat. Wants to lie perfectly still. Better from pressure and warmth on painful part. Joints are hot and swollen. Irritable. Thirsty for large drinks.

***Rhus tox:** Better from continued movement, although painful on first moving. Worse after rest. Attack brought on or worse from cold, damp weather. Very restless. Worse after midnight. Sometimes craves milk.

Lycopodium: Better from motion. Numbness and pain while at rest. One foot hot, the other cold. Worse on the right side. Worse between 4 and 8 p.m. Belching and flatulence. Craves sweets. Lack of confidence and fear of responsibility.

Calcarea carbonicum: Better from continued motion (like Rhus tox). Symptoms occur in a chilly, sweaty, often heavyset person who tires easily. Worse from exertion, cold, and drinking milk. Perspiration from the least exertion. Fear of insects, animals, or poverty. Can't bear to see cruelty.

Silica: Very chilly and feet are freezing cold. Body parts that are lain on go numb. Knee pain. Sensation of a tight bandage around the knee. Foul-smelling foot sweats. Worse from cold, drafts, and dampness. Ailments after vaccination. Averse to meat. Lacks confidence. Conscientious about trifles.

Apis: Stinging, burning pain, which is better from cold. Joints swollen. Thirstless. Given to jealousy. Worse from heat, touch, pressure, and after sleep. Dreams of flying.

Ledum: Chilly, but pain feels better from cold. Pain begins in the ankles and calves and moves upward. Joints are swollen and may feel cold to the touch. Numbness in joints. Worse from motion. Soles of feet painful. Aversion to company and friends.

Causticum: Better in damp or rainy, warm weather. Worse in dry, cold weather. Very chilly. Trembling and weakness of limbs. Restless legs at night. Craves smoked foods. Involuntary urination when coughing or sneezing. Warts around the eyelids, nails, or the tip of the nose. Weeps in sympathy for others. Ailments from long-standing grief.

Aconite: Very anxious, restless, and thirsty. Shooting pains, worse standing, worse at night. Palms of the hands may be red. Feet freezing cold with numbness and tingling. Worse after exposure to cold wind or after a fright.

Kali carbonicum: Sticking, burning pain, which makes the patient shriek. Chilly and worse from cold and drafts. Worse from 2 to 4 a.m. Tearing pain in the big toe. Talks to himself. Fears losing control. Concerned with morality and duty. Aversion to bread. Craves sour foods.

Pulsatilla: Pains change and move about. Worse in a warm room and craves fresh air. Weeps when talking about the pain. Little or no thirst. Worse from rich food, pork, or pastries. Desires sympathy and feels better from it. Affectionate, emotional, or timid. Can't make decisions.

Asphyxia

The inability to oxygenate the body is called asphyxia. Symptoms include pale or blue face and difficulty breathing, or cessation of breathing. The causes include choking, drowning, noxious gases, drugs, anesthesia, electric shock, crushing injuries, nerve damage, tumors, bleeding into the lungs, swelling of the airways due to an allergy, heart problems, and fluid in the lungs.

Take whatever first aid measures are appropriate. This may involve removing any obvious cause of the problem and beginning mouth-to-mouth respiration.

> **Note:** The first four remedies may also be used for "apparent death."

***Antimonium Tartaricum:** Rattling of mucus can be heard in the airways, the face is pale blue, and there is cold sweat on face. Must sit up to breathe. Nostrils flare when breathing. Drowsiness. Quivering of the chin. Worse from warmth.

***Carbo veg:** Craves air and wants to be fanned. Face blue. The head is hot with hot perspiration, but the body and breath are cold. Icy coldness. Burning sensation in chest. Spasmodic cough. Belching.

Camphora: Icy coldness of whole body, but the patient won't be covered. Pupils dilated, breath cold.

Cuprum: Skin blue, cramps, spasms in muscles of hands and feet, jaws contracted, foam at the mouth.

Opium: Drowsy, dull, and sluggish with labored breathing. Skin is hot and sweaty. Face is dark, hot, and may be swollen. Pupils are constricted and don't react to light.

Asthmatic Attack

Asthma involves inflammation of the airways, which restricts the flow of air in and out of the lungs. It is characterized by periodic attacks of wheezing, shortness of breath, a feeling of tightness in the chest, and coughing. The acute symptoms may occur for just a few minutes, or last for days. Asthmatic attacks have many causes including allergens (dust, pollen, foods, smoke, roach droppings, drugs, etc.), respiratory infections, physical or emotional stress, and cold air.

***Ipecacuanha:** *Nausea or vomiting is a key symptom* along with breathing difficulty. Fears suffocation. Feeling of weight on the chest. Cold perspiration. Better from rest, open air. Worse from the slightest motion, warm moist air.

***Nux vomica:** *Begins after meals or in the morning. Oversensitive to noise, light odors, or comments.* Irritable, chilly. *Sense of fullness in the stomach* and clothing feels too tight. Better from damp weather, hot drinks, and belching. Worse in the morning, from cold, after eating, and from uncovering.

***Antimonium tartaricum:** Much thick mucus that can't be coughed up. *Rattling in the chest. The patient feels like he's choking on the mucus.* Despondent. Fears being alone. Better sitting up or after vomiting. Worse in damp cold weather, at night, lying down, being in a warm room, or after vaccinations.

***Pulsatilla:** Gentle, *weepy, clinging. Wants company and sympathy.* Wheezing, coughing up mucus. Hysterical asthma. Better from cool, open air. *Worse in a warm room*, at night, lying on back.

***Arsenicum:** *Extremely anxious, restless, chilly. Worse from midnight to 3 a.m.*, burning in the chest. Doesn't want to be left alone. Wheezing, which is worse when lying down. Better from warmth and moving about, sitting up, or having company. Worse from damp weather, cold drinks, exertion, being alone, or after anger.

Kali carbonicum: *Starts 3–5 a.m.* The patient must sit up or lean forward with the head toward the knees. *Fearful of being alone*, despondent or irritable. Sticking pains. Worse from 3 to 5 a.m.

Carbo veg: *Flatulence with much belching.* Skin is blue and cold. Anxious but not restless. Struggles for air and *wants to be fanned.* Better from belching. Worse sitting or lying down.

Cuprum: *Hiccoughs before the attack. Spasmodic vomiting after the attack. Face is blue with spasms starting in the hands and feet.* Attack comes on suddenly and may last for hours. Better from drinking cold water. Worse from strong emotions, loss of sleep, and hot weather, and also worse at night.

Moschus: Sudden, severe attack with *great fear of smothering*. The chest feels tight. Patient is unable to cough out the mucus. Worse from cold. Life-threatening.

Ignatia: *Often triggered by strong emotions such as anger and grief.* Dry cough. Silent brooding. Worse from consolation and company. Very sensitive to tobacco smoke.

Back Pain from an Injury
(See also "Spine Injuries")

***Arnica:** Pain from any kind of bruising injury, especially to soft tissue.

***Hypericum:** For injuries to the spine or coccyx. Extreme pain, making it impossible to walk or bend over. Pain radiating down the limbs. Twitching muscles.

***Bryonia:** *Pain is worse from the slightest motion*. The patient wants to be perfectly still. Better lying on the painful side. Dry mouth with great thirst. Irritable.

***Rhus tox:** Back feels stiff and is painful when first starting to move, but *continued movement makes it feel better*. Worse in damp or cold weather. Better from warmth. Restless.

Calcarea carbonica: Better from lying on the painful side or on the back. Worse from cold, dampness, lifting, stooping, or walking up stairs. Worries about meeting responsibilities.

Natrum sulph: Pains in the lower back as if from a blow. The whole spine feels sore. Pain radiates upward. Worse from damp weather, lying on the left side, or lying for long in one position.

Magnesia phosphorica: When spasm is the foremost symptom. Better from warmth and worse from cold.

Ruta: Spine feels beaten or lame. Better from warmth, pressure, and lying on the back.

Lycopodium: Better in a cool room, from cold applications, and from warm food and drink. Worse from 4 to 8 p.m., from the pressure of clothes, or from being in a warm room. One foot feels hot, the other cold.

Graphites: Pain in the lower back as if it is broken. Worse from cold and drafts. Also worse from the warmth of the bed. Sad, indecisive.

Kali carbonicum: Worse from 3 to 5 a.m. Pain extends from the buttocks to the thighs. The back feels weak. Worse from cold and better from warmth. Irritable and doesn't want to be alone.

Back Spasm

***Magnesia phosphorica:** Better from warmth and worse from cold.

***Nux vomica:** Must sit up in order to turn in bed. Worse in the morning, after eating, from cold, or while sitting. Emotionally irritable, oversensitive.

Cimicfuga racemosa: Stiffness in the neck and back. Pain in the lower back. Worse during menses, from cold, and in the morning.

Colocynth: Better from warmth and bending over double. Back spasm triggered by anger.

Arsenicum: Anxious, restless, chilly. Better from warmth. Worse after midnight.

Bites and Stings

Note: Some people develop a serious allergic reaction known as anaphylaxis. They may develop difficulty breathing, cramps, vomiting, diarrhea, or hives. If this occurs, see "Anaphylaxis."

***Ledum** (30–200c): An excellent remedy for any puncture wound. The wound may feel cool to the touch.

Apis (30–200c): Bee stings—externally, apply a *diluted* Urtica urens tincture.

Cantharis (30–200c): For wasp stings.

Lachesis: For tarantula bite—skin is hot and looks blue or purple.

Black Widow Spider Bite

The majority of bites occur in outhouses. The bite marks show as two small red spots. There is severe cramping and unbearable pain within one hour. Also, nausea, sweating, and difficulty breathing. Bandage the whole limb with a wide cloth (not a tourniquet).

Ledum (200c), then

Latrodectus mactans (nosode 30c)**:** If you are in a high-risk area, you might want to order this and keep it available. It only works for black widow bites.

Aconite: When fear predominates. Unquenchable thirst.

Hepar (6c)**:** If infection threatens. Every four hours.

Fish Stings

Stonefish, scorpionfish, stingray, weever fish, etc. Agonizing pain. Place limb in water as hot as you can stand to inactivate the poison. Remove and immerse again and again until the pain is gone.

Ledum (200c).

Jellyfish Stings

Symptoms: tingling, swelling. Pour **vinegar** on the tentacles that are still attached to victim. This prevents the discharge of more poison. Do not use alcohol!

Aconite: Use initially, when the victim is frightened.

Ledum: Follows Aconite.

Bleeding

Arterial bleeding is indicated by bright red blood coming out in spurts. Apply pressure just above the wound, between the wound and the heart. Bleeding from veins produces a continuous flow of dark blood. Apply pressure below the wound, with the wound between the heart and your hand.

***Arnica:** Bleeding after an injury.

***Phosphorus:** Bright red blood that won't coagulate, slight wounds bleed too much. Desire for company, great thirst for cold drinks. Phosphorus is excellent for bleeding from dental work.

***Ipecacuanha:** Bleeding with vomiting and nausea. Nosebleeds.

***Lachesis:** Hemorrhage of thin, dark blood that won't coagulate. Patient is weak, talkative, worse after sleep and from heat. Wounds look purplish.

***Cinchona:** For the effects of loss of blood. Helps protect the body until it can recover. Fainting after loss of blood. Internal bleeding. Chilly, abdomen bloated, belching, worse from the slightest touch, sensitive to noise.

Aconite: Bright red blood, fear of death, unquenchable thirst. Skin is hot and dry.

Carbo veg: Blood slowly oozing out from inflamed surfaces. The patient is chilly but craves fresh air. Wants to be fanned.

Millefolium: Active, bright red hemorrhage from nose, lungs, or bowels. Especially for bleeding from injuries.

Crotalus horridus: Blood is black, won't coagulate, and flows from every orifice including the eyes, ears, nose, and anus.

Hamamelis: Oozing of dark red blood. Exhaustion after minor bleeding. Nosebleeds after injuries. Painful wounds.

Blood Poisoning—Septicemia

This condition is due to bacteria in the bloodstream. It can result from an infection anywhere in the body. Infected wounds are a common cause. It may occur after labor from retained placenta or clots. Symptoms include intermittent fever, chills, headache, weak but rapid pulse, exhaustion, sometimes vomiting, and diarrhea. Lymph glands may enlarge at the groin, under the arms, under the jaw, etc. The skin may be hot and dry, or sweaty, cold, and clammy. The patient becomes listless. There may be delirium, followed by coma.

***Pyrogenium:** Especially after labor, but useful in many circumstances. The patient *feels bruised all over* with pain in the limbs. *The bed feels too hard*. Parts lain on become sore, so the patient must constantly change position for relief. *Offensive discharges.* Pulse and fever out of sync, e.g., *high pulse with low fever* or *low pulse with high fever.* Tongue shiny and red. Worse from cold. The patient says she can feel her heart beat. Delusions of having extra limbs. Very talkative during fever.

***Arsenicum:** Extreme anxiety, fear of being alone, great restlessness, great thirst but for small sips of cold water. Burning pains, which are relieved by heat. Offensive discharges. Burning discharges. Very chilly. During headache, wants body warm but head cold. Delusion that he is being watched. Worse from midnight to 3 a.m.

***Lachesis:** Worse after sleep. Extremely sensitive to touch, even from his own clothing. Purplish color to wounds and some areas of skin. Can't stand anything around his neck. Left-sided symptoms. Difficulty swallowing liquids. Worse from hot drinks. Better from open air. Delirium with great talkativeness and delusions. Tendency to bleeding.

***Carbo veg:** A state of collapse. Desperate for fresh air. Much belching with bloated abdomen. Hot sweat on the head, but hands and feet icy cold. Breath cool. Skin cold, clammy, and mottled. Can't stand tight clothing around the waist (also Lachesis and Crotalus). Skin blue or purplish (also Lachesis). Fearful in a dark room or when closing the eyes. Fear of ghosts.

***Crotalus horridus:** Yellow face and/or eyes. Weeping, talkative, delusion that his brain is decaying. Pain in liver. Sensitive to light. Symptoms tend to be right sided (opposite Lachesis). Worse from open air (opposite Lachesis). Tendency to hemorrhage of black blood. Can't swallow solids (opposite Lachesis). Can't stand tight clothing around waist. Bloody or coffee-ground-colored vomit. Worse after sleep (same as Lachesis). Tendency to bleeding.

Anthracinum: Terrible burning pains. Rapid loss of strength, sinking pulse, delirium. Hemorrhage of black, tarlike blood. Edema, foul-smelling pus, hardening of tissue, swollen glands. When Arsenicum seems indicated but fails.

Belladonna: Face red and hot with pupils dilated. Patient can't stand light, noise, or being jarred. Throbbing sensation in the head or other areas. May be irritable, angry, or delirious.

Arnica: Blood poisoning after bruising injuries. The patient doesn't want to be touched and insists she is okay. Complains of the bed being too hard (also Baptisia) and is restless. Discharges smell like rotten eggs.

Apis: Burning, stinging pain relieved by cold. Edema. Thirstless. Worse from heat. Worse from a warm room, touch, pressure, lying down, or after sleep. Better from cold, motion, or sitting up.

Baptisia: Face dusky, dark red. Falls asleep while being spoken to. Feels sore all over. Low fever, delirium in which the patient believes his limbs are scattered about the bed. Foul breath, stool, and urine. Can only swallow liquids; solids gag him.

Echinacea: Used in tincture form, undiluted in 30-drop doses. May be used in addition to other remedies, but not at the same time. It will stimulate the immune system.

Rhus tox: To prevent sepsis after surgery.

Boils: See "Abscess"

Botulism Poisoning

Botulism is a special case of severe food poisoning in which a bacterial toxin called botulin causes paralysis. It is contracted from eating food in which the toxin has formed. Onset of symptoms may occur anywhere from a few hours to eight days. They include double vision, inability to focus, drooping eyelids, difficulty speaking, difficulty swallowing, intense abdominal cramps, vomiting spells, diarrhea, failure of pupils to react to light, and weakness of muscles beginning in the upper limbs and moving downward. Subsequently, difficulty breathing ending in respiratory paralysis.

Most cases result from consuming home-canned vegetables, cured pork and ham, smoked or raw fish, honey, or corn syrup. Sometimes the bacteria enters from an open wound. The toxin is so potent that even a taste of the food could prove fatal. There is a special type of botulism to which infants are particularly susceptible. Do not give corn syrup or honey to infants. Home-canned foods should be cooked for thirty minutes at 250 degrees.

Botulism toxin causes paralysis of the respiratory muscles. If the patient can be placed on a ventilator to breathe for him, the effect of the toxin eventually wears off. When conventional care is available at the onset, treatment involves the administration of antitoxin. However, this is only effective in the beginning, before the toxin has deeply affected the nerve endings.

***Botulinum** (nosode 200c)**:** Difficulty swallowing, breathing, and walking. The patient feels like he's choking. Thick speech, blurred or double vision, stomach cramps, and a masklike expression on the face.

***Gelsemium:** Difficulty swallowing, weak muscles, blurred vision, double vision, eyelids droop, pupils don't respond, speech confused. Thirstless, difficulty breathing, pulse slow. Wants to be left alone.

Belladonna (200c)**:** Sudden intense onset of symptoms. Worse from light, noise, being jarred, being in the sun, drafts on the head, and bright objects. Face is red and feels hot. Hands and feet cold.

Arsenicum: Extremely anxious, restless, weak, and chilly. Fears suffocation and can't lie down. Thirsty for small sips. Fears being alone.

Phosphorus: Sensitive to light, sound, and odors. Startles easily. Afraid to be alone. Thirsty for cold drinks.

Breast Abscess

Such infections occur when bacteria enter the breast through a break in the skin, usually at the nipple. Symptoms include pain and swelling of the breast, discharge from the nipple (sometimes pus), enlarged lymph glands under the arm near the breast, and fever. These abscesses are usually found in women who are breastfeeding. Pain and swelling of the breast when not breastfeeding may indicate other problems, and a medical professional should be consulted.

***Bryonia:** Hot, hard, painful, but not very red. Pain which is worse from the slightest movement.

***Belladonna:** Breast feels heavy, red streaks radiating from one point, throbbing pains. Worse lying down or from being bumped.

***Phytolacca:** Breasts hard and sensitive. Pain radiates from the nipple to rest of the body when nursing. Purple discoloration (also Lachesis). Ulcers with pus. Worse from cold.

Hepar sulph (6x or 6c)**:** When pus begins to form. Worse from the slightest touch, and from cold or draft.

Silica: Ulceration with discharge of pus. The patient is thin, chilly, exhausted.

Mercurius sol: Blood-streaked pus. Perspiration, chills, and excess saliva. Worse in a warm room, at night, and after sweating.

Lachesis: Breast inflamed, purplish color. Worse after sleep. Cold at night but has flushes of heat during day.

Breast, Injuries to

These remedies can be used after any bruising injury or puncture wound to the breast. They can help prevent complications. The remedies are also effective after breast biopsies and mammograms.

Bellis perennis: A good choice for any injury to the breast. Also, if the injury leaves a hardened area beneath the skin that is tender to the touch.

Conium maculatum: The injury leaves a hardened area, which feels better from hard pressure.

Arnica: If Bellis and Conium are not available.

Ledum: After puncture wounds and biopsies. Follow with Bellis or Conium if symptoms indicate.

Breathing, Difficult: See "Asphyxia"

Broken Bones—Fractures

When the skin is intact, the fracture is referred to as "simple." When the skin is broken, it is called a "compound" fracture. For simple fractures, immobilize the area with a splint before attempting to move the person. For a compound fracture, place a sterile cloth over the wound and apply firm pressure to stop the bleeding. If no professional help is available and the person must be moved, apply a splint.

Arnica: First remedy. Use Arnica to minimize pain, swelling, and shock.

Eupatorium perfoliatum: Mostly pain—not much bruising.

Bryonia: Worse from the slightest motion, deep breathing (broken ribs), or a warm room.

Symphytum: Speeds healing of bone after the swelling has lessened. Use a dose of 30c once a day for eight to ten days.

Calcarea phosphorica: Speeds healing of bone when coldness and numbness are present.

Hypericum: For fractures of the spine.

Bronchitis—Acute

Bronchitis is inflammation of the bronchial tree due to infection or irritation (e.g., from dust, chemicals). It often starts with a cold, followed by weakness, chilliness, low fever, sore throat, and back or muscle pain. A dry cough may be followed by congestion with considerable mucus.

> **Note:** Children most often need Ipecac, Kali carb, Antimonium tart, Dulcamara, or Phosphorus. However, any remedy may apply.

***Aconite:** Sudden onset after exposure to cold, dry air. Fearful and restless. Skin is hot and dry. Hard, dry, painful cough.

***Bryonia:** Patient lies perfectly still and is worse from any movement. Dry cough. Dry mouth with thirst for large, cold drinks. Pain on breathing or coughing. Constipation. Irritable.

***Phosphorus:** Yellow, blood-streaked sputum. Great thirst for cold drinks. Better lying on the right side. Burning sensations. Better after a short nap. Desires company and is worse alone. Hoarseness.

***Antimonium tart:** Rattling cough. Thick mucus that the patient is unable to cough up. Worse at night, from lying down, or being in a warm room. Better from sitting up, lying on the right side, moving, or vomiting.

***Ipecac:** Gagging from coughing. Nausea and vomiting accompany respiratory symptoms. Coarse, rattling cough. Symptoms come on quickly. Tendency to bleeding.

***Hepar sulph:** The patient is very chilly and better from warmth. Worse from any draft. Discharges smell like old cheese. Irritable. Better from heat and damp weather. Worse from cold, cold food, and touch.

***Pulsatilla:** Craving for fresh air, even when chilly. Worse from warmth and closed spaces. Craves company and sympathy. Fearful when alone. Quite thirstless even with a dry mouth. Symptoms change in character and from place to place. Bland yellow-green discharges. Better in cool air and from cold food and drink.

Dulcamara: Comes on in damp weather. Worse from weather changes (warm to cold or dry to damp). Patient is chilly and likes being near the radiator or stove. Lots of thick, yellow mucus.

Ferrum phos: Early stages when symptoms are not clear. Slow onset with low fever. Face alternates between red and pale. Sweaty. Nosebleeds. Better from lying down and cold applications. Worse from 4 to 6 a.m., at night, from cold drinks, being jarred, motion, and on the right side.

Arsenicum: Anxious, restless, chilly, thirsty for small sips, exhausted, fearful of being alone. Burning sensations relieved by heat. Worse from midnight to 3 a.m. and from cold. Better from warmth, warm food, and sitting up.

Drosera: Dry cough with gagging, vomiting, or cold sweat. Worse after midnight, from warmth, and from lying down. Better from fresh air, sitting up. Very restless and anxious when alone.

Rumex: Sensitivity to cold air and changes in temperature, tickling in the pit of the throat, and cough from breathing cold air. The patient covers his mouth. Thin mucus followed by thick, yellow, stringy mucus. Foul diarrhea early in the morning. Skin itches when undressing.

Spongia: Dry barking cough, cough like the sawing of a log. Worse after sleep, very chilly, worse lying on the right side, better on the back. The throat and lungs feel dry. Fear of suffocation. Worse after midnight and from cold.

Kali carbonicum: Attack comes on or is worse from 3 to 5 a.m. Sticking pains. Extremely chilly and worse from drafts. Better sitting up with the head bent forward on the knees. Swelling of the upper eyelids.

Bruises

A wound in which the skin is not broken. Pain, swelling, and discoloration.

***Arnica:** First choice.

Bellis perennis: Deep bruises, especially of the breast.

Hypericum: After a crushing blow, intense pain, or injury to parts rich in nerves such as the fingers, toes, and spine.

Ledum: If Arnica doesn't give full relief. Discoloration remaining long after the injury. Wound feels better from cold.

Ruta graveolens: Bruising injuries to bones.

Conium: Tumors or ulcers, which arise after a blow.

Burns

Burns may be caused by the direct effects of heat (thermal burns), and by chemicals, electricity (including lightning), and radiation. Radiation burns can come from sunlight (ultraviolet), X-rays, and other penetrating forms of radiation. Aside from the pain, some other factors to consider are shock, respiratory and/or cardiac arrest (from electric shock), and infection, including tetanus. Homeopathic remedies work to restore balance. They help relieve pain, prevent further tissue damage, promote healing, and stimulate the body to fight infection.

Classification of Burns

First degree: Limited to reddening of the skin. There is tenderness, pain, and sometimes swelling. This burn affects the outer layer of the skin. The tissue usually rebuilds itself in less than two weeks.

Second degree: Reddening plus blistering. The outer and some of the inner layers of the skin are affected. The tissue is still able to regenerate.

Third degree: A deeper burn that damages the full thickness of the skin. Often there is no blistering. After the initial injury, intense pain may not be present because nerve endings have been destroyed. The skin can look scorched and may be insensitive to pinprick.

Remedies for Burns

***Cantharis** (30–200c)**:** First choice. Relieves pain and helps prevent blistering. Also useful for shock triggered by burns, and for when the kidneys are affected with painful urination and bloody urine. The diluted tincture can be used externally (see "External Treatment for Burns" in this section).

Causticum (6–30c)**:** For deeper burns. Also for ailments resulting after burns, or for when the body fails to heal burns quickly. Burns on the tongue (also Arsenicum).

Calendula (30–200c)**:** Excellent for very painful burns.

Urtica urens: Intense burning, stinging, and itching.

Rhus tox: Much blistering, itching, worse from cold, chilly, thirsty.

Kali bichromicum: For deep burns with destruction of skin.

Hypericum (30–200c)**:** For extreme pain. For pain which feels better from cold application or cold air. Mental confusion, irritability. (A diluted tincture can be used externally. See below.)

Echinacea tincture: Ten drops internally every hour to help prevent infection.

Carbo veg: Lungs injured from breathing in hot air.

Hepar (6c)**:** With formation of pus. Administer every four hours for infection after burns. May also be given to prevent infection.

Arsenicum album: To prevent gangrene. Burning pains relieved by warmth, blisters that turn black, exhaustion, anxiety, restlessness, chills, and thirst. Also, burns on the tongue (also Causticum).

Radiation Burns

See "Radiation Burns" and "Radiation Sickness."

External Treatment for Burns

Cantharis tincture: Diluted one part to ten parts of water. A cotton dressing soaked with this is applied loosely to the burn. Keep the dressings wet with this.

Urtica urens tincture: Diluted one part to ten parts of water. A cotton dressing soaked with this is applied loosely. Keep the dressings wet with this.

Hypericum tincture: Diluted one part to ten parts water. When there is much pain. Hypericum oil is another excellent topical treatment.

Hamamelis tincture: For first degree burns. A cotton dressing with a diluted tincture of hamamelis is applied and kept wet.

Calendula tincture (diluted)**:** Bathe the burned area to promote healing and prevent scarring.

Vitamin E oil, or wheat germ oil: Excellent for relieving pain.

Chemical Burns

Cantharis and **Causticum** are useful for chemical burns.

Aside from remedies, there are some first aid measures that can help :he victim.

1. First, bathe the area immediately with large amounts of cold water. Remove any clothing that has the chemical on it. See if the container of chemical has specific directions for first aid.
2. If you know that this was an acid burn, then apply a paste of baking soda, a soap solution, or greatly diluted ammonia. If the burn is from carbolic acid, then bathe the area with diluted alcohol.

If an alkali—such as lye, ammonia, or lime—caused the burn, then diluted vinegar or fruit juice may be applied.

Respiratory and Cardiac Arrest Associated with Burns from Electric Shock

Administer **Arnica** or **Phosphorus** along with the following procedures.

Respiratory arrest: Breathing may stop after burns from electrical shock. Immediately begin mouth-to-mouth resuscitation.

Cardiac arrest: After electrical shock, the heart may stop beating. Immediately begin CPR (cardiopulmonary resuscitation). This involves alternating mouth-to-mouth breathing with pressing sharply on the bottom third of the breastbone to artificially "beat" the heart. Eight presses on the breastbone for each mouth-to-mouth breath is a suggested ratio.

Burns, Shock from

The onset of shock is indicated by restlessness, thirst, increased pulse rate, and faintness when sitting up. If shock ensues the patient will experience pale face, cold sweat, cold hands and feet, weak pulse, anxiety, rapid breathing, restlessness, confusion, and reduced urine output.

Aconite: Shock with great fear of death.

Carbo veg: When there has been great loss of blood.

Arnica: The patient insists he is okay, but refuses to be touched.

Cantharis: Shock after a burn.

Burns—Preventing Tetanus

Hypericum: Has been used for both pain and prevention of tetanus.

Burns, Infection from

Since bacteria thrive on dead tissue and warm places, burns are a fertile field for infection.

Hepar sulph (6c)**:** Three times a day to prevent infection.

Pyrogenium: If infection develops.

Cancer, Pains from

Arsenicum: Sharp burning pains, which are worse from cold and better from applying heat. The patient is restless and keeps moving about. Very thirsty but for small sips. Great anxiety and fear of death. Chilly and exhausted from the least exertion. Diarrhea. Better from warmth, warm applications, and warm drinks. Worse after midnight.

Carcinosin: Especially for cancer of the breast, uterus, or liver. Individuals who are intensely sympathetic and demand much from themselves. People who are worse from heat. Worse from 1 to 5 p.m. or 5 to 6 p.m. Brown spots on skin and blue tinge to the white of the eye. Craves salt, fat, spicy foods, or chocolate.

Apis: Especially for cancers on the right side of the body. Stinging, burning pain better from cold application. Nipples drawn in. No thirst. Worse from heat, touch, pressure, warm closed rooms, and after sleep. Better in open air.

Cadmium sulph: Very chilly even when near a heat source. Blue circles around the eyes. Terrible nausea. Black or coffee-ground-colored vomit. Also vomits green mucus or blood. Weakness with tenderness over the stomach. Bloody-black, offensive stools. Extreme exhaustion. Belching with a salty taste.

Conium: Hardened glands, hardened tumors. Cancer of lip or breast after an injury. Sharp shooting pains in breast. Cancer of stomach with pain extending from stomach to back and shoulders. Burning.

Hydrastis: Especially liver cancer. Sharp, cutting pain like knives. Vomits everything except water. Weak and emaciated. Thick, yellow, stringy discharges. Tongue yellow and indented. Constipation. Weak digestion. Especially left-sided complaints.

Asterias: Breast cancer around the nipple, which is sunk in. Sharp, knife-like pains that go through to the back. Glands under the arms are hard and swollen. Skin hardened. Especially affects the left breast. Stinging pain in the uterus.

Colocynth: Gnawing, boring, or cramping pain followed by numbness. Pain causes the patient to double up and cry out. Bitter taste in the mouth. Better from warmth.

Chemotherapy, Side Effects of

Side effects of chemotherapy include hair loss, nausea, vomiting, changes in appetite, blood-clotting problems, fatigue, and infections. Also kidney, heart, or pulmonary damage.

The following remedies can help the body recover from its toxicity.

***Cadmium sulph:** Main remedy for side effects of chemotherapy—exhaustion, violent nausea, vomiting, and weakness. Craves small cold drinks, which are immediately vomited.

***Ipecacuanha:** Constant nausea not relieved by vomiting. Excess salivation, clean tongue (not coated).

Nux vomica: Nausea and vomiting with an angry, irritable, oversensitive mental state. Chilly and constipated.

Cinchona: Stomach bloated with gas. Vomits undigested food. Worse from drafts and after eating.

Arsenicum: Nausea and vomiting with burning pains. Burning pain relieved by warmth. Extremely anxious and very restless. Exhausted by the least effort. Doesn't want to be alone. Thirsty for small sips.

Chickenpox

Chickenpox is a contagious viral disease characterized by an itchy skin rash of small, reddish bumps, which then become fluid-filled blisters. The blisters arise in small groups, first on the trunk, then spreading to the arms, legs, face, and scalp. The blisters eventually open and form crusts, which darken in time. The virus is spread by airborne droplets or contaminated clothing.

Symptoms include headache, low-grade fever, weakness, and raised blisters on the scalp, trunk, and sometimes in the mouth. As some blisters are crusting over, others are just beginning to appear. Avoid aspirin, which has been associated with Reye's syndrome when used for viral illnesses.

Prevention

Varicella (nosode 30c) or **Antimonium tart**, or **Aconite** and **Pulsatilla**, one dose of each per day.

Remedies for Chickenpox

Aconite: In the early stage with high fever, restlessness, and much anxiety. Sudden onset. Skin is hot and dry. Red face, which may go pale on rising. Desires cold drinks. Worse at night and after midnight.

Belladonna: Throbbing headache, red face, hot skin, bloodshot eyes, drowsy but can't sleep. High fever. Sudden onset. Desires cold water and lemonade. Moans in his sleep. Delirium. Worse from drafts, light, noise, or being jarred. Worse at 3 p.m. and during the night.

Antimonium tart: Bronchitis or rattling cough with thick mucus. Worse from lying down. Must sit up to breathe. Delayed eruption. Eruptions are pus filled or blue. Great drowsiness. Pale face with cold sweat. Tongue is pasty-white with red edges. Craves apples, fruit, and small sips of water. Worse from warmth.

Antimonium crudum: Tongue is coated a thick white, there is a golden-yellow discharge from the blisters, and the patient is worse from warmth. Much belching. Either craves food or has disgust for it.

Extremely irritable. Can't bear to be looked at or touched. Sulks and refuses to talk. Angry or sad with weeping.

Pulsatilla: Worse in a warm room and craves fresh air. Wants a window open even when chilly. Desires company and sympathy. Weeps describing his symptoms. Dry mouth but has no thirst. Bland (non-irritating), yellowish-green discharges. Sleepy in the day, but wide awake at night.

Rhus tox: Intense itching and stiff muscles. The patient is restless and changes position frequently. Worse after rest. Worse in the evening, from cold, dampness, or open air. Anxious in the evening. Thirsty for cold drinks (especially milk). Drowsy after eating.

Bryonia: Dry cough, fever, intense thirst for large cold drinks, worse from any movement and wants to be perfectly still. Very irritable and wants to be left alone. Mouth dry and cracked. Rash develops slowly. Large, dry stools. Better from cool air, pressure, quiet, and rest.

Mercurius solubilis or **Mercurius vivus:** After the fever has abated. Also, when pus fills the blisters. Nasal secretions that burn and smell like old cheese. Much itching, which feels better from scratching and worse from the warmth of the bed. Worse from drafts. Perspires easily and feels worse afterward. Craves cold drinks.

Chlamydia

Chlamydia is a sexually transmitted disease caused by bacteria. It can be acquired and carried by both men and women. Untreated, it can damage a woman's reproductive organs. Untreated chlamydia in men can lead to infertility. Chlamydia can also be passed from a mother to her baby during childbirth. Babies so infected can develop inflammation of the eyes and respiratory tract. Most people with chlamydia show no symptoms. Women may experience vaginal discharge, burning during urination, abdominal pain, low back pain, nausea, fever, pain during sex, and bleeding between menses. Men infrequently exhibit a discharge from the penis, a burning sensation on urinating, itching at the opening of the penis, or pain and swelling in the testicles.

Medorrhinum: In women: thin, burning discharge with fishy odor. In men: yellow discharge, urethra feels sore. In both: worse from damp or cold. Craves fats and sweets, fish, and lemons.

Sulphur: In women: burning and itching of the vagina, worse while sitting, offensive perspiration on thighs. In men: genitals itch, burning in urethra. In both: worse from warmth or heat and from bathing. Craves sweets and spicy foods.

Thuja: In women: thick, greenish discharge, itching of the vagina, vagina very sensitive. In men: Testes feel bruised, offensive odor to semen. In both: worse from coldness or dampness. Craves chocolate and cold drinks.

Choking

If choking is due to something caught in the throat, the Heimlich maneuver is called for. It consists of a quick hard compression under the ribs. When choking is due to a spasm, triggered by something swallowed, the following remedies may help.

Cicuta virosa: After swallowing a sharp piece of bone that injures the throat, the throat closes with danger of suffocation. The object may have been swallowed, but its passage triggers spasm. Inability to swallow. Spasm of the throat on attempting to swallow. The throat feels bruised externally.

Mephitis (1x to 3x)**:** Choking while drinking or talking. Can't exhale.

Hyoscyamus: Choking when swallowing liquids, which come out through the nose.

Cholera

Cholera is an acute bacterial infection of the small intestines. Symptoms appear after one to six days and include profuse diarrhea, vomiting, dehydration, intense thirst, muscle cramps, reduced urine output, and collapse. The patient may exhibit sunken eyes and wrinkled skin. Cholera is usually acquired by drinking contaminated water. Dehydration from diarrhea presents a serious threat. It is important to replace fluids, electrolytes, and sugar.

Prevention

Vibrio cholerae (nosode 30c) once a week or **Veratrum album** and **Cuprum** alternated every four hours. **Camphora** is another option (two drops of a tincture of Camphor on sugar once or twice a day.) Note: Store Camphor well away from other homeopathic remedies, as the fumes can destroy them.

Remedies for Cholera

***Camphora:** First choice at the onset of the disease, when diarrhea is present. Very effective if given early and repeated often. It can be used in the tincture form, two drops (best on sugar to avoid nausea), or in potencies. *Sudden exhaustion, freezing cold but refuses covers,* cramps in calves, burning pain in the stomach and throat, nausea, fingers numb. The patient may feel like he is suffocating.

***Veratrum album:** Diarrhea, *cold sweat especially on forehead, freezing cold,* much thirst, cramps in the legs and fingers, abdomen sensitive to touch. Vomiting, which is worse from motion or drinking. Craves ice water.

***Cuprum:** *Spasms throughout the body, beginning in the hands. Cramps in extremities, thumbs clenched in fists.* Face blue. Cramping and pain in the stomach, spasms in the throat that make speech difficult, vomiting. Feels like she's suffocating and won't let anything touch her face. Craves warm drinks.

***Arsenicum:** *Extremely restless, very anxious, thirsty for small sips, burning pains that are oddly relieved by heat,* cold sweat, black or green vomit, tongue dry and black, wants company. Extremely weak. Great fear of death.

Carbo veg: Abdomen bloated, *much belching* (which gives some relief), head hot but *hands and feet icy cold. Hungers for air* and wants to be fanned.

Podophyllum: Foul-smelling painless diarrhea, which gushes out like a hydrant. Very talkative either during chill or fever. During sleep, the head rolls from side to side. Foul breath with excess salivation and an indented tongue (also Mercurius).

Laurocerasus: Difficulty breathing and worse from any exertion, body cold, lips blue, feels like the throat is closing when swallowing. No vomiting or stool. The condition lingers for days and the patient seems like he won't recover. Patients often fall asleep after taking the remedy.

Phosphorus: Great thirst for ice-cold water, but vomits it shortly after drinking. Profuse diarrhea, which gushes out. Desires company and fears being alone. Sensitive to lights, sounds, and odors. Tendency to bleeding. Hiccoughs after eating.

Cold—Common Cold (Coryza)

Aconite: If the cold started after exposure to cold air or drafts. Symptoms come on quickly and include fever, hot dry skin, great thirst for cold water, red face (sometimes pale on first rising), restlessness, and anxiety. This remedy usually works in the first twenty-four hours.

Belladonna: Symptoms come on rapidly and intensely as in Aconite. The face is hot and red, the eyes are bloodshot and glassy, there is a high fever, and a red, sore throat. The patient may crave lemonade. He is worse from light, noise, or being jarred. He may be thirsty or not. When the fever is very high, there may be delirium. Belladonna often follows Aconite.

Ferrum phosphoricum: The symptoms come on slowly and are rather vague or general. The patient feels ill, but there are no clear symptoms yet. The face alternates between red and pale. Better from lying down and from cold applications. Worse between 4 and 6 a.m., at night, and from cold drinks.

Allium cepa: The nose runs readily with a thin, clear, burning nasal discharge. The eyes water profusely. Much sneezing. Better from cool, fresh air and from moving about. Worse in a warm room and after rest. Tickling in larynx. Colds that started after exposure to damp, cold weather.

Kali bichromicum: Thick, sticky, yellow-green nasal discharge. Sinus discomfort and postnasal drip. Forms mucus plugs in the nose. Violent sneezing that is worse in the morning. Coughs up sticky yellow mucus (worse in the morning). Sensation of a hair on the back of the tongue or in the nostrils. Tired and wants to lie down. Better from heat, motion, and pressure.

Nux vomica: Irritable, chilly, oversensitive to noise, lights, odors, or criticism. The nose runs during the day but is stuffy at night. Chill from uncovering or just moving. Even during fever with a hot body, the patient cannot be uncovered. Tendency to constipation with straining at stool. Can't sleep between 3 and 5 a.m. Better from warmth, covering, and napping. Worse from cold, early morning, uncovering, drafts, noise, odors, and the pressure of clothes.

Pulsatilla: Thick, yellow-green, bland (non-irritating) mucus. Virtually no thirst. Craves fresh air. Can't bear a stuffy room and wants a window open even when chilly. Desires company and sympathy. Wet cough in the morning and dry cough at night.

Arsenicum album: There is a watery discharge from the nose, which irritates the nostrils. The patient is very chilly, restless, anxious, and often wants company. Thirsty for frequent small sips of water.

Mercurius: Foul breath, flabby tongue (sometimes with the imprint of teeth), excess saliva (he may drool), much thirst, yellowish-green nasal discharge that irritates the nostrils. Sometimes there is blood-streaked mucus. The patient perspires a lot and feels worse afterward. Dry cough. Worse at night.

Coldness—Icy
(See also "Hypothermia" and "Frostbite")

Arsenicum: Very anxious, restless, exhausted, and thirsty, but for small sips. Burning pains relieved by heat. Foul-smelling diarrhea. Worse from midnight to 3 a.m. Fear of being alone.

Carbo veg: Top remedy for collapse. Hungry for air and wants to be fanned. Abdomen bloated with much belching. Head hot but breath and body cold. Hot sweat on the head. Pulse feeble, fingertips blue. Feet icy-cold up to the knees. Better from belching and being fanned.

Camphora: States of collapse or shock. Sudden sinking of strength. Freezing cold but absolutely refuses covers, cold perspiration, cold breath. Cramps in calves, coldness followed by burning pain in the stomach, thirstlessness, nausea, fingers numb. The patient may feel like he is suffocating.

Secale: The patient feels hot internally, but the skin is cold to the touch. Even when icy-cold, he can't bear to be covered. Worse from warmth. He feels like ants are crawling on him, especially his hands (so he holds his fingers apart).

Silica: Worse from drafts (opposite Carbo veg), easily exhausted, thirsty, hypersensitive to touch and noise. Better from warmth and covering the head. Worse from cold, drafts, dampness, light, noise, or excitement.

Cuprum: Spasms starting in hands and feet. Face blue.

Bryonia: Lies perfectly still. Symptoms worse from any movement. Thirsty for large, cold drinks. Irritable.

Veratrum album: Freezing cold with profuse cold sweat on the face and forehead. The skin is blue. Extreme weakness. Sudden violent onset of symptoms. The patient wants to be covered. Large stools with straining or painful, watery diarrhea.

Nux vomica: Chill from the slightest movement and from uncovering. Irritable, angry, oversensitive to noise, lights, odors, and imagined insults. Constipation with urging for stool accompanies many complaints. Insomnia 3–5 a.m. Better from warmth, covering, wet weather, and napping. Worse in the early morning, and from cold, uncovering, drafts, noise, odors, and the pressure of clothes.

Colic Pain

Acute abdominal pain due to spasms of internal organs. These can be spasms of the stomach, intestines, bile ducts, ureters, uterus, etc. These remedies are therefore effective in treating pain from kidney stones, gallstones, stomach cramps, menstrual cramps, and more.

***Colocynth:** Pain makes the patient *double over*. Better from touch and hard pressure. Better from heat. Better lying on the abdomen. Pain may come on after anger, or the person may be angry during the attack.

***Magnesia phosphorica:** Pain relieved mostly by heat, but also by bending double. Tendency to right-sided complaints. Chilly and worse from cold. Worse from touch, but better from hard pressure.

Dioscorea: *Pain relieved by bending backward* (opposite of bending double). Worse bending double. Better from motion and hard pressure. Pain radiates in all directions. Sudden pains, which move from place to place.

Chamomilla: *Pain with very angry disposition*, red cheeks, hot perspiration. Can't bear to be spoken to or touched. Very thirsty. Worse at night and from drinking coffee.

Nux vomica: *Irritable, oversensitive* to noise, odors, and lights. Chilly and worse from uncovering. Constipated and strains at stool. Better from hot drinks, warmth, or loosening the belt. Can't stand tight clothing. Worse in the morning. Craves stimulants.

Concussion

A condition resulting from a head injury. Symptoms vary and may include vomiting, flushed face, rapid pulse, confused mental state, restlessness, pupils of unequal size, headache, slight temperature or low-grade fever, loss of consciousness, and coma.

Note: If the patient is unconscious or convulsing, place the remedy between the lips and teeth. This is to prevent the remedy from being inhaled.

***Arnica** (30–200c): First choice. Every half hour for three doses, then every hour until consciousness returns.

***Hypericum:** If convulsions begin. Use as needed. Place the remedy between the lips and teeth.

Cicuta virosa: If convulsions are very violent. Use as needed. Place the remedy between the lips and teeth.

Opium: Use homeopathic opium if the patient is unconscious for protracted periods. Pupils constricted.

Lasting Effects from a Head Injury

Natrum sulph: Aftereffects of a head injury, such as personality changes, confusion, depression, and traumatic epilepsy, have been relieved by this remedy. It works even when taken years after the injury.

Helleborus: The patient becomes mentally slow, answers slowly, concentration difficult, memory impaired, involuntary sighing, chewing motions.

Conjunctivitis
(See also "Neonatal Conjunctivitis")

Inflammation of the outer layer of the eye and eyelid. There are numerous causes of conjunctivitis, including viruses, bacteria, fungi, and various allergens. "Pinkeye" is a very contagious viral conjunctivitis. Newborns are subject to a bacterial form that must be treated, as it can threaten eyesight. (See "Neonatal Conjunctivitis.") The general symptoms of conjunctivitis are redness of the eyes, watery eyes, pain, itching, sensitivity to light, crusts on the eyelids, and blurred vision.

***Argentum nitricum:** With thick, yellow, bland pus. Worse from heat and craves cold, fresh air. Very anxious. Craves sweets, which make him belch. Worse from bright light.

***Pulsatilla:** Yellow-green, bland discharge. Better from fresh air. Worse from heat. Desires sympathy and company. May weep telling of his symptoms. Dry mouth, but no thirst.

***Aconite:** Inflammation after an injury, after removal of a foreign object, or after exposure to cold air. Not much tearing. Eyes feel dry and burn. Very anxious. Thirsty.

***Euphrasia:** Burning hot tears and a desire to blink. Aversion to light. Worse in the evening, from sunlight, and from warmth.

Belladonna: Eyes bloodshot, very red, painful, and hot. Sudden onset. Pupils dilated. Worse from light, noise, or being jarred. Craves lemonade and cold drinks.

Apis mel: Eyelids swollen with stinging pain. Better from cold air and cold application. No thirst. Worse from heat, touch, after sleep, and from 3 to 4 p.m.

Hepar sulph: Thick, foul-smelling pus. Eyes are sensitive to cold and to the slightest touch or draft. Worse from cold and better from warmth. Very irritable. Craves acidic foods.

Sulphur: Eyes hot, dry, and burning. Lids red and swollen in the morning. Worse in a warm room, from bathing, and early in the morning. Craves fats, sweets, spices, or alcohol.

Mercurius corrosivus: Severe burning pain with thin discharge. Very sensitive to light. Burning tears. Swollen lids. Great thirst for cold drinks and cold food. Perspires easily. Use if no other remedy is clearly indicated.

Constipation

(See also "Impaction")

Constipation may involve a lack of bowel movements or difficulty passing stools. Causes include a lack of fiber in the diet, insufficient physical activity, emotional or physical stress, dehydration, bowel disease, neurological problems, and various medications. Along with administering the following remedies, the cause needs to be addressed.

Nux vomica: Constant urging but very little passes. Must strain to pass a small amount of stool. Never feels "finished." Likes spicy foods. Chilly and irritable. Constipation after use of prescription or narcotic drugs (also Bryonia and Opium), or after an excess of food or alcohol. Wakes at 3 a.m. and feels wretched in the morning.

Bryonia: Little or no urging. Stools are large, hard, and dry. Dryness of rectum. Headache. Very thirsty. Irritable (also Nux). After use of drugs (also Nux and Opium).

Alumina: Must strain a lot to pass even a soft stool. No urge to move the bowels. Dryness of the rectum. Stools are hard and sometimes covered with mucus. Constipation lasting for days.

Opium: No urging for stool. Stool starts to come out and then recedes. Constipation lasting for weeks. Loss of appetite. After a fright or from use of opiates. Stools are hard, round, and black. After use of drugs (also Nux and Bryonia).

Sulphur: Constant ineffectual urging to move the bowels. Stools are large and painful. Never feels finished. In people who always feel warm and crave sweets and alcohol. Feet become hot at night and he must uncover them. Anus is sometimes red.

Natrum muriaticum: Craves salt, avoids company, and is irritable and worse from sympathy. Sometimes with rectal pain. Stool starts to evacuate then recedes (also Silica, Opium). During menses, after grief.

Silica: Great urging to stool, but must strain to get stool out. It starts to come out and then recedes (also Natrum mur, Opium). Affects people who are chilly and sweat easily on the head and feet.

Convulsions—Seizures

A convulsion involves a sudden, uncontrollable contraction of the muscles. It can be mild or severe and violent. Most seizures last for a couple of minutes or less. Seizures have many causes, including head injuries, teething in children, hysteria, fevers, epilepsy, neuromuscular diseases, poisoning (from chemicals or foods), tetanus, acute infections, malnutrition, heat prostration, and low calcium levels.

Symptoms vary according to the cause and intensity, but may include momentary loss of consciousness, confusion, drooling, frothing at the mouth, grunting, twitching muscles, incontinence of the bowels or bladder, temporary cessation of breathing, jerking limbs, nausea, and anxiety.

Convulsions in adults are most frequently due to head injury, epilepsy, overheating, and chemical or food poisoning. Convulsions in children are often triggered by teething, eating the wrong foods, infections, or emotional upset.

During some convulsions, the muscles are intermittently contracted and relaxed. These spasms are called *clonic.* When muscles stay contracted, as in tetanus, the contractions are called *tonic. Epileptiform* convulsions are those involving unconsciousness.

Note: Place the remedy between the lips and teeth to prevent it from being inhaled. Convulsions after injuries require Arnica, Cicuta, Hypericum, or Natrum sulphuricum.

***Hypericum:** First choice for convulsions after head injuries. (See also Arnica, Cicuta, Helleborus.)

***Arnica:** After head injuries. The patient avoids being touched. Insists he is okay.

***Belladonna:** Sudden onset with *face bright red and hot, wild staring eyes, pupils dilated*, strong pulse. The body becomes rigid, and sometimes there are violent convulsions. Worse from light, cold, motion, or touch. Especially in infants.

***Calcarea carbonica:** Especially useful in children, if Belladonna doesn't hold. Children with large heads who sweat profusely.

***Cuprum:** May begin with spasms of hands or feet with clenched thumbs, blue face and lips, great nausea with vomiting. Eyeballs roll or become fixed staring upward.

***Stramonium:** Body arches backward, violent convulsions throughout the body, worse from seeing any shiny object, glittering light, or water. Terror. Delirium. Fears darkness and solitude. Triggered by fear, rage.

***Chamomilla:** From anger, or from teething. Angry, uncivil. One cheek red, the other pale. Hot sweat on the face and head.

***Nux vomica:** From exposure to cold air, from abuse of alcohol or food, or after getting angry. All muscles clench, face is purple. Worse from the slightest touch, noise, being jarred, or any draft. Irritable, oversensitive, chilly.

***Hyoscyamus:** May be triggered by a fright. Sudden onset. Patient falls to the ground screaming, delirious. Frothing at the mouth. Muscles twitch. Pupils dilated. Falls asleep after the attack. Different parts of the body twitch. Vomiting, which may give temporary relief.

***Agaricus:** Muscles twitch and jerk, especially those in the face. Frothing of the mouth. Weakness of lower limbs.

***Cicuta virosa:** After a blow to the head. Bending the head, neck, and spine backward. Head twisted to one side, face dark red, arms and legs rigid. Wide-eyed stare. Convulsions spread from above downward. Difficulty breathing.

Ignatia: Convulsions triggered by fear, grief, or other strong emotions. Eyelids and mouth twitch. Cold and pale with a fixed stare.

Causticum: From fright, grief, or being chilled. Involuntary urination during attack. Convulsions during sleep, body icy cold. Craves cold drinks. Right-sided convulsions. Sad, hopeless, sympathetic. Wants company.

Plumbum: Legs feel heavy and numb before the attack. Cramps in calves. Tongue swollen. Paralysis after the attack. Blue line along the margin of gums.

Cina: In children with worms. Face twitches.

Gelsemium: Slower onset than Belladonna. The patient may be drowsy before the attack. May result from fever or fright. Back and neck become rigid. Patient is hot and restless.

Glonoine: From exposure to the heat of the sun.

Helleborus: Automatic motion of one arm and leg. The patient makes chewing motions. Occurs after head injuries.

Opium: In children, from fright. Pupils constricted. *Face dark red and bloated. Head drawn way back.*

Cornea, Scratched

The cornea is the curved, clear covering at the front of the eye. Superficial corneal injuries may be caused by dust, sand, or other particles. Symptoms include eye pain and redness.

***Calendula:** After taking a few pellets on your tongue, dissolve one pellet of Calendula 30c in one ounce of spring water. Place one drop of this in the eye twice a day.

Arnica: A few pellets on the tongue. Do not put Arnica in the eye.

Hepar sulph: If area becomes very sensitive to touch, draft, or cold.

Croup

A condition occurring mostly in young children, marked by a loud barking cough or a metallic cough, hoarseness, difficulty breathing, and fever. It has numerous causes including spasms in the airways, viral infections, swelling of the throat, and diphtheria. If there is a membrane in the throat, see "Diphtheria."

***Aconite:** Use at the first signs of illness. Comes on rapidly (also Belladonna). Frightened, restless, burning in throat, craves cold water.

***Belladonna:** Face red and hot, especially after coughing. Throbbing sensation. Comes on rapidly (also Aconite). Worse from noise, bright light, drafts, and being jarred. Throat bright red. Barking cough.

***Hepar sulph:** Very chilly. Loose, rattling cough. Cough is worse from cold and uncovering. Must sit up to breathe. Worse from draft. Better from warmth. Irritable.

***Lachesis:** Throat pain is worse from drinking liquids or on empty swallowing. Eating solids is not as bad. Throat painful to touch. Ulceration in throat. Worse after sleep, from warmth, from anything around the neck. Better from cold drinks. Talkative. Throat red or purplish.

***Spongia:** Very dry barking cough, or coughing with the sound of sawing through a log. Tickling cough. Better from warm drinks. Can't stand anything tight around the waist. Worse in a hot room or lying down.

***Antimonium tart:** Very thick mucus rattling in the chest, which can't be coughed up. The patient struggles for breath. Face cold, blue, or pale, with cold sweat. Worse from warmth. Better sitting up.

***Kali bichromicum:** Cough has a brassy sound, like air blowing through a metal tube. A membrane may cover the throat. Stringy, sticky, yellow mucus. Extreme weakness.

Phosphorus: Very hoarse, chest tight, worse from lying on the left side, bloody or rust-colored mucus, better from company. Craves cold drinks.

Bromine: Burning in the chest. Coughs every time he breathes. Membrane may line the throat. Worse in the evening, from warmth, and from lying on the left side. Glands swollen.

Cuts: See "Wounds"

Cystitis

Cystitis is an inflammation of the bladder or lower urinary tract. It may be caused by a bacterial infection, or by an irritant, such as a drug, spices, bubble baths, or sanitary napkins. It is most frequently seen in women and the elderly. Symptoms include frequent and/or urgent desire to pass urine, burning or stinging pain, pressure in the lower abdomen, and a strong odor to the urine. Also, pain during intercourse, fatigue, fever, nausea, or vomiting. The elderly may also experience confusion as a symptom.

***Cantharis:** First choice. Scalding pain before, during, and after urination. Constant urge. Urine passed in drops. Sometimes bloody. Urination very painful. Thirsty but worse from drinking. Sometimes fever.

***Staphysagria:** Burning pain when not urinating. Feels like the bladder didn't empty. Worse after intercourse, after catheterization, and after anger.

Aconite: Accompanied by fear, high fever, hot dry skin, great thirst, and restlessness. Comes on suddenly.

Apis: Burning, stinging pain, which is better from cold application. Very little urine, and it is dark and sometimes bloody. No thirst. Worse from heat.

Equisetum: Bladder always feels full, even after urination. Pain at the end of urination. Worse sitting or lying down.

Berberis: Thick mucus in urine. Bright red sediment. Pain in thighs when urinating. Worse from moving.

Lachesis: Worse after sleep, from anything tight around waist, from heat, before menses, lying on the left side.

Belladonna: Urine is dark and cloudy. Sudden onset. Worse around 3 p.m. Worse around menses. Throbbing sensations. Better from pressure.

Dulcamara: After exposure to dampness or damp, cold weather.

Argentum nitricum: Burning, shooting pain and itching. Urine is dark and sometimes bloody. Worse from warmth. Craves sweets, which cause belching. Better from cold and pressure. Anxious.

Causticum: Passes urine when coughing or sneezing. Chilly and worse from cold. Craves bacon and salt. Aversion to sweets.

Death, Apparent: See "Asphyxia"

Dehydration

Loss of fluids may occur from failure to drink, from diarrhea, vomiting, sweating, or excessive urination. The symptoms and signs include sunken eyes, sunken fontanelles in an infant, dry or sticky mouth, skin that flattens out very slowly after being pinched, decreased or absent urine output, decreased tears, and deep and rapid breathing. Severe dehydration may cause sleepiness or coma, and is life threatening. If the person is able to drink, administer fluids orally. Otherwise, intravenous fluids or retention enemas may be appropriate.

***Cinchona:** Dim vision, vertigo, chilly and worse from cold or drafts. Bloating of abdomen. Better lying down or bending double.

Phosphoric acid: Apathetic, listless, seems "burned out," gives one word answers. Craves fruit and juicy things. Chilly, weak, fainting, upset stomach. Crushing headache on top of head. Worse from cold or drafts.

Carbo veg: Craves air and wants to be fanned (opposite Cinchona and Phosphoric acid). Cold body, especially the hands and feet, and cold breath. Fear of darkness. Distended abdomen with much belching. Can't bear tight clothing around his waist.

Calcarea carbonica: Extremely anxious. Worries about her health, about her sanity, about being observed. Dehydration may be preceded by sour-smelling vomit, diarrhea, or perspiration. Especially in heavyset, chilly persons with cold, clammy skin who perspire easily.

Delirium

A state of mental confusion and excitement. It may include illusions of time and space, as well as hallucinations. Delirium may arise from many disorders, both physical and emotional. Fevers, drugs, and infections are just a few causative factors.

***Belladonna:** *Sudden onset. Face red and hot, eyes red, pupils dilated. Feverish. Grinds teeth. Tries to escape from the bed. Worse from noise, light, or being jarred.* Physically strikes out at people, or bites. Better from dark and quiet. Delirious during sleep.

***Hyoscyamus:** *From jealousy or pain. Wants to be naked, attacks with a knife,* talkative (obscene), *suspicious, jealous, shameless, laughing, exposes himself,* mutters. Face pale or red, twitching muscles, pupils dilated. May be feverish.

***Stramonium:** *Goes in and out of delirium. Shy and hides,* or talkative (obscene), swearing or praying. Fearful or violent. Constant hysterical laughter. Plays with genitals. Worse from darkness, solitude, or glittering objects. Better from light and company.

Veratrum album: Restless, *freezing cold, cold sweat on forehead, diarrhea. Craves sour fruit,* salt, or cold drinks. Religious fervor. *Delirious from pain.*

Arsenicum: *During fever. Great fear of death and doesn't want to be alone, especially at night. Great thirst but only for frequent small sips.* Chilly and restless. Very weak.

Baptisia: *Delirious during fevers and infections.* Body feels sore all over. Foul secretions. *Imagines he is broken and his body scattered about the bed.* Tosses around the bed trying to get his pieces together. Falls asleep while being spoken to.

Bryonia: *In delirium, talks about business and says he wants to go home.* Very irritable. *His lips and mouth are very dry* and he's thirsty for large drinks. Worse from warmth and from any motion.

Lycopodium: *Haughty or dictatorial during the delirium.* Envious. Raging and raving, or muttering. Right-sided complaints. Flatulence. Craves sweets. Worse from 4 to 8 p.m. or 3 to 4 a.m.

Rhus tox: *From fear or septic infections. Extremely restless and constantly changes position. Muscles stiff and he stretches often.* Anxiety at night. Imagines he is being watched. Delusion that he is away from home. Afraid to go to sleep. Craves milk or beer. Itching relieved by hot water. Worse from cold or dampness.

Nux vomica: Delirium with sleeplessness. Chilly, irritable, angry. Worse from noise, odors, and light. *Often alcohol related.*

Dengue Fever (Breakbone Fever)

An acute viral ailment contracted from infected mosquitoes. The onset is sudden, with flushed face, headache, pain behind the eyes, fever, chills, great weakness, and stiff, painful muscles and joints. Pain may be experienced as being deep in the bones, thus the name. The initial fever may go to 104 degrees and last two to five days. Often, the fever subsides and the patient feels better for about twenty-four hours. Then, a second, lower fever develops, along with a characteristic measles-like rash everywhere but the face. People who contract the disease twice within two years may suffer an extreme form of the ailment, which includes hemorrhage and shock.

***Aconite:** Fearful, restless, unquenchable thirst, skin hot and dry.

***Belladonna:** Face hot and flushed, throbbing headache. Worse from light, noise, drafts, or being jarred. Better in a quiet, dark room.

***Bryonia:** Pain felt in the whole body, which is worse from the slightest motion. The patient wants to lie perfectly still. Highly irritable. Dry mouth and throat. Thirst for large cold drinks at long intervals. Joints hot and swollen. Worse in a hot room.

***Eupatorium perf:** Pain felt deep in the bones, as if they were broken. Eyeballs painful. Restless. Worse in cold air, but desires cold drinks.

***Rhus tox:** Muscles and joints painful and stiff. Worse after rest, but better from continued motion. Very restless. Worse from cold or dampness. Better from heath and warm drinks. Great thirst. Itching rash which is better from warmth.

Arsenicum album: Anxious, restless, chilly, thirsty for small frequent sips. Burning pain, which is better from heat. Foul diarrhea. Exhausted by the least effort. Desires company. Better from warmth. Worse from midnight to 3 a.m.

Nux vomica: Extreme chill, which is worse from uncovering or even moving. Irritable, snappish, oversensitive to lights, noise, odors, and the pressure of clothes. Pain in the lower back, as if it is breaking. Nausea and vomiting.

Crotalus horridus: Hemorrhage from every orifice. Blood in stool, urine, and perspiration. The patient is irritable, sad, or dwells on death. Weakness and trembling. Cannot lie on the right side. Right-sided complaints. Aversion to light.

Lachesis: Hemorrhages of thin, dark blood. Left-sided complaints. Talkative and intense. Can't bear tight clothing, especially around the neck. Worse from heat and light touch. Better from cold drinks and fresh air.

If shock develops (pale, cold, clammy skin, rapid weak pulse, shallow rapid breathing), see "Shock."

Dental Work: See "Toothache and Dental Work"

Dentition: See "Teething"

Depression

(See also "Depression After Delivery" in the "Pregnancy and Birth" chapter, and "Emotional Remedies")

People suffering from depression often feel worthless, helpless, and hopeless. Their intellectual focus is narrowed, making it difficult for them to "think their way out" of their problems. Chronic depression requires treatment by a professional homeopath. Acute depression is usually a reaction to some life circumstance such as loss of a loved one, disappointed love, or failure at occupation. It can also result from hormonal changes associated with childbirth, menses, or menopause. The following remedies should prove helpful for acute depression.

***Ignatia:** *Top remedy for depression from grief. From the death of a friend, disappointed love*, loss of a job, etc. Silent brooding, much sighing, sometimes hysteria. Changeable moods—laughing then crying. Weeps when alone. Sensation of a lump in the throat, insomnia, or loss of appetite. Worse from warmth, coffee, or the odor of tobacco.

***Aurum:** *Suicidal depression. Takes relief in the thought of suicide.* From grief, failures in business, etc. Feelings of guilt and self-reproach.

Imagines he has neglected his duty, or that he has lost the affection of his friends. Fits of anger at persons not present, or those who have offended him. Worse in the evening.

***Natrum mur:** *Grief that lasts long after the cause.* Desires solitude. Worse from sympathy and company. Silent grief, weeps only when alone. Worse from heat and from the sun. Craves salt. Fear of robbers.

***Phosphoric acid:** *Looks and sounds "burned out."* Apathetic. Gives one word answers when questioned. Craves fruit and juicy foods.

Sepia: Feels no joy in anything. Indifferent to loved ones, to work, etc. Everything, even love, feels like a burden. Drained of physical and emotional energy. Worse from company, but dreads to be alone. May be silent and tearful, or snappish and easily offended. Sees the bad side of everything. Envious and believes everyone is better off than she is. Worse from consolation. Better from dancing or other physical exertion. Craves acidic foods (lemons) and chocolate. Chilly and worse from cold air.

Cimicifuga: Disappointed love. *Extroverted, very talkative, sighing,* pessimistic, sometimes hysterical. Chilly, but better in open air. *Feels like he's in a "black cloud."* Fears insanity. Postpartum depression, depression during menses or at menopause.

Pulsatilla: Gentle, yielding. Weeps easily talking about problems. *Desires sympathy, company, and reassurance. Can't stand being in a warm, closed room.* Craves open air. Changeable moods. Depression before menses, or during pregnancy. Worse in the evening. Fears abandonment.

Calcarea carbonica: Fear of losing his mind. Difficulty concentrating and *fears that people will observe his confusion.* May also fear insects, dogs, or germs. Can't stand to see or hear about violence or cruelty. Wants to hide.

Causticum: *Idealistic, deeply affected by injustice, worries about others, fights for causes.* Anxious at twilight, fears the dark, craves smoked foods. Chilly and better from warmth. Better in rainy weather.

Lycopodium: Goes into depression when something shatters his confidence. Becomes so insecure that he wants to hide and avoid all responsibility. Concerned about how others see him. Self-conscious and uncomfortable around people, yet fears solitude. Much anticipatory anxiety and fear of failure. Weeps when thanked. Craves sweets.

Lachesis: *Extremely talkative, suspicious, jealous.* Hot and worse from heat. Worse after sleeping. Can't bear tight clothing around the neck.

Arsenicum: Grief about himself and what will become of him. *Fears loss of security. Anxious, restless, fastidious, and critical.* Afraid to be alone. Worse from midnight to 3 a.m. Failure to trust those on whom he depends. Worries about the future. Chilly and better from warmth.

Phosphorus: Usually outgoing, sympathetic, better from company. Highly impressionable, and feels other people's pain. Tension between people makes him physically ill. Likes to be hugged. Sensitive to sounds, odors, and lights. Easily startled with fear of thunderstorms. Always better after a short nap. Thirsty for ice-cold drinks. Craves ice cream, chocolate, and spicy food.

Carcinosin: Very sympathetic, intensely caring, and passionate. Overly responsible and feels guilty about being sick. Makes demands on himself rather than on others. Always taking on more work. Loves animals, dancing, travel, and thunderstorms. Craves chocolate. Sensitive to criticism and easily hurt by reprimand. Great anticipatory anxiety. Moved by sad stories. Often has a history of prolonged fear or abuse.

Diarrhea

(See also "Dysentery")

Unless due to a chronic underlying disease, diarrhea is the body's method of ridding itself of some toxin. However, diarrhea can become a threat when it occurs in infants and small children—they can go into a state of dehydration within hours. Critical signs of dehydration are lessened activity, lack of saliva, crying without tears, and a decreased number of wet diapers.

Note: To speed recovery after a bout of diarrhea, use Cinchona.

*__Arsenicum album__ (6x or 6c): From spoiled food. Restless, anxious, chilly, and thirsty for frequent small sips of water. Worse after eating or drinking. Sometimes there are burning pains relieved by heat.

***Cinchona:** Painless, yellow diarrhea. Abdomen is bloated but there is no relief from belching. Thirsty and sweaty.

***Podophyllum:** Diarrhea gushes out like a hydrant after every meal. Weakness after each bout. No thirst.

***Nux vomica:** Chilly, irritable, and oversensitive. Wakes at 3 a.m. Diarrhea from eating badly or using drugs.

Veratrum album: Painful diarrhea, forcibly expelled, exhausting the patient. Feels icy-cold with cold sweat on the forehead. Thirsty and worse from cold drinks. Exhausted. Craves sour fruit.

Colocynth: Severe gripping pains that make him bend double. Better from pressure.

Phosphorus: Craves large, cold drinks. Desires company. Sensitive to light, noise, and odors. Long-standing diarrhea.

Mercurius corrosivus: Hot, bloody, slimy, offensive stools. Perspires before and after stool. Worse after stool.

Baptisia: Sudden, foul-smelling, painless stools. The patient looks intoxicated; eyelids heavy, face dark red.

Carbo veg: Craves fresh air and wants to be fanned. Gas in the upper abdomen with much belching. The hands and feet are cold.

Phosphoric acid: Exhausted but feels better after diarrhea. Craves fruit and juicy things.

Diphtheria

A contagious disease transmitted via droplet infection. It infects the throat but also creates toxins that affect the central nervous system and heart. The incubation period is two to seven days. The symptoms include sore throat, difficulty swallowing, low-grade fever, and fatigue, followed by a *characteristic gray membrane in the throat.* The membrane and swelling of the tissues cause difficulty swallowing and breathing. *The neck may become greatly swollen due to enlarged lymph glands* ("bullneck" appearance).

> **Note:** Don't raise the patient to a sitting position if he is very weak.

Prevention

Diphtherinum (nosode 30c) or Mercurius cyanatus.

Remedies for Diphtheria

***Diphtherinum** (200c)**:** Start with this remedy if available.

***Mercurius cyanatus** (a specific type of Mercurius)**:** Much salivation, perspiration, nosebleed. Membrane is greenish or yellow. Symptoms come on suddenly. Great weakness.

***Apis:** Burning, stinging pain in the throat. Throat is swollen. Eyes may be puffy. No thirst. Drowsiness. Membrane more prominent on the right side (also Lycopodium).

***Lachesis:** Membrane begins or is worse on the left side of the throat. Throat is purplish. Symptoms are worse after sleep. More pain from swallowing liquids. Neck swollen.

***Lac caninum:** *The pain and inflammation shifts from one side of the throat to the other and back again.* Paralysis of the throat prevents drinking. Membrane is shiny and pearly-white colored.

Arsenicum: *Membrane is wrinkled and dry.* Extreme weakness. The patient is chilly, restless, and wants to change position. Anxious and afraid to be alone.

Lycopodium: *Inflammation begins on the right side and may move to the left. Nostrils flap when breathing heavily.* Membrane extends to the nose. Wants warm drinks. Angry on awakening. Drooping of the lower jaw.

Phytolacca: Membrane is gray, white, dark red, or blue. Pain extends to ears when swallowing. Pain also in head, back, and limbs. *Feels sore all over.* Burning in the throat as from a hot coal. *Worse from hot drinks.* Keeps trying to swallow.

Kali bichromicum: *Membrane is greenish* and extends to nose and throat. Pain is in small spots and shifts position. *Thick yellow coat on tongue.*

Crotalus horridus: *Bleeding from all mucous membranes*, hot skin, perspiration, great thirst, and complete exhaustion.

Drowning

Give mouth-to-mouth resuscitation or the Heimlich maneuver followed by mouth-to-mouth. The Heimlich maneuver involves a quick compression of the abdomen. If there is no heartbeat, begin with CPR—compressions of the breastbone followed by mouth-to-mouth resuscitation.

> **Note:** Place the remedy between the lips and teeth to prevent it from being inhaled.

***Carbo veg:** Administer every ten minutes.

***Antimonium tartaricum:** Rattling in the chest. Better sitting up.

Drug Overdose

If the patient is not breathing, make sure the airway is clear and begin mouth-to-mouth respiration. If there is no heartbeat, begin CPR (cardiopulmonary resuscitation).

Gelsemium: Listless, eyelids droopy, limbs heavy, pupils dilated, jaw dropped, eyes glassy.

Nux vomica: Twitching, spasms, seizures, irritability. Worse from noise.

Opium: Stupor, labored breathing, pupils contracted, dry mouth.

Dysentery

Inflammation of the mucous membranes of the intestine. Symptoms include fever, diarrhea, blood or mucus in stool, painful spasms of the rectum. May be caused by protozoa or bacteria.

***Mercurius corrosivus:** First choice. Painful spasms, constant straining at stool with a "never-quite-done" feeling. Bloody stools, which burn and irritate the rectum. Pains in the rectum after stool. Urine also feels hot. Excess saliva, tongue flabby with the imprint of teeth.

***Colocynth:** Pains make the patient double over. Spasms of the rectum before stool. Worse after eating or drinking.

***Arsenicum:** Offensive, foul-smelling stools, sometimes with blood or pus. Great exhaustion. Face pale, sunken. Anxious, chilly, restless. Burning pains relieved by heat, extreme thirst but for small sips. Often comes from eating bad meat.

***Carbo veg:** Much belching with bloated abdomen. The patient is very cold on the outside, but feels burning pains internally. The person's breath feels cold. He is breathless and better from drafts or being fanned. Dark, bloody mucus in stool. Stools smell like a dead body.

***Cinchona:** Abdomen bloated, but belching doesn't relieve it. Worse from drafts. Painless diarrhea, sometimes undigested food.

***Nux vomica:** Spasms of the rectum, which stop after passing stool. Chilly and must be covered. Very irritable, angry. Highly sensitive to odors, lights, and noise. Craves brandy. Wakes at 3 a.m. and can't sleep until morning.

Gelsemium: Looks intoxicated, eyelids droop, limbs feel heavy, chills run up the back. Little or no thirst. Wants to be left alone. Trembles.

Phosphorus: Bright red blood mixed with mucus in the stool. Worse lying on the left side. Desires company. Great thirst for ice-cold drinks. Hypersensitive to odors, lights, and sounds. Painless bloody stools. Better from a short nap.

Sulphur: Diarrhea worse in the morning and after midnight. Anus red, itching, burning, and going into spasms, which stop after stool. Worse from heat in any form.

Ipecacuanha: Nausea and vomiting due to painful straining at stool. Terrible cramping pain. Pain at the navel. Salivation. Clean tongue. Better from open air.

Aloe soc: Abdomen bloated and sensitive to pressure, shooting pains at the navel. Passes urine and stools at the same time. Fainting from stool. Passes stool unconsciously. Spasms and heat in the rectum. Clammy sweat. Headache and nausea. Bloody, jellylike mucus. Passes much gas with stool. Worse after eating and in the morning.

Nitric acid: Extremely chilly, stool irritates the anus, pain after stool that lasts for hours. Splinterlike pains in anus. Rectum feels torn. Violent thirst, anxiety, exhaustion. Worse from touch, cold.

Earache

Inflammation of the Middle Ear (Otitis Media)

Middle-ear inflammation can be caused by viruses or bacteria. It often occurs after measles, mumps, scarlet fever, pneumonia, or influenza. Symptoms are earache, fullness in the ear, impaired hearing, and sometimes ear noises, such as a ringing, crackling, whistling, or roaring sound. Some cases include tenderness in the area, discharge from the ear, fever, and chills.

****Aconite:** Sudden onset after exposure to cold dry air. Patient is restless and scared. The ear is tender to the touch. Sometimes there is a burning pain. Worse at night and from 12 to 2 a.m. Repeat every half hour for several doses.

***Chamomilla:** Unbearable pain with anger. Nothing you do to try to please patients in this state satisfies them. One cheek hot, the other pale. Children needing this remedy like to be carried briskly. Worse from warmth and at night.

***Pulsatilla:** Seeks sympathy, company, and reassurance. Weeps easily. Ear swollen and red. Thick, yellowish-green, bland discharge. Feels stuffy in a warm room and must have fresh air. Worse from warmth or warm application. Thirstless.

***Belladonna:** Often the right ear. Face is red and hot. Pain comes on quickly. Hot, throbbing pain with each heartbeat. Delirious with pain. Cries out in sleep. Better resting in the dark. Worse from light, noise, being bumped, and cold air.

***Hepar sulph:** Ear is extremely sensitive to touch and the patient won't let you near it. Sensitive to cold or the slightest draft. Discharge, which smells like old cheese. Irritable. Better from warmth. Often finishes the cure started by Mercurius.

***Mercurius:** Thick, yellow discharge, sometimes blood-streaked. Worse from the warmth of the bed. Much perspiration and salivation. Bad breath. Thirsty. Tongue shows the imprint of teeth. Pain is worse at night.

Capsicum: Ear is red-hot and bulging. Stabbing pains. Seeks sympathy (as with Pulsatilla). Better from hot application (opposite Pulsatilla). Worse from open air (opposite Pulsatilla). Worse at night.

Kali bichromicum: Discharge of thick, yellow, foul-smelling pus. Stinging pain and itching inside the ear.

Silica: Discharge of blood and pus. Children bore their fingers into their ears. Also, when the ear keeps draining after most symptoms are better.

Apis: Stinging pains. The ear is red, inflamed, and sore. Often right sided. The patient is worse from heat and touch. Restless.

Eardrum Perforation

The eardrum or tympanic membrane lies between the outer and middle ear. It is the organ that vibrates when exposed to sound. It also protects the middle ear from infection.

Perforation can occur from very loud sounds, foreign objects inserted into the ear, or infections. Symptoms include earache, discharge from the ear, hearing loss, and ear noises. Ruptured eardrums usually heal within two months. The following remedies will help with the pain and speed the healing process.

***Calendula:** Once a day for a week. Repeat if necessary.

***Hepar sulph** (6x or 6c)**:** If due to infection. Twice a day for three weeks.

***Silica:** 30c once a week.

Ebola

A severe, highly contagious, often fatal viral disease that first appeared in Africa in 1976. Incubation is three to fourteen days. It is transmitted primarily by touch, but may also be airborne. Initial symptoms include throbbing behind the eyeballs, backache, fever, nausea, vomiting, and diarrhea. This is followed by a raised rash that covers the entire body. There may be bleeding from the mouth, rectum, eyes, ears, nose, and skin. The eyes become bright red like rubies and the face expressionless. Death is usually due to kidney failure and shock.

> **Note:** The cutting down of forests that harbor this disease probably led to its rise. It is believed that the first human case was contracted from a monkey. The importation and use of monkeys as laboratory animals also poses a hazard.

***Crotalus horridus:** General hemorrhage—blood oozes from eyes, ears, nose, mouth, rectum, or skin. Bloody sweat and urine. Skin blisters, yellow face, and fiery-red tongue. Can't swallow solids (opposite Lachesis). Delusions of cerebral decay. Weeps easily from despair. Sleepy but can't sleep. Right-sided symptoms (Lachesis has left-sided). Pains appear and disappear suddenly. Worse after sleep, in the morning and evening, and from exertion.

***Lachesis:** Hemorrhage containing bits of decomposed blood resembling charred wheat. Patient is very talkative, trembling, unable to stick out his tongue because it trembles. Confused or depressed. Can't stand anything tight around his neck. Pulls at his collar. Left-sided symptoms (opposite Crotalus). Worse after sleep, from warmth, pressure, tight clothing, or the slightest touch. Skin looks purplish, and forms ulcers or dark blisters. Face purple, mottled, and puffy. Can't swallow liquids (solids okay). Worse from hot drinks. The liver is sensitive to touch. Breathing stops upon falling asleep.

Phosphorus: Hemorrhages of bright red blood. Extreme sensitivity to light, sound, and odors. Craves ice-cold drinks. Fearful and startles easily. Desires company and is fearful when alone. Blue rings under the eyes. Sees as if through a veil. Feeling of heat in the spine or chest. Feeling of weight across the chest. Pneumonia. Worse lying on the left side. Worse from warm food or drink and in the evening. Better from sleep. Dreams of fire and hemorrhage.

Bothrops: Hemorrhages from every orifice. Face swollen, black vomiting. Shivering followed by cold sweat. Trembling. Unable to talk. Blindness during the day from sensitivity to sunlight. Retinal hemorrhage, pulmonary embolus. One-sided paralysis. Worse on the right side.

Mercurius corrosivus: Much sweating and the patient is worse afterward. He has excess saliva and may drool. Great thirst. Pain behind the eyeballs, sensitivity to light, iris looks muddy and neither contracts nor dilates. Eyelids swollen and red. Violent pulsation in ears. Throat swollen, painful, and burning. Green vomit. Painful spasms of the anus. Abdomen bloated. Hot, bloody, offensive diarrhea. Urine is hot and burning with spasms of the bladder. Worse at night.

Electric Shock/Lightning

After removing the source of the shock, perform artificial respiration if the person is not breathing, or cardiopulmonary resuscitation if there is no heartbeat. Electric current can cause the heart to stop, or it can burn and destroy tissues. Internal burns may be more serious than outward appearance suggests. After giving the following remedies, consult the "Burns" section.

***Phosphorus:** Pale face, weak pulse, fear of death, won't be left alone.

***Arnica** (30–200c)**:** Fear of being touched. Says he is okay.

Morphinum or **Opium:** Difficulty breathing, face pale or bluish, dreamlike state, shock from terror.

Emotional Remedies

These remedies are useful for people who are "stuck" in certain emotional states, or who have developed physical ailments after being in those states.

Ignatia: *Top remedy for grief and the effects of grief, loss, or disappointed love. For the aftereffects of any strong emotion. Silent brooding, much sighing,* sometimes hysteria. Changeable moods—laughing then crying. Weeps when alone. Sensation of a lump in the throat, insomnia, or loss of appetite. Hysterical paralysis. Worse from warmth, coffee, or the odor of tobacco. For physical ailments that began after grief or other strong emotions.

Aconite: *Panic, anxiety attacks, and terror* accompanied by racing pulse, hot flushed face, and extreme thirst. Predicts the time of his own death. Hypersensitive to pain, sound, light, and odors. Worse from warmth. Ailments after terror.

Aurum: *Suicidal depression.* Desires death due to hopelessness or to physical pain. Has an excessive sense of duty and feels overwhelmed by conscience. Believes he is a failure and has lost the affection of his friends. Sudden fits of anger, especially if he is contradicted.

Arsenicum: *Anxious, insecure, and afraid to be alone. Fears disease, poverty, and death.* Restless, exhausted, perfectionist, suspicious, and controlling. Worse after midnight. Chilly and thirsty for small sips. This remedy can also help ease fear in the last moments of life.

Stramonium: *Frightened and physically strikes out violently.* Fears darkness and desires light. Fear of and worse from being alone. Worse from seeing shiny objects. Kicking and biting, delusions about dogs (also Belladonna). The patient is extremely thirsty but has difficulty swallowing. Better from warmth, light, and company. Often triggered by a frightful experience.

Belladonna: Striking, biting, or kicking. Red-faced, hot, pupils dilated. Worse from touch, noise, light, or being jarred. Throbbing headache.

Delusions about animals and insects. Belladonna is a major remedy for delirium.

Phosphoric acid: *Listless, apathetic, burned out,* and very chilly. *Takes a long time to answer questions* and gives one word answers. Craves fruit. From grief, emotional shocks, exhausting illness, or loss of fluids (also Cinchona). Night sweats. Passes large amounts of clear urine.

Staphysagria: *Suppressed anger* and emotional states or ailments resulting from suppressed anger. After insult or humiliation. For victims of rape or other crimes where the person was abused.

Nux vomica: *Angry, irritable, impatient, malicious,* worse in the morning, awake from 3 to 5 a.m. Craves stimulants and alcohol. Feels the ill effects of drugs and alcohol (such as nausea, vomiting, and vertigo). Ambitious, jealous. Angry when obliged to answer or when interrupted.

Pulsatilla: *For feelings of abandonment or helplessness.* Weeps easily and wants reassurance. Better from sympathy and company. Craves open air and can't bear a stuffy, warm room. Thirstless. Ailments that occur after being left alone or feeling abandoned.

Cimicifuga: *Grief. Similar to Ignatia with sighing, sadness, jerking of muscles, hysteria,* and ailments from disappointed love. Extroverted and talkative, jumping from one subject to another (see also Lachesis). More fearful than Ignatia. Fear of insanity. Chilly but better from cold air. Stiff neck, which is worse from drafts.

Chamomilla: *Angry and uncivil.* Pushes you away. Extreme sensitivity to pain, which the patient describes as unbearable. Angry at every trifle, at being spoken to. Cheeks red and hot.

Argentum nitricum: *Anticipatory anxiety, phobias (e.g., claustrophobia, agoraphobia).* Feels hurried. Fears her impulses and losing control. Worse from warmth or closed rooms. Desires company, but experiences anxiety in a crowded room. Diarrhea from anxiety.

Gelsemium: *Anticipatory anxiety* leads to an almost paralyzing fear. Feels drowsy, weak, or leaden. Flushed face, droopy eyelids. Wants to be alone. Thirstless. Better from alcohol.

Lachesis: *For extreme jealousy* and ailments resulting after periods of jealousy. Very talkative and jumps from one subject to another. Worse after sleep, from heat, and from anything touching the neck. Left-sided symptoms.

Coffee: *Ailments from excitement, excessive joy, and surprises.* Mentally overactive and can't shut it off. Memory active. Makes lots of plans. Insomnia. Oversensitive to pain, with despair from pain. Hypersensitive to sound, light, odors, touch, and flavors. Aversion to open air.

Encephalitis

Inflammation of the brain. Many cases are due to viral infection such as mumps, measles, and herpes simplex. Other causes include bacterial infection, vaccination, reactions to drugs, and stroke. Symptoms: stiff neck and back, drowsiness, stupor, face looks expressionless, fever, headache, vomiting. Can progress to convulsions, paralysis, and coma.

***Belladonna:** Sudden onset. Face red, hot, and perspiring. Throbbing sensation, pupils dilated. Hands and feet cold. Sensitive to light, noise, or being jarred. Spasms and pain of neck muscles. The head tends to bend backward. Tendency to bite or physically strike out. Worse from anything cold on the head. Sudden onset.

***Aconite:** Sudden violent onset, great fear of dying, unquenchable thirst, skin hot and dry, burning pains in the brain. Face red and bloated. Often followed by Belladonna.

***Apis:** Cries out with a shriek, especially in sleep. Burning and throbbing in the head, sense of suffocation, pupils dilated, hands and feet cold. Thirstless, apathetic during fever. Worse from heat, after sleep, and from touch. Stiff neck and pain in the back of the head. Better from cold application.

***Bryonia:** *Worse from any motion* (increases pain). Wants to lie perfectly still, has great thirst with dry lips and mouth, sudden starting from sleep, has cold sweat on the forehead, makes chewing motions. Squinting of eyes, stiff neck, pain in the joints and limbs, white tongue, stupor. Worse from heat and from sitting up. Follows Belladonna after fever is reduced.

***Gelsemium:** Eyes droop, arms and legs feel heavy. Face flushed, severe headache, chilliness down the back yet worse from heat, vision dim, neck muscles sore.

Helleborus niger: Head hot, forehead wrinkled, shooting pains in the head, automatic movements of one arm or leg. Severe headache, *rolls head and bores it into pillow*. Sighing, picks at clothing mindlessly. Sudden screams during sleep.

Cuprum: Screaming and convulsions, face pale to blue with blue lips, eyes rolling. Cold sweat, twitching limbs, craves ice-cold drinks, bites glass when drinking. *Thumbs curl in*, looks frightened on waking.

Opium: Coma. Prior to that, labored breathing, pupils constricted, eyes half closed and looks intoxicated, vomiting. Patient does not complain.

Hyoscyamus: Delirium, talking, singing, laughing, speaking obscenities. Twitching muscles. Involuntary diarrhea. Worse at night and when lying down.

Camphora: Head tilted to one side, extremely pale, freezing cold but refuses covers, cold sweat, pulse slow and weak, teeth clenched.

Mercurius: Worse at night and from lying on the right side. Much perspiration and worse afterward. Foul breath with drooling. Lengthwise groove in the tongue. Tongue shows the imprint of teeth. Craves cold drinks. Greenish bloody stools. Creeping chilliness.

Epileptic Attack

An epileptic attack involves seizures in which the patient falls to the ground with contractions of the arms and legs. Other symptoms include sudden crying out, twitching muscles, numbness or tingling, chewing movements, hallucinations of sight or odor, incontinence, and loss of consciousness. Seizures usually occur without warning, although some people get a sense that they are about to occur.

Note: In any situation where the person is convulsing or unconscious, place the remedy between the lips and teeth to prevent it from being inhaled.

***Causticum:** *From fright, grief, being chilled, cold drinks.* Often occurs during adolescence, or is associated with menses. Screams and grits teeth. Violent movements of the arms and legs. Involuntary urination. Vertigo. *Especially in people who are intensely sympathetic, idealistic, or rebellious.* Generally chilly.

***Bufo:** *Cries out and then goes into spasms, with distortion of the face and foaming mouth.* Head drawn to one side or backward. Face drenched in sweat. Headache after fit. Falls asleep, snoring after fit. Worse at night, during sleep, after a fright, or after masturbation or intercourse.

***Cuprum:** Face pale or blue. *Violent convulsion, which may begin with the patient crying out. Spasms of the hands or feet with clenched thumbs*, and blue lips. Attacks may occur at night or at fixed intervals. Cold hands and feet. Better from cold drinks. Affects serious, introverted, self-critical people with intense unexpressed emotions.

***Hyoscyamus:** *May be triggered by fright, grief, or alcohol. Feels dizzy, sees sparks, hears ringing noises.* Twitching and jerking motions. *Screaming*, frothing at the mouth, grinding teeth. Passes urine or stool. Falls asleep after the attack. Vertigo. *Affects jealous, suspicious, talkative people.*

***Cicuta virosa:** *After a blow to the head, from worms, during childbirth, from strong emotions. Body rigid and arches backward.* Head twisted to one side, face blue or dark red, arms and legs rigid. Screaming. Convulsions spread from above downward. Difficulty breathing.

Ipecacuanha: Convulsions triggered by digestive problems. Persistent nausea, excess salivation, and nosebleeds. Worse from damp warmth and overeating, especially rich foods and pork.

Belladonna: The patient senses the attack coming on. *Convulsions begin in the face and upper extremities. The patient clutches his throat due to spasms.* Face is blue. Unable to swallow. Involuntary passage of urine and stool. Vertigo. Worse from light, cold, motion, and touch.

Nux vomica: *From digestive problems, abuse of alcohol or after getting angry.* The patient senses the attack coming on and may feel as if ants were crawling over his face. Twitching limbs, body may arch backward. Involuntary passage of urine and stool. Worse from the slightest touch, noise, being jarred, or from any draft. Affects ambitious, perfectionist, or irritable individuals who hate to be contradicted.

Note: Epilepsy caused by a blow to the head can sometimes be relieved by Natrum sulphuricum.

Exhaustion

***Arnica:** After extreme physical effort. Muscles feel sore, and the bed feels too hard.

***Cinchona:** After loss of body fluids (blood, sweat, stool, etc.) and acute illnesses. Chilly and worse from cold. Very hungry at night. *Abdomen full of gas, much belching, which doesn't help.* The mind is most clear in the evening.

***Carbo veg:** *Craves open air and wants to be fanned. Much belching.* Hands and feet freezing cold. Digestion weak and slow. Aversion to darkness. From loss of fluids, exhausting diseases, etc.

***Kali phos:** *Nervous exhaustion from overwork*, worry, or exhausting diseases. Insomnia from nervous exhaustion. Hungry at 5 a.m. and better from eating. Yellow coating on the tongue. Worse from cold.

***Phosphoric acid:** After loss of fluids, sexual excesses, grief, etc. *Mind feels exhausted, can't think of words.* Confused. Takes a long time to answer. Listless. Chilly and *better from warmth.* Passes great quantities of clear urine.

Picric acid: Brain fatigue after mental or physical exertion or loss of fluids. *Better from cold and worse from heat* (opposite Phosphoric acid).

Cocculus indicus: After loss of sleep or from jet lag.

Arsenicum: Extremely weak, chilly, very anxious, and restless. After illness. Constantly moves about in spite of exhaustion. Thirsty for small sips. Worse at midnight. Fear of death and better from company. Desires warmth.

Calcarea carbonica: Weakness after illness, exertion, or sex (also Staphysagria). Feels confused and wants to hide. Afraid people will observe his incapacity. Can't bear to hear about cruelties. Aversion to coffee and meat. Very chilly. Perspires from the least exertion and during sleep.

Alfalfa: The tincture stimulates the appetite and improves nutrition to help recover strength after acute illnesses.

Eyes

This section includes injury, scratched cornea, conjunctivitis, stye, and uveitis.

Eye Injuries

***Arnica** (30c or 200c)**:** First choice.

***Hypericum:** Follows Arnica if there is much pain.

Symphytum: Injury from blunt object with pain in the eyeball. Blood in eye.

Aconite: Inflammation of eye from injury, after removal of foreign object, or from exposure to cold air. Worse from cold air. Great anxiety.

Ledum: Black eye from a blow.

Scratched Cornea

The cornea is the curved, clear covering at the front of the eye. Superficial corneal injuries may be caused by dust, sand or other particles. Symptoms include eye pain and redness.

***Calendula:** In addition to the usual pellets on the tongue, this remedy can also be used topically. Dissolve one pellet of Calendula 30 in one ounce of spring water. Place one drop of this in the eye twice a day.

Arnica: A few pellets on the tongue. Do not put Arnica in the eye.

Hepar sulph: If area becomes very sensitive to touch, draft or cold.

Conjunctivitis ("Pinkeye")

Inflammation of the outer layer of the eye and eyelid. There is a contagious form called pinkeye, which is caused by bacteria. Inflammation can also be caused by irritation from wind, dust, smoke, or bright light. See also "Neonatal Conjunctivitis."

***Argentum nitricum:** With thick, bland, yellow pus. Worse from heat.

***Pulsatilla:** Yellowish-green, bland discharge. Better from fresh air. Desires sympathy.

***Belladonna:** Eyes bloodshot, very red, painful, hot. Sudden onset. Pupils dilated. Worse from light.

***Euphrasia:** Burning hot tears, desire to blink.

***Aconite:** Inflammation after an injury, after removal of a foreign object, or after exposure to cold air. There is not much tearing and the eyes feel dry and burn. Anxious.

Apis mel: Eyelids swollen with stinging pain. Better from cold application. No thirst.

Hepar: Thick, foul-smelling pus. Eyes sensitive to cold, touch, draft.

Mercurius corrosivus: Severe burning pain, burning tears, puffy red irritated lids.

Sulphur: Eyes hot, dry and burning. Lids red and swollen in the morning.

Stye

Also called a "hordeolum," a stye is an infection of the oil glands in the eyelid. They ordinarily drain and heal by themselves and it is best not to squeeze them.

A warm compress several times a day will assist the draining process. Symptoms include swelling of the eyelid, eye pain, tearing, and a sensation as if something were in the eye.

Pulsatilla: For beginning stage.

Staphysagria: If Pulsatilla fails or if the stye leaves a hard nodule after healing.

Uveitis

Very painful inflammation of the middle layer of the eye, between the sclera and the retina. It has been associated with numerous chronic health problems, but the cause in many cases remains obscure. Symptoms include intense pain, which may come on rather quickly, redness of the eye, blurred vision, and light sensitivity.

***Aconite:** Rapid intense onset. Fearful, restless, worse from cold air, thirst for cold water.

Bryonia: Dryness of eyes, worse from any movement and wants to lie still. Thirsty.

Gelsemium: Twitching of eye muscles. Eyelids may droop. Pain in back of the eye. Worse from heat and hot weather.

Rhus tox: Hot tears, lids may swell, worse after exposure to cold or damp weather, or at night. Restless.

Arnica: Bruised feeling. Fear of being touched. Can't bear pain. Worse from heat, motion, after sleep.

Hepar sulph: Extremely sensitive to touch, cold, or any draft. Pus may be present.

Mercurius (sol or vivus): Worse at night, in a warm room, from heat, light. Perspires easily and feels worse afterward. Burning pain.

Silica: Great sensitivity to light. Thin, chilly, better from covering the head. Sweats profusely on the head and feet. Worse from cold weather, drafts, dampness.

Fears

This section includes panic attacks, fear of open spaces (agoraphobia), fear of closed spaces (claustrophobia), fear of heights (acrophobia), fear of bridges, fear of airplanes, fear of darkness, and fear of disease or contamination.

Panic Attack

***Aconite** (30c or 200c)**:** General remedy for panic. Fear comes on suddenly and with great intensity. Restless, afraid of death, thirsty. Skin hot and dry. Palpitation. Better in open air. Predicts the time of his death. Worse from cold, or cold dry wind. Worse at night.

***Argentum nitricum** (30c or 200c)**:** Fear of his own impulses (e.g., fear that he would throw himself off a bridge). "What if" fantasies ("What if the cable on the bridge broke as we drove over it?"). Better from fresh, cool air. Worse in open spaces or a crowd. Craves sugar, which causes belching.

Phosphorus: In the sensitive, warm, outgoing person. Always better from company and reassurance. Startles easily. Anxious during thunderstorms. Sensitive to sounds, odors, and lights. Thirsts for ice-cold drinks. Craves ice cream, spicy food, or chocolate.

Kali ars: Fears about health, especially of heart attack. Worse at night (1–3 a.m.). Sleeps with a hand over the heart. Chilly and can't get warm. Persistent thoughts at night. Aversion to going to bed.

Arsenicum: Especially at night and when alone. Fastidious, perfectionist, critical. Fears disease, robbers, or death. Very restless and chilly.

Agoraphobia (Fear of Open Spaces)

***Argentum nitricum** (30–200c)**:** Feels hurried and may walk fast. Fear of his own impulses (e.g., fear that he would throw himself off a bridge). "What if" fantasies ("What if the cable on the bridge broke as we drove over it?"). Better from fresh, cool air. Worse in open spaces or a crowd. May crave sugar, which causes belching.

Aconite (30–200c)**:** Fear comes on suddenly and with great intensity. Great restlessness, fear of death, palpitation. Better in open air. Worse from cold or cold dry wind. Worse at night. Worse from open spaces, narrow places, or in a crowd.

Kali arsenicum: Is sure he is going to have a heart attack.

Phosphorus: In the sensitive, warm, outgoing person. Always better from company and reassurance. Startles easily. Anxious during thunderstorms. Sensitive to sounds, odors, and lights. Thirsts for ice-cold drinks. Craves ice cream, spicy food, or chocolate.

Claustrophobia (Fear of Closed Spaces)

Fear of being trapped or shut in, as in elevators, trains, boat cabins, or planes.

Argentum nitricum: Worse from being in a confined, hot place. Fear of losing control. Anticipatory anxiety.

Pulsatilla: Better from sympathy, company, and fresh air. Worse in a stuffy room, especially cellars and vaults. Weepy, timid. Moods constantly changing. No thirst.

Aconite: Sudden attack. Fear of death. Worse around crowds. Waves of fear. Very thirsty.

Acrophobia (Fear of Heights)

***Argentum nitricum:** Fear of his own impulses, e.g., fear that he would throw himself off a bridge. "What if" fantasies. (*What if the cable on the bridge broke as we drove over it?*) Better from fresh, cool air. Worse in open spaces or a crowd. May crave sugar, which causes belching.

Aconite: General remedy for panic. Fear comes on suddenly and with great intensity. Restless, afraid of death, thirsty. Skin hot and dry. Palpitation. Better in open air. Worse from cold, or cold dry wind. Worse at night.

Aurum: For serious people with a strong sense of duty who judge themselves harshly and who are quick to anger. Workaholics. Sometimes deep depression.

Sulphur: For shaggy-looking, unconventional, independent, philosophical people who love to pontificate. For a person who has an answer for everything, but often does more talking than doing. A collector who never throws anything away. Craves sweets. Likes a cool environment and can't stand heat.

Phosphorus: Outgoing, needs other people, loves to be the center of attention, very sensitive to others' feelings. Highly impressionable. Also sensitive to odors, lights, and loud noises, especially thunder. Craves ice-cold drinks, ice cream, and spicy food.

Pulsatilla: Gentle, emotionally dependent, insecure, weeps easily, looks for someone strong to lean on. Can't stand a warm, closed room.

Staphysagria: Timid and lets people walk over him. Holds a lot of anger while being too nice. Feels much resentment.

Fear of Bridges

Argentum nitricum: Fear of losing control, with lots of "what ifs" ("What if I get a flat in the middle of the bridge?"). This remedy can be used before the event, in order to prevent anxiety.

Aconite: Sudden panic, with fear of death, dry mouth, and pounding heart.

Fear of Airplanes

***Argentum nitricum:** He starts to feel afraid long before the flight. Fears he will panic or lose control during the flight. Worse in a closed warm space. Has lots of "what if" disaster fantasies.

***Aconite:** Sudden fear of death with dry mouth and pounding heart. Intense thirst. Skin hot and dry. Repeat this remedy as needed.

Calcarea carbonica: May also fear insects, dogs, or insanity. The mind gets tired, it becomes difficult to concentrate, and the individual fears that people will observe his confusion. Can't stand to see or hear about acts of cruelty. Wants to hide. Chilly and worse from cold.

Arsenicum: *Anxious, restless, chilly, fastidious, critical.* Fears being alone and is better from company. Imagines people are looking at him. Chilly and worse from cold.

Fear of Darkness

Stramonium: This person has never recovered from some terrifying event. Worse from darkness, being alone, and seeing any shiny object. Thirsty. Dreads the sight of running water.

Phosphorus: In the sensitive, warm, outgoing person. Better from company and reassurance. Startles easily.

Arsenicum: Grief about himself, and what will become of him. *Fears loss of security and support system. Anxious, restless, chilly, perfectionist, critical.* Failure to trust those on whom he depends. Worries about the future.

Aconite: Intense fear, which comes on suddenly. Dry mouth and pounding heart. Extremely restless. Certain he is about to die.

Fear of Disease

Arsenicum album: The person who needs this remedy is generally anxious, very controlling, cautious, fastidious, and selfish due to insecurity. Fears poverty and being alone. Often (not always) slender. A chilly person. Better from warmth.

Argentum nitricum: Much anticipatory anxiety, fear of losing control, imagines horrible outcomes and "what if" scenarios. Fear of closed or open spaces. Impulsive and hurried. Craves sweets, which cause belching. Always needs fresh, cool air.

Phosphorus: Sensitive, warm, spontaneous, outgoing person. Better from company. Highly suggestible and better from reassurance. Oversensitive to lights, odors, and sounds. Startles easily.

Calcarea carbonica: May also fear insects, dogs, or insanity. His mind gets tired, it becomes difficult to concentrate, and he fears that people will observe his confusion. Can't stand to see or hear about acts of cruelty. Wants to hide. Chilly, tires easily, and sweats from the least exertion. Often—but not always—heavyset.

Kali carbonicum: He prides himself on being logical, even when he should be emotional. He likes rules and regulations and lives by them. Concerned with duty and right and wrong. Fears spontaneity and losing control. Fears to be alone, but then treats people badly. Feels his fear in his stomach. Wakes at 3 a.m. and can't sleep again. Very chilly.

Nux vomica: Irritable and oversensitive to everything. A high-energy person, who thrives on responsibility and often lives on stimulants. Wants to be in charge and doesn't take well to criticism. Anger is the first response to stress. Very fault-finding and can be abusive, both mentally and physically. Very chilly. Wakes up at 3 a.m. and can't sleep again until morning.

Fear of Germs, Contamination, or Contagious Diseases

Calcarea carbonica: May also fear insects, dogs, or insanity. His mind gets tired, it becomes difficult to concentrate, and he fears that people will observe his confusion. Can't stand to see or hear about acts of cruelty. Wants to hide. Chilly, tires easily, and sweats from the least exertion. Often—but not always—heavyset.

Arsenicum album: Anxious, insecure, or afraid to be alone. Very controlling, perfectionist, cautious, fastidious. Suspicious and not easily reassured. Selfish due to insecurity. He may also fear poverty, robbers, or death. Worse at night. Restless, chilly, and better from warmth.

Sulphur: Shaggy-looking, unconventional, independent, philosophical. Loves to pontificate. Has an answer for everything, but often does more talking than doing. A collector who never throws anything away. Craves sweets. Likes a cool environment and can't stand heat.

Lachesis: Intensely talkative and changes the subject constantly. You don't get a word in and can't tell where the conversation is going. Can't stand heat, or having anything tight around the neck. Vivid imagination and is given to fits of suspicion and jealousy. Fear of snakes, of evil, of being poisoned, of going to sleep.

Thuja: Imagines his body is very delicate, thin, or brittle. Well mannered, indirect, and manipulative. He never says exactly what he means. Can't stand cold, damp weather. Gets sick from onions.

Fevers

Because fever is such a general category, there are many remedies listed here. At the end of this list, see "Some Distinguishing Features of Fevers," which can help in your choice. If the fever is associated with or looks like a particular ailment, try looking up the ailment first.

***Aconite:** Sudden, violent onset with extreme anxiety and restlessness. Unquenchable thirst for cold water. Skin hot and dry, or cold sweat with an icy-cold face. Waves of coldness pass through him. Chilly if uncovered. Sweats on the parts that are lain on. Worse at night. For early stages of illness.

***Belladonna:** Sudden, violent onset with face red and hot, hot perspiration. Burning heat with ice-cold hands and feet. No thirst during fever stage. Pupils dilated. Throbbing pains. Sometimes has a hot head with a cold body. Worse from light, noise, cold air, or being jarred.

***Ferrum phos:** At the beginning of an illness with no clear symptoms. Face is either flushed or pale. Perspiration. Worse from cold air, at night or from 4 to 6 a.m., from exertion or strong emotions.

Arsenicum: Anxious, restless, chilly, thirsty for frequent small sips. Doesn't want to be alone. Foul-smelling diarrhea. Fevers coming on or worse from midnight to 3 a.m. Burning pains relieved by heat. The fever may come and go at regular intervals. Cold sweats. Better from warm drinks.

Bryonia: Worse from any motion. Wants to lie still and not be disturbed. Thirst for large, cold drinks. Dry cough, dryness of mucous membranes. Pulse full and hard. Profuse, sour sweat.

Gelsemium: Looks drowsy or intoxicated, with drooping eyelids. Limbs feel heavy. Wants to be held because he shakes so badly. Chill up and down the back. No thirst.

Lachesis: Ailments that come on or are worse after sleep. Worse also from hot drinks, tight clothing, light touch, and warmth. Hot perspiration and icy-cold feet. Left-sided symptoms. Feeling of a lump in the throat. Lesions look purplish.

Lycopodium: Chill between 3 and 4 p.m., followed by sweat. Right-sided symptoms, or they go from right to left. Worse from warmth except for the throat and stomach, which are better from warm drinks. Worse from 4 to 8 p.m., from tight clothes, and after sleep. Better from motion, after midnight, from getting cold, and from being uncovered.

Nux vomica: Angry, irritable, and oversensitive to noise, lights, odors, or comments. Body burning hot, yet he's chilly if uncovered. Chill from moving. Aching in the back and limbs. Wakes at 3 or 4 a.m. and cannot sleep. Worse after eating and at 3 a.m. Constipated, and strains at stool.

Baptisia: Low fever. The whole body feels stiff and sore. Putrid odor of bodily discharges. Face or throat is dark red. Slurred speech; he looks intoxicated. Falls asleep while being spoken to. Can only swallow liquids. Delusion that he is broken and tosses around the bed trying to get the pieces together. Fears to sleep because he might suffocate. Hunger and thirst during fever. Baptisia is followed well by Bryonia or Arsenicum.

Apis: Little or no thirst except during chill. Burning or stinging pain better from cold application. Cries out. Worse from any kind of heat. Worse after sleeping, from touch, motion, or being in a warm room. Better from open air, uncovering.

Opium: Unconscious or drowsy with deep snoring. Labored breathing. Hot perspiration. Face dark red, swollen, and hot. Pupils constricted. Pulse full and slow. No pain in spite of illness. Thirsty. Worse from heat.

Phosphorus: Desires company and fears to be alone. Cannot lie on the left side. Better after short naps. Chilly in the evening, with cold knees. Normally thirsty for large cold drinks, but may be thirstless. Sensitive to lights, odors, and sounds. Worse from warm food or drink. Better from cold and cold food. Craves salt and cold drinks. Startles easily. Bright red bleeding from small wounds.

Pulsatilla: Desires company, sympathy, and reassurance. Chilly in a warm room, yet craves cool, fresh air. Wants the window open. Can't bear external warmth. Usually thirstless, but better from drinking and from cold food. Burning hot at night. One part of the body feels hot, the other cold. Weeps easily. Worse at 4 p.m.

Pyrogenium: Fever associated with blood poisoning. Infections related to childbirth. Foul-smelling discharges (breath, stool, sweat, or vomit). High fever with slow pulse or vice versa. The bed feels too hard. Parts lain on become sore and the patient must constantly change position for relief. Tongue shiny and red. Chill with hot sweat. Worse from cold. The patient says she can feel her heart beating. Delusions of having extra limbs. Very talkative during fever.

Rhus tox: Restless and constantly changing position. Muscles stiff and better from stretching. Worse during rest. Skin red with intense itching. Skin painful from cold air. Great thirst. Worse from cold or dampness. Anxious at night. Better from warmth. Dreams of great exertion.

Cinchona: Abdomen bloated with no relief from belching. Fever and chills come and go at regular intervals. Great exhaustion. Perspiration and diarrhea may accompany the fever. Bitter taste in the mouth and circles under the eyes. Worse from drafts, the slightest touch, and noise.

Agaricus: Twitching and jerking motions along with vertigo and delirium. Twitching eyeballs. Burning, itching sensations as if frostbitten. Chilly. Delirium goes from singing and rhyming to screaming and raving.

Echinacea: Use as a tincture in 30-drop doses, especially for fevers from blood poisoning. Foul discharges, extreme weakness, arms and legs ache. Chilliness with nausea. Tongue dry and swollen.

Sulphur: Burning pains, especially in the face, palms, and feet. Offensive discharges, itching and burning sensation of skin, redness of orifices (lips, nostrils, eyes, anus, etc.). Diarrhea in the morning. Patient has difficulty breathing and craves fresh air. Desires sweets.

Stramonium: Face red, bloated, and hot with a terrified expression. Violent fever with much perspiration. Aversion to fluids. Dread of darkness. Desires light and company. Devout, earnest, beseeching, and ceaselessly talking. Worse from seeing shining objects.

Some Distinguishing Features of Fevers

The remedies with an asterisk (*) have the symptom most strongly.

Fever without thirst: *Pulsatilla, *Gelsemium, Apis, Lycopodium (in peritonitis), Ignatia.

Fever with thirst: *Arsenicum, *Bryonia, *Phosphorus, Cinchona, Eupatorium per, Hepar, Nux vomica, Sulphur, Chamomilla, Veratrum album, Hyoscyamus, Stramonium.

Fear with fever: Aconite, Arsenicum, Baptisia, Belladonna, Hyoscyamus, Stramonium.

Coldness (external) with fever: *Arsenicum, *Carbo veg, Belladonna, Bryonia, Cinchona, Phosphorus, Pulsatilla, Rhus tox, Veratrum album.

Fever from bacterial infections: *Arsenicum, Baptisia, Echinacea, Nitric acid, Pyrogenium, Silica, Thuja.

Cold, clammy sweat with fever: *Arsenicum, *Camphora, *Carbo veg, *Antimonium tart, *Veratrum Album, Ignatia, Ipec, Lachesis, Lycopodium, Mercurius cyan, Pyrogenium.

Hot sweat with fever: *Chamomilla, *Lachesis, *Carbo veg, *Opium.

Fever better after sweating: Aconite, Arsenicum, Veratrum album.

Fever worse after sweating (or if there is no relief): *Mercurius, *Hepar, Pyrogenium, Belladonna, Antimonium tart.

Vomiting during fever: Natrum mur, Arnica, Arsenicum, Crotalus horridus, Cactus grand, Cina, Ipec.

Vomiting of bile with fever: *Baptisia, *Chamomilla, *Mercurius, *Mercurius cyan, *Eupatorium perf, Cinchona, Gelsemium, Ipec, Nux vomica.

Stomach symptoms with fever: *Bryonia, Hydrastis, Nux vomica, Mercurius, Carbo veg, Pulsatilla, Cantharis.

Headache with fever: Belladonna, Bryonia, Gelsemium, Nux vomica, Hyoscyamus, Rhus tox.

Fevers in children: Aconite, Belladonna, Chamomilla, Coffea, Ferrum phos, Stramonium.

Convulsions with high fever: Belladonna, Cicuta, Hyoscyamus, Stramonium, Opium.

Delirium with high fever: Apis, Arsenicum, Belladonna, Opium, Pulsatilla, Stramonium.

Low fevers: *Baptisia,*Arsenicum (can also be used for high fevers).

Weakness during fever: Arsenicum, Phosphorus, Baptisia, Bryonia, Eupatorium per, Ignatia, Muriatic acid, Natrum mur, Phosphoric acid, Pulsatilla, Rhus tox.

Worse from warmth during fever: Apis, Pulsatilla.

Talkative during fever: *Lachesis, *Gelsemium, Baptisia (sometimes).

Flu

The flu (influenza) is a contagious viral disease characterized by sudden onset of fever, chills, weakness, aching muscles or joints, sore throat, cough, headache, and loss of appetite. With some flus, there is abdominal pain and diarrhea. Body temperature can be 101 to 104 degrees, and usually breaks in four to five days. If the fever or cough continues beyond that, consult the "Pneumonia" section. Also, see "Post-Influenza Remedies" at the end of this section.

> **Note:** Many ailments, including serious ones, begin with flu-like symptoms. For this reason, it is sometimes possible to abort the

ailment by catching it in the flu-like stage. Therefore, treat flus aggressively.

Prevention of Flu

Most patients in a particular epidemic will experience similar symptoms. The remedy that matches the symptoms most people are getting will also be the best preventive.

Here are a few examples of remedies that can be used for prevention. However, any of the following flu remedies might be the one that fits this season's flu.

Influenzinum (200c)**:** Once a week may help prevent the flu. Use 30c more often if 200c is not available.

Arsenicum album: When most people getting the flu feel weak, anxious, chilly, thirsty for small sips, and are worse at night and when alone. They may have burning pains relieved by heat. A burning throat may be relieved by hot drinks.

Gelsemium: When most people getting the flu look drowsy or intoxicated, with drooping eyelids and flushed faces. Limbs feel heavy. Want to be left alone. Chills run up and down their backs. No thirst during the fever. Pain in the eyeballs or in the back of the head. Pulses are slow.

Flu Remedies

The following remedies will be useful for everything from common influenza to the most virulent forms, including avian flu.

***Oscillococcinum:** General flu symptoms. Use it in the first twenty-four hours.

***Aconite:** *Use at the first sign of the flu*, especially after exposure to cold air. It will often abort the disease. *Sudden violent onset with dry red face*, great anxiety, restlessness, unquenchable thirst, dry painful cough, racing pulse. Repeat the remedy at least three times; every three hours is good.

***Bryonia:** *Lies perfectly still, worse from any motion, very irritable, wants to be left alone.* Thirsty for large, cold drinks. Dry cough, headache (worse when coughing), and muscle and joint pain. Sharp pains when moving or coughing. Holds the chest when coughing. Dry mouth and lips.

***Eupatorium perfoliatum:** *Deep aching pains in the bones or back.* Restless, but moving about doesn't help. Intense thirst for cold drinks. Hacking cough.

***Rhus tox:** Restless with stiff muscles. Must keep changing position, which gives some relief. Worse after lying still. Worse when first starting to move, but better after moving. Anxious, chilly, and thirsty. Red triangle at the tip of the tongue. Craves milk. Desires cold drinks but is worse from them.

***Arsenicum album:** *Anxious, restless, and thirsty for small sips. Extreme weakness from the start.* Chilly and craves warmth. Worse after midnight. Restless with frequent changes of position (similar to Rhus), exhausted from the least exertion. Burning pains in the throat, chest, and abdomen, which are relieved by heat. Diarrhea.

***Gelsemium:** *Looks drowsy or intoxicated with drooping eyelids and flushed face.* Limbs feel heavy. Wants to be left alone. Chills up and down the back. No thirst during the fever. Pain in the eyeballs or the back of the head. Pulse slow.

Belladonna: *Sudden onset with hot, red face. Dilated pupils, red throat, high fever, and throbbing headache.* Worse from noise, being jarred, from stooping, or from light. Sometimes delirious.

Baptisia: *More serious cases. Face is dark red to purplish.* Dirty tongue with a darker streak in the center. The patient complains that the bed is too hard, and is curled up like a dog. Looks confused or intoxicated. Falls asleep while talking. Delirious and thinks his arms and legs are scattered about the bed.

Mercurius (Vivus or Solubilis): *Sweats profusely and feels worse afterward. Foul odor to breath and perspiration.* Tongue flabby, with the imprint of teeth. Excess saliva (may drool), but great thirst for cold drinks.

Blood-streaked secretions (mucus, stool, etc.). Creeping chilliness. Better from rest, moderate temperature. Worse at night, after sweating, lying on the right side, from the warmth of the bed, from drafts, and from hot or cold.

Nux vomica: *Extremely chilly, chill from uncovering or just moving.* During a fever with a hot body, the patient cannot uncover. Irritable, angry, oversensitive to noise, lights, odors, or imagined insults. Constipation with urging for stool. Worse after eating, in the morning, from cold or drafts. Insomnia from 3 to 5 a.m. Better from warmth, covering, napping, and passing stool.

Antimonium tart: Thick secretions in the lungs that can't be coughed up, but can easily be heard when coughing. Choking, very drowsy, perspiring, nauseous. Worse from lying down, at night, or in a warm room. Better from sitting up, lying on the right side, moving, or vomiting.

Phosphorus: *Especially when pneumonia threatens. Great thirst for cold drinks. Burning sensations (anywhere). Worse lying on the left side. Afraid to be alone* and desires company and reassurance. Easily startled and afraid of thunderstorms. Hypersensitive to odors, sounds, and lights. Tickling cough with tightness in the chest. Craves salt, spices, or ice cream. Pneumonia with burning in the chest—worse lying on the left side. Bloody sputum. Better from short naps, eating, cold food and drink, company, sitting upright, and lying on the right side. Worse from being alone, warm food or drink, evening, and lying on the left side.

Pulsatilla: *Weepy and desires company and sympathy. Fearful when alone. Great craving for fresh air, even when chilly. Worse from warmth or being in a closed room. Thirstless even with dry mouth.* Bland greenish-yellow discharges. Cough, which is worse when lying down. Better from company, sympathy, cool open air, sitting upright, and cold food and drinks. Worse from warmth, a closed room, being alone, and warm food or drink.

Sulphur: When other remedies fail. The patient feels very hot and his feet burn. Worse from heat. Burning pains. Redness of lips, ears, eyelids, and anus. Worse at 11 a.m. Diarrhea in the morning.

Camphora: State of collapse. Icy coldness of body, but the patient refuses covers.

Pyrogenium: Foul odor to discharges (breath, stool, sweat, or vomit). Black stools. High fever with a slow pulse or low fever with a fast pulse. The patient is exhausted, restless, or talkative. He says the bed is too hard and that he feels bruised all over. Imagines that his body covers the whole bed.

Post-Influenza Remedies

For symptoms that remain after the flu, you may try any of the above flu remedies. For weakness after the flu, Gelsemium or Phosphoric acid may help.

Gelsemium: Body feels leaden and the patient can barely keep his eyes open. He may feel a chill up the back. No thirst. Looks drowsy or intoxicated.

Phosphoric acid: Seems both mentally and physically burned out. Blue circles around the eyes. Gives one word answers. Craves fruits and juicy things. Pressing headache on top of the head.

Food Poisoning

(See also "Botulism" and "Mushroom Poisoning")

Nausea, vomiting, abdominal cramps, bloating, diarrhea (sometimes bloody), weakness, fever, and chills are the common symptoms. Induce vomiting unless the person is unconscious or convulsing.

***Nux vomica:** Vomiting, nausea, or pain in the stomach. Very cold, chilly from moving, highly irritable, and sensitive to light, sound, and odors. Cramping pains.

***Carbo veg:** Much belching, abdomen bloated, violent burning from abdomen to chest, and cramping pains. Ice-cold hands and feet, but the head is warm. Hungry for air and wants to be fanned. Especially after bad meat or fish.

***Arsenicum:** Nausea and vomiting. Frightened and doesn't want to be alone. Restless, exhausted, and chilly. Burning pains that are better from heat. Offensive-smelling stool, especially after bad water or meat. Worse from midnight to 3 a.m.

Pulsatilla: Better from cool, open air, though the patient may be chilly. Can't bear a stuffy room. Better from sympathy, company, and reassurance. Dry mouth but no thirst. Heartburn. Tongue coated furry white, especially after eating fatty food or meat.

Cinchona: The whole abdomen is bloated, but belching gives no relief. Painless yellow diarrhea, vomiting of undigested food, worse from any draft or from the slightest touch. Better from warmth.

Colocynth: Cramping pains, which cause the patient to double up. Better from warmth.

Ipecacuanha: Nausea not relieved by vomiting. Clean tongue. Excess saliva.

Pyrogenium: Feels bruised all over and the bed feels too hard. High fever with low pulse or vice versa. Delirious. Symptoms occur after eating bad meat.

Lycopodium: Much flatulence. Chilly. Worse from the pressure of clothes. Especially after eating shellfish.

Urtica urens: Preceded by burning, stinging rash. Especially after eating shellfish.

Argentum nitricum: Black vomiting, convulsions, green stool, loss of consciousness.

Frostbite

(See also "Hypothermia")

Freezing of tissues. Symptoms are burning pain, tenderness, numbness, redness, and swelling. There are three degrees of frostbite, just as there are three degrees of burns. In the first degree, the skin is white, cold, and wrinkled, with loss of sensation. In the second degree, blisters form, which may be filled with bloody serum. In third degree frostbite, the tissue starts to die. For third degree frostbite, see "Gangrene." For minor frostbite, gently massage with cold (never hot!) water. Apply Calendula ointment.

***Agaricus muscarius:** *Burning and itching*, redness, and swelling. Feels like ice-cold needles. *Worse from cold air and from touch.*

***Secale:** *Aversion to heat or touch.* Doesn't want the painful part covered. Burning sensation, better from cold. Feels like ants crawling under the skin. Tiny hemorrhages on the surface of the skin. More anxious than the Agaricus state.

Hepar sulphuricum: If pus forms. Skin sensitive to cold, draft, or touch.

Crotalus horridus: If gangrene threatens.

Gallstone Pain

Gallstones may block the duct through which bile drains from the gallbladder. Bile becomes concentrated behind the stones, causing irritation and pressure in the gallbladder. The pain often comes on after a meal, especially a fatty one. It is usually in the upper right side of the abdomen, but may extend to the right shoulder or to the back. The pain is generally constant and may be accompanied by fever, chills, nausea, bloating, and yellow discoloration of the skin. Such pain that is worse from motion is usually due to gallstones. With urging to urinate, more likely it's kidney stones.

Note: One method of passing gallstones, which is often recommended, is to drink half a cup of olive oil mixed with one-third cup of lemon juice. This mixture is consumed one tablespoonful every fifteen minutes. It can be repeated daily for two or three days if necessary.

***Cholesterinum:** If you tend to have gallstone problems, order this and keep it on hand. It is specific for gallstone pain. If the remedy picture is unclear, or if the symptoms are very general, this should be the first choice.

***Chelidonium:** *Better from hot applications or drinking hot water. Chill during the attack.* Pain just below the right shoulder blade. Pain extends downward across the navel into the intestines. The face is sometimes yellow. Vomiting. Clay-colored stools. Chelidonium has been reported to assist in expelling gallstones and to prevent their formation. A 6c potency two to three times a day for a couple weeks may be most effective.

***Berberis vulgaris:** *Pain radiates in all directions from a small, central point.* Often right sided. Shooting, burning pain. Urine has grayish-white deposit.

***Colocynth:** *Patient doubles up with pain. Better from steady pressure.* Impatient, irritable, or angry. Coated tongue.

***Dioscorea:** *Pain is better from straightening up* and bending backward (hyperextending). Worse from doubling up. Flatulence.

***Belladonna:** Face hot and red or yellow. Strong pulse. Comes on suddenly. Sense of fullness in the area of the stomach. Worse from drinking anything. Worse from light, noise. Repeat every half hour.

***Ipecacuanha:** *Nausea accompanies the pain.* Tongue is clean (not coated). Excess saliva, even drooling. No thirst. Worse from heat.

***Cinchona:** *Face and eyes are yellow. Bloating and constipation.* Worse from light touch, but better from pressure. Chilly and worse from cold and drafts, but craves cold drinks. Attacks occur periodically, sometimes every day at the same hour. Cinchona has been reported to prevent stone formation.

***Nux vomica:** *Face yellow. Chilly, constipated, irritable*, and hypersensitive to noise, odors, or criticism. Can't stand anything tight around abdomen. Aversion to food. Worse in the morning.

***Chionanthus:** Helps expel stones and prevent their formation. Clay-colored stools, constipation, black urine, yellow skin. Tongue is heavily coated with greenish-yellow fur. Sensation of a string tied around the intestines. Better lying on the abdomen. Worse from motion, jarring, or cold.

Lycopodium: Intense pain with tenderness in gallbladder area. Flatulence, bloated abdomen, constipation, and heartburn. Worse from 4 to 8 p.m. Worse from the pressure of clothes. Better from warm drinks and food. Chilly but wants fresh air.

Calcarea carbonica: Very cold with cold sweat especially on the head, hands, and feet. Bends double, clenches hands, writhes with pain. Worse from cold and the pressure of clothes.

Bryonia: Worse from the slightest movement, even deep breathing. Lies perfectly still on painful side. Mouth and lips dry, thirsty for large, cold drinks. Worse from heat. Irritable.

Veratrum album: Freezing cold with cold sweat on the face. Vomiting and diarrhea. Face is pale or blue. Worse from the least motion, and from drinking, especially cold drinks. Cold feeling in the abdomen.

Aconite: *Comes on suddenly with intense pain. Fear of death.* Feels very cold, but can't stand a hot room. Feels faint from sitting or standing. Often useful in the first attack. Repeat every fifteen minutes.

Gangrene

Tissues die and begin to putrefy. It can be caused by infections, or anything that obstructs circulation, such as crushing injuries, frostbite, or blocked blood vessels. Two types of gangrene, dry and moist, have somewhat different appearances. In dry gangrene, the tissue is cold and black and begins to whither. Often the toes are affected, but it may spread to the knees. The dry type is associated with advanced diabetes and arteriosclerosis. In moist gangrene, the tissues are hot and red at first, but later become cold and blue. The gangrenous area spreads and there is an offensive odor, due to putrefactive bacteria.

***Lachesis:** From wounds that have become infected. *Tissue looks purple and oozes dark blood.* Cold extremities, but worse from heat. Ice-cold feeling in the affected part, with tingling, itching, and sometimes burning. Fever and thirst. Worse from touch, warmth, and after sleep. Can't bear tight clothing.

***Secale:** Extremities cold, numb, or tingling. *Feels better from cold and worse from being covered.* Toes and fingers turn dark, dry, and fall off.

***Arsenicum album:** *Chilly, restless, very anxious,* burning pains relieved by warmth. Foul diarrhea. Exhausted from the least exertion. Thirsty for small sips.

***Crotalus horridus:** Moist gangrene. After an injury or infection. Offensive odor, spreads rapidly. Black blisters on a swollen limb. Patient may look yellow, and the skin may be cold and clammy. Mentally can't focus and weeps easily. Right half of the body feels tender.

***Cantharis:** Raw burning pains, frequent urination, great mental excitement. Delirium with barking and biting. Worse from seeing bright objects or from drinking cold water.

Anthracinum: Foul secretions, horrible burning pains, black or blue blisters, great exhaustion, restlessness. Boils or ulcers that have become infected.

Carbo veg: Ice-cold extremities, skin blue, burning pains. Near a state of collapse, short of breath, much belching. Boils that haven't healed and the inflammation has spread.

Echinacea tincture: For gangrenous ulcers. Ten drops every two hours. Also, diluted tincture applied locally.

Sulphuric acid: Bruises or other mechanical injuries gone bad. Better from warmth, worse from cold.

Gingivitis

Inflammation of the gums.

***Mercurius (sol or vivus):** Bad odor in the mouth, metallic taste, excess saliva. Tongue coated. In people who are sensitive to both hot and cold, are worse at night, after sweating, and from lying on their right sides.

Kreosotum: Painful, swollen, or spongy bleeding gums. Foul odor to the mouth. Along with gingivitis, the teeth may decay quite rapidly.

Hekla lava: Gum is hard like rock. Worse on the right side.

Natrum mur: Cracks in the corners of the mouth and the middle of the lower lip. Craves salt. Eruptions on the lower lip. Affects people who like solitude and shun the limelight.

Phosphorus: Gums bleed easily, with bright red blood. Tongue is dry and smooth. Patient is thirsty for ice-cold drinks. Craves ice cream. Affects people who love company, like being the center of attention, are very sensitive to feelings, and bleed easily from small wounds.

Silica: Sensitive to cold water. Often in people who are slender, chilly, who perspire easily (especially from their feet), get infections from minor wounds, are fastidious, and have difficulty being assertive.

Nux vomica: Gums swollen, white, and bleeding. Back of the tongue coated white or yellow. In people who are perfectionist, irritable, ambitious, often constipated, and who may crave coffee, beer, tobacco, or spicy food.

Grief

For grief and ailments from grief. Grieving is a natural means of discharging emotional trauma. However, sometimes a person becomes stuck in the grief without any resolution. The following remedies will be helpful. Empathic nonjudgmental listening is another effective tool.

***Ignatia:** Top remedy for effects of grief, loss, and disappointed love. Silent brooding, much sighing, sometimes hysteria. Changeable moods—laughing then crying. Weeps when alone. Sensation of a lump in the throat. Insomnia, loss of appetite. Worse from warmth, coffee, and the odor of tobacco. For physical ailments that began after grief.

***Natrum muriaticum:** When grief becomes chronic. The patient is solitary, introverted. Lives inside his head, rather than relating to people. Worse from sympathy (gets angry or cries). Worse from company. Self-reliant and will rarely ask for help. Self-condemnation and pervasive guilt feelings. Flies into a rage over trifles. Holds a grudge forever. Sensitive to sunlight. Craves salt.

***Aurum:** When grief turns to thoughts of suicide. Great sense of duty that he feels he didn't fulfill. Guilt feelings, self-condemnation. Talks about suicide. Disgust of life. Hurried and can't do things fast enough. Uncommunicative, angry, worse from contradiction. Sobs in his sleep. Better from music and from thinking about dying.

***Phosphoric acid:** *Apathetic, gives one word answers, emotionally and mentally burned out.* Poor memory and aversion to thinking. Blue rings around the eyes. Craves fruit, juicy things, or cold drinks. Crushing headache on top of the head. Better from warmth. Worse from exertion or being talked to.

***Ambra grisea:** Loss of love of life. Can't stand the presence of strangers. Very shy and thinks people are laughing at her. Worse from the presence of strangers, conversation, and music. Better from cold food and drink.

Cocculus: *This state often results from prolonged periods of dedicated caretaking for loved ones.* Physically and emotionally drained. Suffers horribly from loss of sleep. When spoken to, the individual takes a long time to answer. Vertigo and motion sickness. Chilly.

Causticum: *Idealistic, deeply affected by injustice, worries about others', fights for causes.* Anxious at twilight, fear of the dark, craves smoked food. Chilly and better from warmth. Better in rainy weather.

Gums, Abscess of

***Mercurius (sol or vivus):** Bad odor in the mouth, metallic taste, excess saliva. Tongue coated.

***Hepar sulph** (6x–6c)**:** Extremely sensitive to touch or cold. Pockets of pus. Hepar sulph helps the pus to find a vent, so it can drain.

***Silica:** Abscess on the gum or at the root of a tooth. Sensitive to cold, but not as sensitive to touch as Hepar. Use after Hepar if the abscess fails to drain fully.

Belladonna: Use before abscess forms, when there is redness and throbbing pain, but no pus yet.

Hekla lava: Abscess feels hard like a stone. Abscess after tooth extraction.

Gunshot Wounds

This is a surgical problem and needs professional attention. However, homeopathic remedies can reduce tissue damage, help stem bleeding, reduce pain, and help prevent shock.

***Arnica** (200c)**:** Give this first to prevent further tissue damage, reduce pain, help control bleeding, or prevent shock.

Ledum (200c)**:** To prevent tetanus, especially in wounds that don't bleed much.

Hypericum (30–200c)**:** To help heal injured nerves. Especially when there is much pain.

Cinchona: If there has been much loss of blood, this can help sustain the body.

To Prevent Infection

Hepar (6x, 3c, or 6c)**:** Three times a day along with other remedies.

Hantavirus

A serious viral disease carried by rodents, especially the deer mouse. It is contracted by inhaling the droppings of rodents, or by contact with their urine, saliva, or feces. The disease is not passed between humans. Onset is sudden and intense. Symptoms begin one to five weeks after exposure. The initial symptoms are flu-like, with fever, chills, intense muscle aches, nausea, and vomiting. There is a constant dry cough with severe sore throat. Flushed face and red rash on the neck or armpits. The patient seems intoxicated and confused, with slurred speech. Bruising all over the body. Eyes bloodshot and face dark and puffy. There is a brief period when the person seems to be recovering, but this is followed in one or two days by rapid breathing, fluid in the lungs, internal hemorrhage, and respiratory failure.

***Aconite:** *Sudden, violent onset of symptoms. Very fearful and predicts the time of his death.* Restless. Unquenchable thirst for cold water. Hypersensitive to noise and odors. Eyes dry, hot, red, and inflamed. Face is red, hot, dry, and swollen, but may become icy cold. Face turns pale on rising. Stool is green like chopped herbs. Spasms of the bladder, urinary retention with screaming and restlessness. Pulse is rapid, full, and hard. Numbness in extremities. Cold waves pass through him. Worse at night and from cold.

***Belladonna:** *Sudden, intense onset. Face is red, hot, swollen, and shining. Pupils dilated*, eyes may protrude. Throbbing headache. Worse from light, noise, being jarred, and from lying down. Delirium, furious rage with striking, and biting. High fever, but no thirst during the fever. Hands and feet icy cold. Spasms of limbs. Thirst for cold water but with dread of drinking. Violent palpitation of the heart is felt in the head. Worse from drafts of air, especially on the head. Worse from looking at shiny objects. Better sitting up, or being in a darkened, quiet, warm room.

***Pyrogenium:** *Rapid pulse with low body temperature or slow pulse with high temperature. Great soreness with aching in all the limbs.* Profuse hot sweat. Bodily discharges have offensive odor (breath, vomit, diarrhea, etc.) Bursting headache, vomit resembling coffee grounds. Anxious, talkative, restless. Delusion he is "crowded" with arms and legs.

***Baptisia:** Has some similarities to pyrogenium. Sore muscles and putrid odor of bodily discharges. Legs and back feel sore and bruised. *Flushed face and looks intoxicated. Falls asleep while being spoken to.* Slurred speech. Can only swallow liquids. *Throat dark red.* Delusion that he is broken and tosses around the bed trying to get the pieces together. Fears to sleep because he thinks he might suffocate.

***Rhus tox:** *Extreme restlessness and constantly changes position.* Needs to stretch. Muscles stiff and better from motion. *Worse during rest.* Palpitation of the heart when sitting still. Joints hot, painful, and swollen. Skin red with intense itching and painful from cold air. Great thirst, craving for milk. *Worse from cold or damp environments.* Anxious at night. Better from warmth. Dreams of great exertion.

Arsenicum album: *Fearful and restless. Body cold as ice. Fears death and being left alone. Exhausted from the least exertion. Constant thirst for small sips of water. Burning pains relieved by heat.* Burning sensation in the throat, chest, stomach, and abdomen (which feels like hot coals). Vomiting of blood, bile, or mucus. Short of breath, fears suffocation, and cannot lie down. Better sitting up, from heat, and from changing position. Worse from cold, being alone, and from midnight to 3 a.m.

Gelsemium: *Looks drowsy or intoxicated. Eyelids droop, limbs hang down, face is dark red.* Much weakness and trembling. Slow breathing with long inspiration and sudden forcible expiration. Blurred eyesight with vertigo. Chilliness up and down the back. Thirstless. Pulse slow and weak. Better after urination.

Bryonia: *Worse from any motion, wants to be quiet and lie still. Irritable if disturbed. Great thirst for large, cold drinks.* Can't sit up in bed (feels like he'll faint), dry painful cough, dryness of all mucous membranes. Lips parched, dry, and cracked. Bursting headache, liver swollen and sore, dry hacking cough, stitching pain in the chest, pulse full and hard. In delirium, says he wants to go home and talks about business. Better from pressure and lying on the painful part. Worse from warmth, motion, rising, eating, and coughing (holds his chest).

Arnica: Low fever, head hot with cold body. Body aches as if beaten, the bed feels too hard, skin is black and blue, whole body is sensitive. Fears being touched or approached, cannot bear pain. Says there is nothing the matter with him. Feeble pulse, stitching pain in the heart, nose bleeds dark blood, vomiting of blood, stomach bloated. Brown, bloody, putrid diarrhea. Worse from the least touch. Better lying with the head low. Dreams of death and mutilated bodies.

Echinacea (tincture, 30- to 40-drop doses)**:** Mentally confused, great drowsiness, chilliness with nausea, tongue dry and swollen, tingling sensation in the tongue, lips, and throat. Face flushed with fast pulse. Throat purple or black and ulcerated. Nausea that is better lying down, aching in limbs, recurring boils, enlarged lymph nodes. Pains in the abdomen, which come and go suddenly and are better from doubling over. Dreams of dead relatives.

Headaches

This list includes migraine headaches. These are distinguished by recurrent attacks often on one side of the head, which may include visual disturbances and nausea or vomiting. The headache may last from hours to days.

See "Some Distinguishing Features of Headaches" at the end of this list of remedies.

*__Bryonia:__ Worse from any movement and lies perfectly still. Constipated. Thirsty for large, cold drinks. Bursting headache (pressure from the inside out). Worse from moving, even from moving the eyeballs. Also worse from stooping, opening the eyes, or being jarred. Better in a dark room.

*__Nux vomica:__ Often from overeating, or from spices, alcohol, coffee, or drugs. Chilly and irritable. Worse in the morning, after eating, from the sun, or from cold. Sometimes with vertigo. Constipated but with frequent urging. May feel like a nail has been driven into the top of the head. Worse around 3 a.m. Worse in sunshine. Oversensitive to lights, sounds, odors, and criticism.

*__Belladonna:__ Sudden, violent headache with throbbing. Face red and hot. Pain is often on the right side or in the temples. Worse from stooping, light, noise, being jarred, or drafts on head. Better from bending backward and being in a dark, quiet room.

*__Antimonium crudum:__ Tongue coated thick white and the patient is very irritable. From disordered stomach, bathing in cold water, grief, sun exposure. Belching and bloating. Nausea and vomiting. Vertigo, nosebleed. Worse from overeating, damp cold, or summer sun. Better from open air, lying down, and moist warmth.

*__Gelsemium:__ Preceded by dim vision, double vision, or blindness. Dull, heavy ache. Limbs feels heavy and eyelids droop. Looks intoxicated. Starts in the neck and ends in the eyeballs. Soreness in the neck and shoulders. Pain in the temple extending into the ear. No thirst. Worse from heat. Drowsy and wants to lie quietly. Better with head held high, from open air, or from moving. Sometimes better from passing urine.

***Pulsatilla:** Craves fresh air and must have a window open. Sometimes comes from overeating fatty or rich food. Tongue coated white. Pain moves about. Thirstless. Desires company and sympathy. Weeps easily.

Sanguinaria: Pain settles above the right eye. Better from lying down in a dark room or sleeping. Sometimes with nausea or vomiting. Pain sometimes like a flash of lightning or an electric current. Headache every seventh day. Veins and temples distended. Better from vomiting, sleep, or passing urine. Worse from sweets.

Spigella: Above the left eye. Better lying on the right side with the head high. Better from cold wraps on the head. Worse in stormy weather, from tobacco smoke, stooping, or moving.

Cocculus indicus: From motion sickness, loss of sleep, or the stress of caring for loved ones. Can't stand the smell of food. Headache in the back of the head, worse from lying on the back. Pain in the eyes. Worse after eating, from open air, after loss of sleep, or from touch, noise, or being jarred.

Ignatia: From grief, worry, or anger. Feels like a nail has been driven out through the side of the head. Worse in the morning, from stooping, open air, coffee, cigarette smoke, and warmth. Changeable mood.

Ipecacuanha: Constant nausea not relieved by vomiting. Excess salivation, clear tongue. Brain feels bruised. Suppressed anger. Anger followed by calm. Worse from the least motion and from lying down. Better from open air.

Iris versicolor: Preceded by blurred vision, pain may extend to the teeth. Sour vomiting. Sometimes nosebleed. Vomiting of bile, which gives some relief. Headache in front or in the right temple. Sometimes burning in the throat or stomach. Aversion to company. Sadness during headache. Worse from eating sweets, cold air, evening and night, and rest. Better from continued motion.

Natrum mur: Starts in the morning. Nausea and vomiting of clear fluids. Worse from coughing. Craves salt. Better from open air, cold bathing, and lying on the right side. Worse in the morning and from heat and sun. Worse from company and sympathy.

Natrum sulph: Sometimes triggered by head injuries, even months or years before. Diarrhea and vomiting of bile. Feeling of heat on the top of the head. Sometimes boring pain in the right temple, preceded by burning in the stomach. Scalp sensitive to touch. Worse during menses, or from noise, stooping, light, eating, or damp weather.

Phosphorus: Headache located above the left eye; the patient sees black spots. Worse in the morning and evening. Worse lying on the left side. Worse in a warm room. Desires cold drinks, ice cream, or salt. Burning sensation in the palms of the hands. Startles easily.

Sepia: Often left sided, with pain from within seeming to move outward. Pain comes on suddenly along with hot flashes, stiff neck, and nausea. Worse indoors and when lying on the painful side. Often associated with menses. Irritable or weepy. Aversion to company but dreads to be alone. Craves chocolate or lemons. Worse from cold, before menses, and in the evening. Better from exertion, firm pressure, and naps.

Silica: Very chilly. Hair feels sensitive, head perspires. Pain begins in the back of the head and extends to the eyes. Headache recurs once a week. Sensitive to every impression. Worse from the slightest jar, from cold, stooping, dampness, bathing, drafts, touch, or consolation. Better lying on the left side. Better from warmth and wrapping up the head. Chilly, but has an aversion to warm food.

Agaricus: Headache on the side, as if from a nail. Sometimes with nosebleed. Twitching of the eyelids, tongue, and muscles. Talkative. Worse in the morning, from cold, or from touch. Better from gentle motion.

Cinchona: The patient feels like his head would burst, like his brain is bumping into his skull. Throbbing pain. Sensitive scalp. Headache after loss of body fluids. Abdomen bloated and belching doesn't help. Oversensitive to light. Worse from drafts, light touch, after eating. Better from warmth and firm pressure.

Coffea: From becoming overexcited. Sleepless from excitement. Worse from noise, odors, open air, and coffee. May seem like his brain is being torn to pieces or a nail was driven in. Despairing and weeps from pain.

Eupatorium: Throbbing pain, as if a heavy cap is pressed over the skull. Pain in the back of the head when lying down. Aching in bones. Restless from pain. Great thirst for cold drinks. Worse from cold air and motion. Headache every third and seventh day.

Some Distinguishing Features of Headaches

Must lie down: Bryonia, Natrum mur, Nux vomica, Sepia.

Better lying with head high: Arsenicum, Gelsemium, Phosphorus, Pulsatilla, Spigella.

Better from motion: Arsenicum, Iris versicolor, Lycopodium, Rhus tox, Pulsatilla.

Better in a dark room: Belladonna, Bryonia, Sanguinaria, Silica.

Worse in a dark room: Carbo veg, Silica.

Better from open air: Pulsatilla, Carbo veg, Cimicifuga, Glonoine, Natrum mur, Phosphorus, Sepia, Arsenicum.

Throbbing: Belladonna, Glonoine, Lachesis, Cinchona, Phosphorus, Argentum nitricum.

Left-sided: Spigella, Sepia (also right), Mercurius, Phosphorus, Arsenicum.

Right-sided: Chelidonium, Belladonna, Carbo veg, Iris versicolor, Ignatia, Lycopodium, Bryonia, Sepia (also left).

While constipated: Bryonia, Nux vomica, Natrum mur, Natrum sulph, Pulsatilla, Aloe.

After overeating: Nux vomica, Pulsatilla, Nux moschata.

With exhaustion: Arsenicum, Cinchona, Gelsemium, Ignatia.

Cries out with pain: Bryonia, Sepia, Arsenicum.

Hot flushed face: Aconite, Belladonna, Glonoine, Gelsemium, Chamomilla.

After head injury: Arnica, Natrum sulph, Helleborus, Hypericum, Natrum mur, Belladonna.

Worse from reading: Natrum mur, Ruta, Sepia.

Worse from odors: Ignatia, Sepia, Belladonna, Coffea, Phosphorus, Lycopodium, Silica, Colchicum, Sulphur, Aurum.

Worse from noise: Belladonna, Bryonia, Nux vomica, Spigella, Arsenicum, Cocculus, Lachesis, Coffea, Silica.

Every seven days: Iris vers, Phosphorus, Sanguinaria, Silica, Sulphur.

Every two weeks: Arsenicum, Chelidonium, Sulphur, Ferrum, Cinchona, Ignatia, Pulsatilla, Sanguinaria.

During perspiration: Arsenicum, Bryonia, Sulphur, Mercurius, Carbo veg, Pulsatilla.

During cold sweat: Gelsemium, Veratrum alb.

After breakfast: Iris vers, Nux vomica, Lycopodium.

Better from wrapping something tight around the head: Pulsatilla, Silica, Argentum nit.

Begins at 3 p.m.: Belladonna.

From anger: Staphysagria, Ignatia, Bryonia, Nux vomica, Chamomilla, Phosphorus, Natrum mur, Lycopodium.

Worse from light: Belladonna, Bryonia, Cocculus, Gelsemium, Ignatia, Natrum mur, Phosphorus, Sanguinaria, Sepia, Silica, Sulphur.

Head Injuries: See "Concussion"

Heart Problems

Included here are heart attack, gradual cardiac failure, and angina.

Heart Attack

The patient may experience nausea, followed by chest pain or pressure, pain down one or both arms, difficulty breathing, vomiting, cold sweat, and blue face. (See also "Angina.") Repeat the remedy every ten to fifteen minutes. If the victim is not breathing and there is no heartbeat, begin cardiopulmonary resuscitation.

***Arnica** (200c)**:** every fifteen minutes.

***Aconite** (200c)**:** *If fear is predominant. Predicts the time of his death.*

***Latrodectus mactans:** *Extreme pain in the chest extending down the left arm to the hand.* Gasps for air. Numbness of extremities. Weak but rapid pulse. Skin cold.

***Arsenicum album:** *Extremely anxious, chilly, restless, thirsty for small sips of cold water.* Doesn't want to be alone. Feeling of a weight on or constriction in the chest. Burning pains. Face gray to blue. If there is no response after a few doses, try another remedy. *Note: Arsenicum will only work for three to five hours for heart attack.* After that, another remedy must be used (often Sulphur if the patient feels waves of heat, or Phosphorus if he craves large cold drinks, can't lie on his left side, and wants company.)

***Antimonium tartaricum:** Less anxious than Arsenicum, face and fingernails blue, not much thirst, more hopeless than scared. Ankles may swell, *tongue is coated thick white. Lungs may have fluid that can be heard rattling.* Differs from Arsenicum in that there is *no thirst*, and the patient is *worse from warmth and worse from draft.* Sense of fullness in the chest.

***Carbo veg:** *Craves air, wants to be fanned, abdomen bloated with much belching*, no thirst. Face pale, hands and feet freezing cold. Mentally dull or foggy. *Note: Carbo veg may not hold and should be followed by another remedy.* Sometimes Sulphur follows, if the patient experiences waves of heat. Kali carb may follow if he is cold, worse from drafts, leans forward to breathe, or can't lie on his right side.

Oxalic acid: *Skin is cold and has a mottled appearance, extreme exhaustion,* numbness of hands and feet, fingernails blue, sharp pains in the chest. Wants to lie perfectly still.

Gradual Cardiac Failure

Heart failure is a condition where the heart loses its ability to pump blood effectively. This results in a deficit of oxygen and nutrients for the tissues. The condition is usually chronic and develops over time. When the left side of the heart fails, it can lead to fluid in the lungs, called pulmonary edema. When the right side fails, fluid may collect in the hands, feet, or abdomen.

Symptoms include swelling of the hands, feet, or abdomen, bulging of neck veins, shortness of breath, palpitations, rapid or irregular pulse, weakness, cough, and decreased urine production.

Naja: *Stitching pain in the chest, radiating to the nape of the neck and the left shoulder, with numbness of the left arm and hand.* Pain goes through to the back. Fear of death. Feels like a weight on the heart. Face looks purplish, can't stand clothing around the neck, worse lying on the left side.

Lachesis: *Feeling of constriction in the chest.* Can't stand clothing around the neck. Face looks purplish. Worse lying on the left side. Feels like he is suffocating when falling asleep. Worse after sleep.

Lycopus: *Horrible pounding feeling in the heart with a throbbing feeling in the head and neck.* Worse lying on the right side (opposite Naja and Lachesis). Can't stand the smell of food.

Laurocerasus: Face looks purple, lips blue, gasping for air. Worse if totally sitting up or lying down. Best when just reclining. Very cold. Worse from motion.

Latrodectus mactans: Extreme irritability with numbness of the left hand and arm. Gasps for air. Weak but rapid pulse.

Crataegus: Use in low potency (3x) every three or four hours for several weeks. When the heart is failing steadily, with rapid pulse, difficulty breathing (which is worse from exertion), a blue tinge to the face, and some swelling of the ankles.

Angina

Severe pain near the heart radiating to the left shoulder and arm. Face pale or blue, much perspiration. Fear of death. Sometimes there is difficulty breathing. The symptoms resemble a heart attack, except the episode only lasts a few seconds or minutes and does not produce permanent damage to the heart. Usually due to atherosclerosis, it is caused by inadequate blood flow through the coronary vessels. The attack may be triggered by physical exertion or emotional stress. Chelation therapy may be the long-term solution.

***Aconite:** For the first attack. Intense fear of death, restlessness, great thirst, skin is hot and dry. Aconite doesn't have the weakness or exhaustion of the Arsenicum state.

***Cactus grand:** *Feels like an iron band around the chest being drawn tighter.* Pulse fast but feeble. Worse lying on the left side.

***Arsenicum:** Tightness in the chest with *burning sensation*. Very chilly and better from warmth and covers. Fear of death and being left alone. Restless, thirsty for small sips, face pale. Profound weakness and exhaustion from the least effort.

***Latrodectus mactans:** *Pain extends down left arm to fingers* with numbness. The patient screams with pain. Gasping for breath. Skin cold. Constriction in the chest.

Iodum: Feels *like a tight band around the heart itself* (as opposed to the whole chest). Face flushed, worse from heat. Patient is usually very thin. Restless and anxious.

Spongia: *Heart feels as if it is getting bigger*, too large for chest, as if it might burst out. Worse lying down. Chilly and worse from any draft. Numbness in the arm or hand.

Heat Stroke: See "Sunstroke"

Hepatitis—Acute

Inflammation of the liver. It can be caused by infection with viruses, bacteria, or protozoa. It can also result from toxic chemicals like solvents, insecticides, anesthetics, antibiotics, and other medicines.

Hepatitis begins with flu-like symptoms: weakness, drowsiness, chills, sore throat, nausea, vomiting, headache, stupor, and sometimes coma. The liver is located on the right side of the trunk from a few inches above the hip to a couple inches below the nipple. It may become enlarged and tender to the touch. Jaundice may develop, although it is absent in most cases, especially in infants and children. Enlarged spleen (lower left side of trunk), swelling of lymph glands under the jaw. It can take anywhere from eight weeks to twelve months to fully recover.

Prevention

A timely dose of homeopathic **Phosphorus** may prevent or reduce severity of infectious hepatitis. The **Hepatitis nosode**, available from some homeopathic pharmacies, may also help. The herb **Milk thistle** offers some protection to the liver during exposure to chemicals.

Remedies for Hepatitis

Aconite: Great fear of death, unbearable pain, moaning, and tossing about. Sudden high fever. The patient's face is red, hot, and dry. Much thirst.

Belladonna: Pain in the liver is worse from pressure, breathing, coughing, or lying on the right side. Face red with hot perspiration. Pupils dilated. Can't bear light, noise, being jarred, or cold air.

Cardus marianus: Face yellow, headache, nausea and vomiting, urine and stool golden yellow. Hard, difficult stools alternating with diarrhea. Worse from eating (opposite Chelidonium). Worse when moving. Lower potencies are best, but give what you have.

Chelidonium: Pain in the upper right side of the back, face yellow, liver area is painful to touch. Much nausea and sometimes vomiting.

Temporarily better from eating. Better from hot drinks. Lower potencies best (6c–12c), but give what you have.

Cinchona: Abdomen bloated with much belching, which gives no relief. Liver is enlarged, hard, and sensitive to the slightest touch. Face yellow, bitter taste in the mouth, constipation or painless diarrhea. Circles under the eyes, ringing in the ears.

Lycopodium: Dull, aching pain in liver. Worse after eating, Much gas. Feels full after a few bites of food. Desires sweets. Worse from 4 to 8 p.m. Can't stand tight clothes. One foot cold, the other warm. Better from warm drinks.

Natrum sulphuricum: Sharp pains in the liver. Worse from lying on the left side, from moving, and in the morning. Vomits bile. Stools dark green. Diarrhea when first standing. Depressed and dislikes to be spoken to, especially in the morning. Suicidal thoughts. Worse from dampness.

Nux vomica: Angry, irritable, oversensitive to noise, odors, and light. Very chilly. Dislikes the pressure of clothing. Liver enlarged and hard. Wakes 3–4 a.m. Constipation with straining.

Phosphorus: Unquenchable thirst for cold drinks, tendency to hemorrhage of bright red blood, perspiration during sleep, fear of being alone, worse lying on the left side, burning sensations. Desires company. Startles easily.

Hernia

A hernia is a condition in which some part of the body projects itself outside of its natural cavity. In a *strangulated* hernia, the projected organ is tightly pinched by surrounding tissues. This is a serious matter, which usually needs surgical intervention, as it can lead to gangrene.

Types of Hernias

Hiatal hernia: Sometimes called diaphragmatic, where the stomach protrudes through the diaphragm. Burping up acid, heartburn, pain just below the breastbone. Abdomen bloated, gurgling sounds, cramping pain, constipation, nausea, and vomiting.

Inguinal: Where the intestines protrude through the scrotum. This is usually a surgical problem. It may be life threatening if strangulated. Pain and hardening in lower abdomen.

Umbilical: Protrusion through the bellybutton. The remedies that apply here are usually Nux vomica, Plumbum, Calcarea, Lachesis, and Opium.

Remedies for Hernias

Calcarea carbonica: Good remedy for umbilical or hiatal hernias. For hernias in children (see also Aurum). Abdomen bloated, gurgling sounds, cramping pain. Chilly, fearful. Worse from cold and drafts. Perspires on the head.

Lycopodium: Inguinal, strangulated. Often right sided. Abdomen bloated with gurgling sounds, flatulence, and cramping pains. Feet cold. Irritable. Worse from tight clothes and after sleep (also Lachesis) and from 4 to 8 p.m. Craves sweets.

Nux vomica: Protruding inguinal hernia, *strangulated*, often left sided (but can be right sided.) Bowels feel bruised. Constipation, nausea, vomiting, very chilly. Chill from uncovering.

Cocculus: If Lycopodium and Nux fail. Strangulated. Worse on the right side. Bloated abdomen, nausea and vomiting, abdomen feels bruised, constipation. Unable to stand.

Aurum: Inguinal hernia in children. Cramplike pains.

Lachesis: Strangulated. Hernia threatening gangrene. Skin over hernia is mottled and dark. Often left sided. May come on during or just after sleep. Can't stand constrictive clothing around the neck or waist. Very talkative. Worse from warmth.

Belladonna: Strangulated. Throbbing pain, face red and hot, pupils dilated. Constricted feeling around the navel. Feels like a hard ball pressing outward. Worse from light, noise, being jarred, and cold air.

Opium: Strangulated. Face dark red, swollen, and hot. Pupils constricted. Foul-smelling vomit, intestines feel lacerated. Worse from heat, and better from cold.

Plumbum: Strangulated. Extreme cramping pains that radiate, vomiting of stool. Abdomen feels drawn in as if by a string, abdomen retracted, pain around the bellybutton.

Herpes Labialis (Cold Sores on the Lips)

This is an infection caused by the herpes simplex virus, type one. Small, usually painful blisters form on the lips and sometimes inside the mouth. The virus can spread to other parts of the body by contact. The blisters usually last from a week to ten days.

Natrum mur: Worse from heat, especially from the sun. Craves salt. Often appears after emotional stress.

Rhus tox: Better from heat and moving about. Restless and thirsty. Worse at night.

Herpes Simplex (Genital)

This is a sexually transmitted viral infection, characterized by recurrent eruptions of small, painful blisters on the genitals, around the rectum, or in adjacent areas. It is caused by the herpes simplex virus, type two. It is contagious and may be spread even in the absence of symptoms. The virus can be passed to a baby during childbirth, with serious results. Latex condoms are an effective barrier. The first outbreak of symptoms may include fever, weakness, muscle aches, and lessened appetite. Burning and itching may precede the blisters. The blisters turn into ulcers, which heal in one to two weeks.

Natrum mur: *Worse from heat, especially the sun. Craves salt.* Often triggered by emotional upset. Wants to be alone, may feel depressed.

Sepia: *Worse before menses or before or after pregnancy.* Worse from birth control pills. Feels better from exercise. Often depressed or irritable. *Craves lemons and sour foods.*

Rhus tox: *Very restless. Worse from cold and damp weather. Worse at rest.* Worse in the winter. Thirsty. Better from warmth and moving about.

Dulcamara: *Triggered by exposure to damp weather* or when getting cold. Very sensitive to cold. Worse during rest. Worse in the summer and fall. Quarrelsome. Worries about others.

Petroleum: *Affects people with very dry skin, which cracks. Worse in the winter.* Aversion to fatty food. Excitable. Can't make decisions.

Herpes Zoster (Shingles)

Herpes zoster is an acute infection, which triggers a painful rash. It is caused by the same virus that causes chickenpox. After getting chickenpox, the virus stays dormant and emerges years later. The attacks are often triggered by stress or anything that compromises the immune system. At that time, the virus travels up the nerve tract, causing pain and burning sensations. Chickenpox-like blisters form over three to five days, ulcerate and then form dry crusts. The crusts fall off after two to three weeks. Chills, fever, and weakness may occur for three to four days before the rash. Sometimes the pain continues after the rash is gone. This condition is called postherpetic neuralgia.

***Arsenicum album:** When rash first shows. *Burning pain, which is better from heat.* Skin is very dry. Worse from midnight to 3 a.m. Large crusts that bleed when peeled. Anxious, chilly, and restless. Pain persists after rash. Thirsty for frequent small sips of water.

***Rhus tox:** Often found on the right side. *Continuous itching and burning. Worse during rest, cold, rainy weather, and at night. Chilly, restless.* Better when moving. Pain persists after rash. Thirsty for large drinks.

***Mezereum:** *Sharp lightninglike pains. Chilly but worse from warmth* (opposite Arsenicum). *Worse from touch.* Burning and itching. Brownish scab. Pain persists after rash. Anxious.

***Ranunculus bulbosus:** Sharp pains similar to Mezereum. *Burning and itching blisters filled with irritating fluid.* The blisters show up in clusters. Worse from cold, dampness, and touch. Pain persists after rash. Worse from moving (opposite Rhus tox).

Natrum muriaticum: After grief or emotional upset. Worse from heat, from sun. Better in open air. Craves salt.

Mercurius: Blisters with dry scales, which burn or bleed when scratched. Worse at night. Perspires easily. Excess saliva, but thirsty.

Hives—Allergic

Hives are raised red welts, which often itch. There are numerous causes including medicines, foods, pollen, insect bites, exposure to chemicals, and sunlight.

***Apis:** Burning stinging pain, worse from heat and better from putting cold on it. Swelling of tissues. No thirst. Worse from touch, pressure, after sleep, or from lying down.

***Urtica urens:** Burning, stinging, itching. Better from rubbing. Worse after bathing and exercise.

***Rhus tox:** Skin red, burning, and itching. Better from warm water. Patient is extremely restless and constantly shifts position. Stiffness and pain in the joints and muscles. Worse from cold, dampness, and getting wet. Unquenchable thirst. Chilliness. Worse at night. Better from heat and warm drinks. Craves milk.

Arsenicum: Anxious, chilly, and restless. Burning pain, which is oddly better from heat. Thirst for small sips. Exhausted. Worse after midnight.

Natrum mur: Itching and burning. Worse after exertion. Craves salt. Oversensitive to sunlight. Worse from consolation and company. Deep crack in the middle of the lower lip.

Sulphur: The patient feels hot. Worse from heat, craves fresh air. Burning sensations, red itching skin that is worse from heat and bathing. Bodily discharges smell foul and irritate the skin. Sudden diarrhea in the morning. Craves sweets.

Mezereum: Intense itching. Very chilly but worse from warmth. Chilliness follows eruption. Coldness or numbness after scratching. Anxiety felt in stomach and when alone. Craves bacon, ham, and fat.

Antimonium crudum: Tongue coated white. Aversion to being looked at or touched. Craves pickles and acidic foods. Constant belching and bloating after eating.

***Histaminum:** If other remedies fail or if symptoms are not clear.

Hookworm: See "Worm Infestations"

Hydrophobia: See "Rabies"

Hypothermia

A condition arising from exposure to cold, in which the body temperature drops to below 95 degrees. Symptoms may come on gradually, with the individual being unaware of the problem. Symptoms include drowsiness, confusion, lack of coordination, uncontrollable shivering, slurred speech, delirium, and coma. Cover the patient and apply warm compresses to the neck, chest, and groin. Excessive use of heat can cause heart failure or shock. If the person is not breathing, institute mouth-to-mouth resuscitation. If there is no heartbeat, begin cardiopulmonary resuscitation.

Prevention

If you know you will be exposed to cold for lengths of time, take **Aconite** every four hours.

Remedies for Hypothermia

***Aconite:** Every fifteen minutes. If unconscious, alternate Aconite and Carbo veg. Place the remedies between the lips and teeth. The patient is frightened, thirsty.

***Calcarea carbonica:** From exposure to cold and wetness. Worse from any draft.

Rhus tox: From exposure to cold and wetness. Aching muscles, restlessness. Worse at night, thirsty.

Arsenicum: Anxious, won't be left alone, thirsty for small sips of water, restless in spite of great weakness.

Hepar sulph: Worse from the slightest touch or any draft. Irritable.

Bryonia: Worse from any motion.

Carbo veg: Craves air and wants to be fanned. Belching.

Immunization: See "Vaccination, Treating the Effects of"

Also see "Preventing Illness with Homeopathy" for homeopathic alternatives to vaccination.

Impaction—Fecal

Impaction is overloading of the feces in the bowel, so that they are unable to pass. This may be accompanied by pain and spasm of the rectum. Manual removal of the stool may be necessary. Warm mineral-oil enemas are sometimes helpful. Symptoms include frequent straining with passage of liquid stools, abdominal cramps, or sudden diarrhea in a person with chronic constipation.

***Belladonna:** Skin dry and hot, throbbing sensations, stinging pain in the rectum. Worse from light, noise, or being jarred. Craves lemonade.

***Opium:** No urging to stool. After operations on the abdomen, after use of drugs, from lack of exercise, during pregnancy, or after a fright. Stool comes out as black round balls. Warm and worse from heat.

***Plumbum:** Constant ineffectual urging to move the bowels. Stools are hard black balls, similar to the Opium symptom. Chilly. Better from doubling over.

Lachesis: Worse after sleep, from light touch, and from heat. Can't bear tight clothing, especially around the neck. Often very talkative.

Causticum: Heartburn with sour belching and vomiting. Craving for smoked foods (meat, fish). Ailments from long-standing worry, grief, or fright. Ill effects from burns. Anxious at twilight. Impaction is sometimes due to large hemorrhoids. The patient finds it easier to pass stool when standing.

Infections

Homeopathic remedies have been used to treat infections for two hundred years. Antibiotic-resistant infections can be treated with homeopathic remedies. Local infections are listed alphabetically in this book according to type, such as "Abscess," "Wounds—Infected," "Lymphangitis," or body part, such as "Sore Throat," "Earache," and "Eyes." Infections throughout the whole body (systemic) will be listed under the name of the disease, such as "Pneumonia," "Cholera," "Anthrax," or "Measles." There is a listing for "Blood Poisoning," also called septicemia. See also "Gangrene."

Influenza: See "Flu"

Injuries

For cuts, blows, and punctures see "Wounds."

See also "Animal bite," "Back Pain," "Bleeding," "Breast, Injuries to," "Broken Bones," "Burns," "Concussion," "Cornea, Scratched," "Eardrum perforation," "Electric Shock," "Eyes," "Gunshot Wounds," "Lyme Disease," "Radiation, Exposure to," "Shock," "Snakebite," "Spine Injuries," "Sprains," "Splinters," "Sunburn," "Sunstroke," "Surgery," "Toothache and Dental Work," and "Vaccination."

Insanity: Psychoses—Acute

Psychosis is a loss of contact with reality. Symptoms may include delusions, hallucinations, disorganized thought, confusion, depression, and unfounded fears. While some people suffer these symptoms chronically, a healthy person can temporarily evolve to such a state from great stress (grief, fear, jealousy, anger, pain), from a high fever, or from toxicity (drugs or other chemicals). The following remedies will be most helpful in the temporary states. There are homeopathic psychiatrists who treat chronic illness with homeopathy.

Note: All of these remedies have multiple uses and are often called for in physical problems that have little or no mental aspect. For example, a person needing Belladonna for an abscess will not exhibit any of the Belladonna symptoms described below.

***Belladonna:** Sudden violent onset. Face red and hot. Striking, biting, kicking. Neck veins bulging. Extreme sensitivity to light and noise. Strength increased. Hallucinations, which frighten the patient. Delusions of animals, fear of animals, especially dogs. Loves to make animals suffer, wants to set fires, jumps out of bed, pulls the hair of bystanders. Worse from seeing shining objects.

***Stramonium:** Intense fear of darkness and the night. Sees animals, ghosts, angels, and the dead. Violent rage alternating with convulsions. Laughing, biting, violent sexual fantasies. Sleeplessness. Excitement triggered by seeing shining objects. Impulse to kill with a knife.

***Hyoscyamus:** Extreme jealousy, suspicion. The individual thinks people are trying to trick him. Violent outbursts, wants to kill everyone he sees, exposes himself, plays with his genitals. Thinks he is possessed by the devil. Picks at his fingers and lips. Gestures as though he is grasping for something. Very talkative or silent for hours, has convulsions, refuses to eat.

***Anacardium:** The patient feels caught in a battle between his "good" and "bad" sides. He may see it as God and the devil. Sees devils, or hears the voices of dead people. Hatred, violent cursing, laughing, rage. Anger when contradicted. Delusion that he is two people. Sad but cannot weep. Worse in the morning. Wants to kill from anger.

***Veratrum album:** Believes he is Christ, believes he is appointed by God to convert others. Spits in people's faces. Critical, always finding fault, cursing all night. Delusions that he is talking with God in heaven, or that he is a prince or a person of rank. Despair of his social position. Embraces inanimate objects. Feigns deafness. Chases his family out of the house. Very chilly.

***Nux vomica:** Delusion that people are questioning him and he must answer. Irritable when questioned. Delusion that people are carrying on pranks behind his back. Fear of terrible dreams, quarrelsome, sudden impulse to kill for a slight offense. Chilly, worse in the morning, oversensitive to stimuli and criticism. Wakes at 3 a.m.

Mercurius: The patient feels hurried inside (like the feeling of rushing to make a deadline). Always discontented. Has a desire to kill loved ones, or a desire to kill anyone who contradicts him. Commits criminal acts without remorse. Delusions that he is surrounded by enemies, or that he has ruined the health of his loved ones. Worse at night. Perspires without relief, excess saliva and drooling, flabby tongue with the imprint of teeth. Confused and loses his way in well-known streets.

Lachesis: Extreme talkativeness and constantly changing subjects. Delusion that he is under superhuman control. Makes prophesies. Has insane jealousy, sees frightful images, and tears out his hair. Strikes out physically from jealousy. Desires to kill by poison. Delusion that he is charmed and cannot break the spell. Hot and worse from heat. Can't bear anything to touch his neck. Worse after sleep. Tongue trembles.

Arsenicum: Anxiety drives the patient out of bed. Restless, chilly. Worries about his salvation. Fear of death, feels guilty of a crime, aversion to solitude and desires company. Worse after midnight. Delusions that he has offended people, a friend met with an accident, he contaminates everything he touches, his bed is covered with rats, he is being watched, or a dead friend is on the sofa. Loves to make animals suffer. Has sudden impulses to kill.

Tarentula hispanica: A state of extreme excitement with a desire for wild dancing and constant movement. Desires loud music and feels better from it. Destructive, impatient, violent anger when touched. Threatens destruction and death. Laughing and mocking. Aversion to or desire for certain colors. Desires to lie in the dark and not be spoken to.

Insomnia

Homeopathic remedies for insomnia are best taken a couple times a day and again at bedtime. They are correcting the underlying problem. The following are remedies for the most common types of acute insomnia. Chronic insomnia may need the care of a professional homeopath.

***Kali phosphoricum:** Nervous exhaustion from mental exertion or worry. Chilly, nervous, startles easily. Wakes hungry at 5 a.m. Better from eating and gentle motion.

***Nux vomica:** Tends to be more awake and mentally active in the evening. The patient may overindulge in food, drink, or stimulants. Chilly, irritable, angry, oversensitive, or constipated. May wake at 3 a.m. unable to sleep. Insomnia from overuse of coffee (also Coffea and Chamomilla) or after using sleeping pills or drugs.

***Coffea:** Wide awake and excited by good news, surprises, or just excitement. The mind won't shut off, as if from drinking too much coffee. Insomnia from drinking too much coffee (also Nux and Chamomilla).

***Cocculus indicus:** Insomnia from prolonged loss of sleep. For people who have been staying up all night caring for someone. Also for insomnia from jet lag (Melatonin may work better). Feels worse from fresh air.

***Chamomilla:** For people who are oversensitive to pain and in a snappish mood (e.g., children who are teething). For people who can't sleep because they have gotten used to sleeping pills. When coffee drinkers drink too much coffee (also Coffea and Nux).

***Arnica:** Insomnia after physical exertion. Too physically exhausted to sleep. Complains of sore muscles and says the bed feels too hard.

Aconite: Insomnia after terrifying experiences. Restless, very thirsty. Skin hot and dry.

Ambra grisea: Loss of love of life. Tired but unable to sleep due to worry. Feels embarrassed in company, especially around strangers. Very nervous and perspires during conversation. Sleepy until he lies down, and then is wide awake.

Belladonna: Throbbing head, face red and hot, pupils dilated. May see faces in the dark, or frightful images upon closing the eyes.

Arsenicum: Very anxious and extremely restless. Great fatigue, sometimes fear of death. Can't stay in bed and moves about even though exhausted. Chilly, better from company, and thirsty for frequent small sips. Worse from midnight to 3 a.m.

Capsicum: From homesickness, especially in children.

Gelsemium: From anticipation. Also, insomnia from exhaustion or overthinking.

Lachesis: The patient's breathing stops as soon as he falls asleep. Afraid he will die if he sleeps. Worse after sleep. Can't stand anything tight around his neck.

Sulphur: Sleepy during the day but awake at night. Abundance of thoughts. Awake from 2 a.m. to 5 a.m., then falls asleep in the morning. His feet burn at night and he puts them out of the covers.

Jellyfish Stings: See "Bites and Stings—Jellyfish"

Kidney Stones, Pain from

(See also "Nephritis," "Uremia," and "Organ Remedies—Kidney" in chapter 4)

Kidney stones are insoluble substances that crystallize out into the urine. These stones may not produce symptoms until they begin to move down the ureter. Symptoms include excruciating, intermittent pain in the kidney area or lower back. The pain may radiate to the abdomen, genital area, or thighs. Nausea, vomiting, bloating, chills, fever, and frequent urination are also seen.

> **Note:** Pain that is worse from motion is usually due to a gallstone. With urging to urinate, more likely it's a kidney stone. Most of the remedies that apply to kidney stone pain also work for gallstone pain.

***Berberis vulgaris:** Pain radiates in all directions from a central point. Urging to urinate with pain on urination. Urine has grayish-white deposit. Kidney area is sensitive to touch. Bubbling sensation in the kidney region. Worse from moving. Face gray.

***Dioscorea:** Pain is less from straightening up and bending backward. Writhing and twitching with pain. Pain may also be felt at the navel, which is relieved by pressure. Worse from doubling up.

***Aconite:** Patient feels frightened, experiences extreme pain, is very cold but can't stand a hot room, and feels faint from sitting or standing. Sudden onset. Aconite is often useful in the first attack. Repeat every fifteen minutes.

***Belladonna:** Red face, dilated pupils, strong pulse. Comes on suddenly. Sense of fullness over the stomach. Worse from drinking anything. Sensitive to light, noise, or being jarred. Repeat every half hour.

***Magnesia phosphorica:** Patient doubles up with pain (also Colocynth). Better from heat and rubbing. Sensitive to cold or any draft.

***Colocynth:** Patient doubles up with pain. Better from steady pressure, bending over, and warmth. Impatient, irritable, and angry. Coated tongue. Passes much urine.

Nux vomica: Often the right kidney with pain extending to the genital area and legs (also Causticum). Painful urging to urinate, with urine passing in drops. Chilly, irritable. Worse in the morning, from uncovering, and from the pressure of clothes.

Calcarea carbonica: Pressing pain in the kidneys and lower back. Chilly and worse from cold. Perspires easily. Hands and feet cold and damp. Worse from the pressure of clothes.

Benzoic acid: Pain extends to the chest when breathing deeply. Burning pain in the left kidney. Urine is dark with a strong odor of ammonia. Lower back sore and stiff.

Ipecacuanha: Nausea accompanies the pain. Tongue is clean (not coated). Pain shoots from the kidneys to the thighs and knees.

Sarsaparilla: Pain at the end of urination, from the right kidney extending downward. The patient screams when passing urine. Better from warmth. Urine cloudy.

Ocimum canum: Right-sided pain. Vomits every fifteen minutes. Writhing in pain, screams. Restless. Urine cloudy or red. Better from warmth.

Causticum: Pain from the kidneys to the genital area. May begin during sleep. Better from cold drinks.

Calcarea renalis: May help relieve pain as well as pass the stones.

Hydrangea arbores: Soreness over the kidneys with bloody urine. Sharp pain in the lower back. Hydrangea may help break up the stones.

Pareira brava (Tincture: five drops in hot water): If all else fails.

Lead Poisoning

Symptoms are somewhat different in children and adults. In children: abdominal pain, vomiting, drowsiness, irritability, weakness, convulsions, or coma. In adults: loss of appetite, constipation, abdominal cramps, weakness, pale face, or paralysis of muscles. There may be a metallic taste in the mouth. In chronic cases, there is often a blue line along the margins of the gums.

> **Note:** Before giving homeopathic remedies for lead poisoning, have the patient drink Epsom salts dissolved in water. This binds to the lead and helps remove it.

***Causticum:** Chilly, worse from drafts. Constant desire to clear the throat. Craves salt and smoked meats. Aversion to sweets. Progressive paralysis.

***Alumina:** Great constipation, pain in the abdomen, painful urging long before stool. Fear of knives. Mouth and throat feel dry. Limbs feel heavy. Experiences vertigo when closing the eyes.

***Colocynth:** Painful spasms, which make him bend double. Better from pressure, warmth, or bending forward.

***Alumen:** Weakness of the arms and legs. Abdomen feels retracted. Spasmodic pains worse from walking. Extreme constipation with marble-like stools. Sensation of a band around the limbs.

Opium: Pupils contracted. Deep snoring during sleep. Hot perspiration. The patient feels like there is a stone in his abdomen. Better from cold. Worse during and after sleep.

Petroleum: Internal spasms better from bending double. Deep cracks in skin that bleed. Nausea with bitter green vomiting. Motion sickness from riding in cars. Worse from dampness or cold. Gets hungry after passing stool. Feels death is near.

Kali iodatum: Flatulence, craving for fresh air, clucking noises in the abdomen. Weeps during sleep, pain in the small of the back. Better from motion and fresh air. Worse at night, from cold food, or from being in a warm room.

Kali bromatum: Wringing of hands, trembling, confusion, numbness of the body.

Belladonna: Pupils dilated, delirium, sensitivity to touch, light, and noise. Worse from the sun and from drafts. Better in a dark room.

Lyme Disease

The disease is named after the town of Old Lyme, Connecticut, where it was identified by researchers in 1975. It is a tick-transmitted disease caused by *Borrelia burgdorferi*, a spiral-shaped bacterium. The disease has three stages:

Stage 1: In three to thirty days, a skin rash may appear where the person was bitten. It expands and clears in the center to form a ring or "bulls eye" appearance. You can't depend on that symptom alone, because 20% of cases do not produce a rash. Another indication is flu-like symptoms, including weakness, fever, headache, and muscle and joint pain.

Stage 2: Weeks or months later, neurological problems or cardiac disorders may develop. Facial paralysis or heart rhythm disorders are typical. Joint and muscle pain can also occur. The rash may return, but in other parts of body.

Stage 3: Months to years later, chronic debilitating problems occur, such as arthritis, extreme fatigue, cognitive disorders, sleep disturbance, and personality changes.

Homeopathic treatment of the later stages is complex and requires a professional homeopath. The best approach is prevention, and the following remedies may provide protection after a bite.

To Help Prevent the Disease After a Tick Bite

1st day: **Ledum** 200c.

2nd day: **Hypericum** 200c.

3rd day: **Borrelia burgdorferi** (nosode 30c). One dose a day for one week, then one dose a week for one month.

See a homeopathic professional as soon as possible.

> **Note:** Dr. Stephen Tobin, DVM, states that he has cured dogs, cats, and horses of Lyme disease with Ledum in the 1M potency. He states that the remedy has worked for both recent and old cases. He has gotten feedback from people who tried it for their own Lyme disease with positive results. He stated that one MD gave blood tests before and after treatment with Ledum and found the blood levels of Lyme disease had declined.

Dr. Tobin's treatment of animals involves giving one pellet of Ledum 1M three times a day for three days. Ledum 1M is the equivalent of a 1000c potency, or five times stronger than a 200c. Such potencies are best used by professionals.

> **Note:** There is a combination remedy called LymePlex which may help some cases of lyme disease. I know of one woman who was cured by it after conventional treatment failed. It contains ten remedies covering the various stages of Lyme disease. The remedies are Baptisia, Belladonna, Bryonia, Calcarea carbonica, Calcarea fluorica, Eupatorium perfoliatum, Gelsemium, Kali carb,

Mercurius v, and Rhus tox. It is available, by prescription, from King Bio Pharmaceuticals at 1-800-543-3245.

Lymphangitis

This is another variation on an infected wound. After a wound, a red line or streak runs up the limb from the injury. This is an inflammation of the lymphatic channels, often with streptococcus or staphylococcus bacteria. It is sometimes accompanied by fever and chills (a serious development). The wound should be soaked in hot salt water. The following remedies may assist the body in fighting off this infection.

***Belladonna:** Hot, red, with throbbing sensation. Relatively sudden onset. Patient is worse from touch, noise, being bumped, draft of air, or lying down.

***Apis:** Burning, stinging pain, which feels better from cold. Skin red with swelling as if from a bee sting. No thirst.

***Lachesis:** Blue, purple, or black appearance to the inflamed area. Tendency to bleeding of dark blood. Discomfort from light touch or from warmth. Can't stand tight clothing, especially around the neck. Worse after sleep.

***Mercurius:** Blood-streaked pus. Perspires easily and feels worse afterward. Excess saliva but great thirst. Bad breath, and foul odor to the wound. Worse at night and from the warmth of the bed.

Arsenicum: Burning pain, which feels better from warmth. Anxious, chilly, restless, and thirsty for small sips. Worse after midnight.

Hepar sulph: The wound is worse from cold, draft, or the slightest touch. The patient feels very cold and wants to be covered. Feels as if a breeze is blowing on him or on the wound. Irritable.

Pyrogenium: Wound has an offensive odor. The site of the injury is swollen and inflamed.

Rhus tox: Itching and burning, which is worse from cold and better from warmth (opposite Apis). Restlessness and thirst. Worse at night.

Anthracinum: Burning pain. Tendency to bleeding of thick, dark blood. Black or blue blisters. Sleepless from pain. Very anxious.

Bufo: Pain goes up the arm from the injury. Itching and burning. Feels better from hot water. Yellow, irritating pus. Worse from moving. Sleep disturbed and unrefreshing.

Malaria

Malaria is caused by a parasite carried by the anopheles mosquito. It can also be acquired from transfusions or infected needles. Symptoms include sudden recurring attacks of chills, shivering, high fever, sweating, headache, diarrhea, bloody stools,vomiting, weakness, cough, muscle pain, jaundice, and coma. The chill, fever, and sweating occur in distinct stages.

Prevention of Malaria

Malaria officinalis: Use 30c, two doses a week. Continue for four to eight weeks after exposure.

Cinchona: If Malaria officinalis is not available.

Arsenicum album: If neither Malaria officinalis nor Cinchona is available.

Remedies for Malaria

***Cinchona:** Attacks are preceded by nausea, headache, and hunger. There is no thirst during the chill phase of the attack. Bloated abdomen not relieved by belching. Hypersensitivity of the senses. Worse from light touch, but better from pressure. Worse from cold and drafts. Profuse sweat during sleep. Symptoms are worse every third day.

***Arsenicum:** Great fear, afraid to be alone, restless, thirsty for frequent but small sips of water (except during the chill, when he is thirstless). Alternately feels as if there is ice water or boiling water in his veins. Burning pains, which are paradoxically relieved by heat. Worse from midnight to 2 a.m. Foul-smelling diarrhea.

***Pulsatilla:** Predominately thirstless. Craves open air and can't bear a warm, closed room. Desires company and sympathy. Sour vomit. Worse from eating fat or rich food.

***Nux vomica:** Cramping in abdomen and legs. Irritable and hypersensitive. Wakes at 3 a.m. and can't sleep. Worse in the early morning. Worse from cold, drafts, noise, odors, being touched, or tight clothing around his waist.

***Eupatorium:** Pain in his bones as if they were broken. Attacks preceded by extreme thirst. Chill starts in the small of the back and is followed by nausea and vomiting. The chill is worse from drinking, moving, or uncovering. Very restless and constantly moving, which does not bring relief. Craves cold drinks. Worse from cold air and the smell of food.

Natrum muriaticum: Attack often begins between 9 a.m. and 11 a.m. It is preceded by headache as if hammers were in the head. Green vomit. Chill begins in the fingers and toes. The patient may experience blindness or unconsciousness during the chill phase. General aversion to company and consolation. Fever blisters on the lip. Craves salt but has an aversion to bread. Cold feeling in the heart.

Gelsemium: Faced flushed with a drowsy look. Eyelids droop. Limbs feel heavy. Mostly thirstless. Chill felt up the back. Muscles feel bruised. Pulse full but slow.

Rhus tox: Thirsty, restless, and constantly changing position. Stiff muscles and aching joints. Intense itching of the skin with rash during fever. Worse at night, after rest, during damp weather, and from cold.

Apis: Vomiting before chill. Burning, stinging rash partially relieved by cold. Swelling of the eyelids, lips, or face. Mostly thirstless.

To Prevent Relapses of Malaria

Cinchona.

Mammograms, Effects of

Breasts get rather rough treatment during a mammogram. A single dose of either of these remedies can help the body deal with the trauma. Best used either just before or immediately after the mammogram.

Bellis perennis or

Conium maculatum

Arnica: If the above remedies are not available.

Measles

Measles is a very contagious viral illness that is spread by droplets from the nose, mouth, or throat. Symptoms include fever, cough, inflammation of the throat, inflammation of the eyes with sensitivity to light, and a rash. One characteristic sign is the appearance of tiny white spots like grains of salt inside the mouth (Koplik's spots). This is followed three to five days later by the characteristic rash beginning in front of and below the ears and on the neck, soon spreading to the trunk and extremities. The fever may reach 104 degrees.

Prevention of Measles

Morbillinum nosode (30c once a week), or **Malandrinum** (30c once a week), or **Pulsatilla** (12c once a day).

Remedies for Measles

*__Aconite:__ Use when symptoms first appear. Sudden high fever, hot dry burning skin, dry cough, extreme thirst, restlessness, great anxiety, and aversion to light. Pulse full and rapid. Better after sweating.

*__Belladonna:__ In the beginning, with sudden onset. Skin red, hot, eyes bloodshot, hot perspiration. Drowsy but can't sleep. Dry cough. Sometimes has spasms of the limbs or convulsions.

*__Ferrum phosphoricum:__ Slow onset, low fever. Face alternating between red and pale. Restless. Weary but talkative. Thirsty, sweaty. Worse at night and from 4 to 6 a.m. When no other remedy is clearly indicated.

*__Pulsatilla:__ Low fever, worse in a warm room, craves fresh air. Thirstless. Desires company and sympathy. Weeps readily. Watery eyes. Greenish-yellow bland discharge from the nose.

Bryonia: Rash is pale or doesn't fully develop. Patient is worse from any motion and wants to lie perfectly still. Respiratory symptoms with dry, painful cough. Thirst for large drinks. Irritable.

Gelsemium: Drowsy, limbs feel heavy, eyelids droop, face flushed, thirstless. Wants to be left alone. Better after perspiring.

Sulphur: Rash appears late. Itching and worse from heat. Better from open air. Diarrhea around 11 a.m. Redness around the eyes, mouth, and nose. White tongue with red tip and edges.

Euphrasia: Hot, burning tears with a bland discharge from the nose.

Rhus tox: Great restlessness, very thirsty, feels sore all over. Chilly and better from warmth. Feels temporarily better from moving around.

Arsenicum: Exhausted, chilly, restless, and very anxious. Frequent thirst for small sips. Worse from midnight to 3 a.m. Burning sensations relieved by heat.

Kali bichromicum: Throat pain extending to the ears. Worse from 2 to 5 a.m. Very chilly. Thick, stringy yellow mucus.

Silica: Persistent cough after measles.

Apis: If meningitis occurs as a complication. Worse from heat. Lets out a shrill cry.

Meningitis

Meningitis is an inflammation of the membranes around the brain and spinal cord. It may be caused by a bacteria, a virus, a fungus, chemicals, drug allergies, tumors, or a blow to the head. Meningitis may be cerebral, spinal, or cerebrospinal.

Symptoms differ somewhat in adults and young children. In adults: *Stiff neck*, fever, headache, vomiting, confusion, muscular rigidity, arching of the back, drowsiness, or coma. In children (three months to two years old): Fever, vomiting, convulsions, high pitched-cry. May be caused by infection or a blow to the head.

***Arnica:** *If caused by a blow to the head*. Face red and hot with cool body. Heavy sleep, pupils contracted, twitching muscles, refuses to be touched. Passes stool and urine involuntarily.

***Belladonna:** *Face red and hot, bloodshot eyes, pupils dilated,* extremities freezing cold, headache, throbbing sensation. Face distorts, grinds teeth. Violent delirium alternating with coma, biting, pulse full and fast. Can't bear noise, light, touch, draft, or lying down. Better semi-erect.

***Apis:** Face hot, red,.puffy, eyelids swollen. Throbbing or sharp pain in the head. *Lets out a shrill scream, often during sleep.* Worse from the slightest touch, from heat, and after sleep. Sleepy, but restlessness prevents sleep. Thirstless but may crave milk.

***Helleborus:** *Patient is very dull, groggy, and has a vacant expression.* The neck is rigid and bent backward, the limbs move unconsciously, and there is great pain in the back of the head and neck. Pupils are dilated but he's not bothered by light (opposite Belladonna). Shrieks in sleep.

***Gelsemium:** *Mentally dull, staggers, limbs feel heavy, eyelids droop.* Thirstless, trembling and wants to be held, profuse urination. Difficulty breathing, nausea, and severe chill. Totally exhausted. Numbness.

***Stramonium:** *Very fearful and worse from darkness, from being alone,* from seeing shining objects, and after sleep. Better from light and company. Awakens screaming.

Bryonia: *Worse from any motion as it increases the pain.* Stiff neck, pain in the joints and limbs, nausea, white tongue, stupor. Worse from heat and from sitting up. Dry lips and mouth with great thirst. Follows Belladonna after fever is reduced.

Aconite: *Great fear, predicts time of death.* Restless, thirsty. Skin hot and dry. Sudden onset.

Hypericum: *From concussion or an injury to the spine.* Dread of moving, numbness in limbs, desires warm drinks.

Veratrum album: Vomiting if the head is lifted, convulsive shocks, pale and freezing cold, collapse.

Plumbum: Limbs painfully contracted, gas pains in stomach, retraction of abdomen.

Opium: Coma, pupils constricted. Stupefaction. Mania.

Rhus tox: Vertigo, bleeding of the ears and nose, dry cough, stiff muscles. Restless and can't get comfortable. Worse after rest. Thirsty.

Hyoscyamus: Grinds teeth. Hands and feet thrash about. Delirium. Unconscious after convulsions.

Mercury Poisoning

Mercury is extremely poisonous and can be absorbed through the respiratory tract, the gastrointestinal tract, or the skin. Some sources of mercury contamination are coal-fired power plants, incinerators, dental amalgams, thermometers, certain pesticides, some vaccines, and certain fish.

Acute mercury poisoning is due to exposure to a high dose over a short period of time. Symptoms of acute mercury poisoning include cough, tightness in the chest, difficulty breathing, nausea, vomiting, and diarrhea. Pneumonia and kidney damage are serious immediate consequences.

Treatment of acute mercury poisoning: Immediately after ingestion, give an emetic to induce vomiting. Then administer egg white and water. Beat three egg whites into twenty-four to thirty-two ounces of water. Have the person drink it. Seek professional medical help as soon as possible.

Chronic Mercury Toxicity

Symptoms of chronic mercury poisoning include tremor, memory loss, insomnia, inflamed gums, excess salivation, foul breath, a metallic taste in the mouth, blue rims on the gums, mouth ulcers, loose teeth, eczema, great fatigue, diarrhea, loss of appetite, weight loss, great sensitivity to heat or cold, and profuse perspiration. Personality changes may also occur. These include loss of willpower, timidity, indecision, lack of confidence, apathy, suicidal thoughts, and violent impulses. Chronic mercury poisoning produces nonspecific symptoms and may resemble any number of other ailments.

In children, mercury poisoning can result in a condition called acrodynia, which is characterized by painful leg cramps, irritability, numbness or tingling of the skin, perspiration, itching, and red, peeling skin on the palms of the hands and soles of the feet.

Remedies for Chronic Mercury Toxicity

***Hepar sulph:** The chief antidote. Very chilly and worse from cold, the slightest draft, and uncovering. Quite sensitive to touch. Sticking sensation in the throat. Ulcerated gums, excessive saliva, headache, painful lumps on the head, inflamed eyes, swollen glands in the neck and arms, spasms of the rectum, paralysis (also Nitric acid and Sulphur).

***Mercurius vivus:** Taking Mercurius 30c once a day for six to ten days may stimulate the body to excrete the mercury stored in the tissues. During this procedure, the mercury in the tissues is released and excreted with the stool, urine, and perspiration. If the process becomes too uncomfortable, then stop. Before using this method, it is wise to do a kidney/liver cleanse. There are numerous herbal blends just for this purpose, available at health food stores.

***Phytolacca:** Rheumatic pain with a constant desire to move, but worse from motion. Neuralgic pains, shooting pains like electric shocks, dark red throat with enlarged uvula, swollen glands under the jaw. Stony-hard lumps in the breast, breast abscesses, great exhaustion, and vertigo when rising. The patient feels indifferent to life and is sure he will die. Worse in damp, cold weather and at night.

***Belladonna:** Abscesses that develop rapidly, with redness, heat, and throbbing. Difficulty swallowing fluids. Worse from noise, light, heat of the sun, drafts on the head, and being touched or jarred. Fear of dogs. Bangs his head. Feels an impulse to set fires.

***Nitric acid:** Chilly and worse from cold. Splinterlike pains (also Hepar). Bodily discharges irritate the openings through which they pass (nose, mouth, and rectum). Worse from touch and being jarred. Bad tempered and unmoved by apologies. Anxiety about health with fear of death. Perspiration smells like urine. Paralysis (also Hepar sulph and Sulphur).

***Aurum:** Pain in bones, especially at night. Trembling from anger. Loss of confidence and sees himself as a failure. Weary of life with suicidal depression. Better from fresh air or hearing music.

Carbo veg: Hungry for air and wants to be fanned. Bloating of abdomen with much belching. Feet icy cold. All food disagrees.

Cinchona: Very chilly and worse from cold. Bloating of abdomen, not relieved by belching or flatulence. Painless diarrhea. Mentally apathetic or sad. Extreme sensitivity of all senses. Sensitive to cold, drafts, noise, light touch, and odors. Headache with throbbing pain and red face. Worse from drafts, cold, motion, loss of fluids, and light touch.

Sulphur: Burning sensations, red itching skin (worse from heat and bathing). Bodily discharges smell foul and irritate the skin. Redness and itching of anus, lips, nose, and eyes. Sudden diarrhea in the morning. Craves sweets and spices. Worse from bathing, being in a warm room, at 11 a.m., and from standing. Paralysis (also Hepar sulph and Nitric acid).

Miscarriage

See chapter 6, "Pregnancy and Birth."

Morning Sickness

See chapter 6, "Pregnancy and Birth."

Motion Sickness (Sea, Car, Air)

All of these remedies can be used preventively.

Petroleum: Stomach pain, which is better from eating, from warm air, and from keeping the head high.

Tabacum: Nausea, vomiting from the least motion, salivation, cold sweat, fainting. Better from fresh air.

Cocculus indicus: Worse from fresh air and from eating. Irritable. Worse from the smell of food.

Nux vomica: Angry, constipated, chilly, irritable, oversensitive, and critical. Worse from noise, light, odors, and cold. Craves fats and spices.

Ginger, the herb, is also very effective.

Mumps

Mumps is a contagious viral disease characterized by painful inflammation of the salivary glands, which are between the ear and the jaw. Symptoms include painful swelling of the salivary glands, fever, headache, loss of appetite, fatigue, and pain on chewing or swallowing. Possible complications include swelling of the testicles, pancreatitis, and encephalitis.

Prevention of Mumps

Parotidinum (nosode 30c) or **Pilocarpus (Jaborandi).**

Mercurius vivus may also be effective if the above remedies are not available.

Remedies for Mumps

***Aconite:** Sudden onset, skin dry and red, unquenchable thirst, very restless, extremely anxious.

***Belladonna:** Sudden onset, hot perspiration, high fever, red face, throbbing sensations. Worse from light, noise, cold air, or being jolted.

***Mercurius solubilis:** Foul breath, excess saliva, tongue shows the imprint of teeth, perspires freely but is worse afterward. Worse at night, and from the heat of the bed.

***Pulsatilla:** Inflamed testes or breasts. Can't stand being in a warm, closed room. Craves fresh air. Asks for the window to be opened. Better from company and sympathy. Thirstless.

Jaborandi: Profuse, thick saliva and much perspiration with a flushed face.

Parotidinum: This nosode can be used one day a week as a preventive or to speed recovery.

Phytolacca: Pale skin, hard glands, can't swallow anything hot. Pain radiating to the ears. Body feels stiff, worse from hot drinks and better from cold drinks.

Abrotanum: Inflamed testes or breasts. If Pulsatilla fails.

Mushroom Poisoning

Even one or two bites may be sufficient to cause poisoning. Symptoms can begin from a few minutes to fifteen hours after ingestion and vary depending on the variety of mushroom. They include watery eyes, salivation, perspiration, cramps, diarrhea, nausea, vomiting, vertigo, convulsions, and coma. Induce vomiting unless the person is unconscious or convulsing.

Absinthium: Trembling followed by convulsions. Excited, restless, delirious. Hallucinations, giddiness, vertigo on rising, spasmodic twitching of the face. Tongue trembles.

Arsenicum: Fear of death, extreme restlessness, great thirst but for small sips. Burning pains relieved by heat, chills, weakness, and fear of being alone.

Belladonna: Sudden intense onset of symptoms. Burning pain, throbbing, spasms, delirium (biting, spitting, or kicking). Face is red and feels hot. Hands and feet cold. Pupils dilated. Better in a quiet, dark room. Worse from light, noise, being jarred, being in the sun, drafts on the head, or seeing bright objects.

Agaricus: Twitching, jerking, spasms, exaggerated involuntary movements, extreme chills, burning and itching of the skin. Worse from cold, pressure, and touch.

Pyrogenium: Exhausted but extremely restless. Feels bruised all over. High fever with slow pulse or vice versa. Aware of his heart beating. Foul-smelling discharges (breath, stool, sweat, and vomit). Better from moving about, warmth. Worse from becoming cold.

Camphora: Freezing cold and shivering, but won't be covered. Extremely weak pulse. Face cold and blue, cold breath, grinning expression.

Nausea

(See also "Motion Sickness," as well as "Morning Sickness" in chapter 6)

***Ipecacuanha:** Nausea not relieved by vomiting. Clean tongue (not coated). Excess saliva, and patient may drool. Cough with nausea. Worse from motion. Sometimes with diarrhea. Vomits food, mucus, bile, or blood.

***Antimonium crudum:** Heavy white coating on the tongue. Nausea right after eating or drinking. Worse from eating fats, pastries. Worse being touched or looked at. Better from lying down and from warmth.

***Antimonium tartaricum:** Nausea, retching, vomiting, deathly faintness. Thick, white coating on tongue. Craves small frequent sips of cold water. Fear from nausea. Must lie on the right side to avoid vomiting. Thick mucus rattling in chest. Cold sweat, drowsiness.

***Nux vomica:** Tongue coated in back. Feels like a stone is inside the stomach. Constipated and strains at stool. Very chilly and better from warmth. Hypersensitive to noise, odors, lights, or criticism. Anxious, irritable, or angry. Worse from overeating, spices, coffee, alcohol, or drugs. Worse in the morning in bed. Sometimes unable to vomit.

***Iris versicolor:** Vomiting very sour material that burns the throat. Feeling of heat inside. Vomits bile. Nausea with headache or alternating with headache. Worse after exertion. Lots of thick, stringy saliva. Worse from sweets and milk.

***Tabacum:** Constant nausea, which is worse from moving and opening the eyes. Wants to uncover his abdomen, which decreases the symptoms. Better from fresh air. Watery diarrhea, weakness, and cold sweat accompany the nausea and vomiting. Worse from the odor of tobacco.

Phosphorus: Craves cold drinks, which are vomited when they become warm in the stomach. Vomits food by the mouthful. Worse from warm food. Worse lying on the left side. Sensitive to light, odors, and sounds. Desires company. Burning in the stomach extending to the throat and bowels. Better from a short nap.

Cadmium sulphuricum: Intense nausea and retching with black vomit. Everything eaten is vomited. If anything touches the lips, it triggers vomiting. Burning pain in the stomach. Desires sips of cold water, which also stimulate vomiting. Includes nausea from cancer, chemotherapy, and radiation poisoning.

Argentum nitricum: Vomits sticky mucus. Much belching with bloating of the stomach. Burning pain. Pain that radiates from a point in the stomach. Green diarrhea like chopped spinach. Worse from warmth, sweets, at night, and on the left side. Better from cold. Very anxious.

Colchicum: Nausea on looking at, smelling, or even thinking about food. Worse from motion, cold, strong odors, bright light, and touch. Wants to lie perfectly still. Chilly. Discouraged.

Pulsatilla: Worse from eating fatty or rich food. Worse in a warm room and craves fresh air. Desires sympathy and may weep describing the pain. No thirst. Vomits food long after it was eaten. Sensation as if there is a stone in the stomach.

Bryonia: Worse from the least motion and lies perfectly still. Dry mouth with dry, cracked lips. Thirst for large, cold drinks. Worse from warm drinks. Nausea and faintness when rising up. Stomach sensitive to touch. Sensation as if there is a stone in the stomach.

Crotalus horridus: Abdomen hot and tender. Can't bear clothing around the stomach. Vomits food, bile, and blood. Vomit that is black or looks similar to coffee grounds. Can't lie on the right side. Bleeds dark blood from any orifice. Bloody sweat. Worse after sleep. Hypersensitive to light. Eyes yellow.

Arsenicum album: Burning pains, sometimes like hot coals, which are oddly relieved by heat. The patient feels chilly, terribly anxious, and exhausted. Wants frequent sips of water. Fears death or serious illness. Foul-smelling vomit and diarrhea. Can't stand the sight or smell of food. Vomits blood, bile, or green mucus. Exhausted by the least effort. Worse after midnight.

Veratrum album: Violent retching and forcible vomiting. Freezing cold with cold sweat on the forehead. Thirst for cold water, which is vomited immediately afterward. Copious, painful watery diarrhea. Worse from drinking or moving.

Cocculus: Nausea from riding in cars or boats. Nausea from watching moving objects. The patient has an aversion to food or drink, but may crave cold drinks. Profuse salivation. Worse when cold, and from loss of sleep or the odor of food. Aversion to fresh air (opposite Tabacum).

Cinchona: Weakness after vomiting, diarrhea, and other loss of fluids. Yellow, painless diarrhea. Vomits undigested food. Worse from the slightest touch and after eating. Abdomen bloated. Cold feeling in abdomen after drinking. Profuse perspiration at night. Chilly and worse from cold.

Necrotizing Fasciitis

A rare but particularly virulent form of streptococcus can produce a condition called necrotizing fasciitis. The streptococcus produces a toxin that kills and digests tissues at a rapid rate. A minor wound produces a painful reddish bump, which becomes golden-brown or purple. The area enlarges and the center turns black. Other symptoms include fever, perspiration, chills, nausea, vertigo, weakness, and shock.

Belladonna: In the beginning when there is a red, hot, throbbing sore on the skin. Sudden intense onset of symptoms. In systemic infections, the face is red and hot, the pupils are dilated, and the hands and feet are cold. Worse from light, noise, drafts on the head, being jarred, being in the sun, seeing bright objects. Better from quiet, being in a dark room, standing or sitting up, and bending the head backward.

Tarentula cubensis: In the beginning, when there is a burning, stinging, painful, hard sore on the skin. Fever, chills, perspiration, reduced urine output.

Lachesis: Purplish color to wounds, which may ooze dark blood. Cold extremities but worse from heat. Ice-cold feeling in the affected part, with tingling, itching, and sometimes burning. The patient can't stand anything around his neck. Extremely sensitive to touch even from his own clothing. Left-sided symptoms. Difficulty swallowing liquids. Worse after sleep, from warmth, and from hot drinks. Better from open air. Delirium with great talkativeness and delusions.

Crotalus horridus: Yellow face, eyes, and skin. Right half of body is very sensitive to touch. Hemorrhages of black, stringy blood. Weeping, talkative, has a delusion that his brain is decaying. Sensitive to light. Symptoms tend to be right sided (opposite Lachesis). Worse from open air (opposite Lachesis). Can't swallow solids (opposite Lachesis). Can't stand tight clothing around the waist. Bloody or coffee-ground-colored vomit. Worse after sleep (same as Lachesis).

Rhus tox: Extremely restless and constantly changing positions. Muscles stiff and better from stretching. Worse during rest. Skin red with intense itching. Very chilly and skin painful from cold air. Great thirst for cold drinks. Worse from cold or dampness. Anxious at night. Better from warmth. Dreams of great exertion.

Arsenicum: Very fearful and restless, chilly, thirsty for small frequent sips, and exhausted from the least exertion. Burning pains like fire, which are better from warmth. Foul-smelling diarrhea. Afraid to be alone. Worse midnight to 3 a.m., from cold, cold drinks, and when alone. Better from warmth, warm drinks, sitting up, and company.

Neonatal Conjunctivitis

This condition may be caused by irritation, a blocked tear duct, or infection. When due to an infection, it can cause serious eye damage. The baby's symptoms include watery, bloody drainage from the eyes, thick puslike drainage, and swollen, red eyelids. This typically occurs anywhere from one day to two weeks after birth.

While various bacteria can cause this problem, the bacteria responsible for gonorrhea and those which cause chlamydia create the most serious problems. They are acquired from the mother during childbirth. The viruses of both genital and oral herpes are other offenders.

*__Argentum nitricum:__ Thick, yellow, bland pus. Worse from heat. Eyelids swollen.

*__Pulsatilla:__ Yellow-green, bland discharge. Better from fresh air. Worse from heat. Wants to be held.

*__Aconite:__ Very anxious. Condition comes on abruptly. Great thirst. Eyes red, lids swollen, discharge of pus.

*__Thuja:__ Greenish-yellow discharge from eyes. Chilly and worse from cold.

*__Nitric acid:__ Chilly, sensitive to noise, and may have strong-smelling urine. Watery eyes.

*__Sulphur:__ Eyes hot, dry, red, and burning. Lids red and swollen in the morning. There may be redness of the anus or mouth as well. Hot and worse from heat. Doesn't like to be bathed.

*__Mercurius corrosivus:__ Thin, burning discharge from the eyes. Perspires readily. Sensitive to draft. Worse at night.

*__Euphrasia:__ Great excess of burning-hot tears, which irritate the eyes and cheeks. Desire to blink.

Rhus tox: Very restless and thirsty. Hot, scalding tears or yellow pus. Swollen lids.

Apis mel: Eyelids are very puffy but there is not much discharge. Better from cold application. No thirst. Hot tears. Sensitive to light.

Hepar: Thick, foul-smelling pus. Eyes sensitive to cold, touch, and draft. Blood seeps between swollen lids. Better from warmth. Very sensitive to light.

Belladonna: Eyes bloodshot, very red, painful, and hot. Sudden onset. Pupils dilated. Worse from light.

Arsenicum: Chilly, anxious, restless, and thirsty. Better from warmth and warm applications. Worse after midnight.

Chamomilla: Very angry and crying. Hot and better from cold. Eyelids swollen. Blood seeps out from between lids.

Calcarea carbonica: Swollen lids, much mucus in eyes. Chilly but sweats profusely, especially about the head. Sour-smelling perspiration. Affects large babies with big heads.

Nephritis—Acute

Inflammation of the kidneys. There are numerous causes including infections, drugs, alcohol, heavy metals, malnutrition, and exposure to cold. Symptoms may include blood in the urine, reduced or increased volume of urine, change in the color of urine, nausea and vomiting, and edema. (See also "Uremia.")

***Apis:** No thirst. Pain in the kidneys. Edema of the face and limbs. Passes urine but in small amounts. Worse from heat and better from cold. Puffy under the eyes. Skin is sensitive to touch. Difficulty breathing, which is better from sitting up. Worse from heat, touch, or lying down.

***Berberis:** Kidneys are sensitive to touch. Pain with numbness. Burning pain, with the sensation of boiling water. Pains that radiate from one point at or near the lower back to the hips and legs. Pain and stiffness in the lower back, along with numbness. Frequent, strong urge to urinate. Worse from moving. Dry mouth with sticky saliva.

***Natrum sulph:** Urination frequent but scanty, dark. Brown, bitter coating on the tongue. Sour vomiting. Very chilly with profuse sweats at night. Loose stools in the morning. Very large stools. Very sensitive to light. Worse in the morning and in damp weather. Skin itches while undressing.

***Terebinthina oleum:** Very cold with burning sensations. Pain causes the patient to urinate. Urine has the odor of violets. Burning pain in the kidneys extending to the bladder. Urine is smoke colored, thick, and slimy. Bloody urine. Coughs up mucus. Worse from cold, pressure, urinating, and at night.

***Arsenicum:** Restless, anxious, thirsty for small frequent sips of water. Chilly and craves warmth, weak, afraid to be alone. Watery diarrhea, swelling of the face.

Belladonna: Sudden and violent onset. Pain extending from kidney to bladder. Sensation of burning and heat. Worse from touch, noise, light, being jarred, or cold drafts. Pains come and go quickly. Craves lemonade. Starts in sleep.

Cantharis: Violent, sharp, burning pains in kidney area. Kidney area is sensitive to touch. Pain before, during, and after urination. Intense urging to pass urine, which feels hot and scalding. Worse after drinking cold water or coffee. Better from warmth, rubbing, and cold. Restless and excitable, furious delirium. Worse from being approached or touched. Shreddy burning stools. Pupils dilated.

Helleborus nig: Slow in answering questions. Involuntary sighing. Picks at lips and clothes. Abdomen distended. Moaning and rolling the head from side to side. Bores head into pillow. Horrible smell from the mouth. Lower jaw falls. Muscles twitch and the patient cries out in his sleep. Urine scanty with coffee-ground sediment.

Phosphorus: Blood in urine. Great thirst for cold drinks. Desires company and fears being alone. Worse lying on the left side. Better after short sleep. Very sensitive to odors, light, and noise.

Hepar: Very chilly and worse from cold, any draft, and touch. Coughs when uncovered. Feels as if a wind were blowing on him. Urine has a putrid odor. Irritable. Profuse sour sweat.

Veratrum album: Restless, weak, freezing cold. Cold sweat on the forehead, large quantity of watery diarrhea. Craves cold drinks, sour fruit, or salt. Vomiting with diarrhea. Worse from cold drinks, from exertion, and during stool.

Neuralgia

Neuralgia, severe stabbing or lightninglike pains along the course of a nerve, often affects the face, neck, or chest. Certain areas of the face may become sensitive and trigger an attack when touched. It has many causes including inflammation of a nerve, toxins, pressure on a nerve, and nutritional deficiencies. Tincture of *Plantago major* can be applied externally, undiluted, for temporary relief.

***Aconite:** From exposure to cold drafts, accompanied by a feeling of tingling or numbness. Often left sided.

***Belladonna:** On the right side of the face, often caused by cold. Throbbing pain. Face red and hot.

***Colocynth:** After exposure to cold, damp weather. Better from warmth and pressure. Tearing pain extending to the eye. Often left sided.

***Magnesia phosphorica:** Better from warmth and usually right sided. Stabbing pain, worse from moving the face, or from any draft. Tenderness over the affected part.

***Spigella:** Often left sided. Pain like a red-hot needle that radiates down the nerve. Sometimes feels cold after being touched. Worse from the least motion and in the daytime. Better from pressure.

***Arsenicum:** Terrible burning pain, restlessness, and great anxiety. Thirsty, but for small frequent sips. Chilly and worse from cold. Better from warmth. Worse from rest and better after exercise. Exhaustion.

***Chamomilla:** Unbearable pain with great anger. Worse from warmth, and at night. Face is hot, sweaty, and flushed. Great thirst.

***Hypericum:** When the condition is due to an injury.

Cinchona: Extreme pain brought on and made worse by the slightest touch. Better from firm pressure. In people weakened by ailments and loss of fluids.

Lycopodium: Sudden pains, usually right sided. Worse from moving, talking, eating, or touch. Worse from 4 to 8 p.m. Craves sweets. Flatulence after eating.

Pulsatilla: Weepy. Worse in a warm room. Craves cool, fresh air and feels better from it. Pain as if the nerve were a rubber band stretched and suddenly let go. Desires company and sympathy. Often right sided.

Staphysagria: Often from decaying teeth, with pain extending to the eyes. Better from warmth and in the morning. Worse at night and after anger. Pain triggered by touching the lips with a spoon.

Phosphorus: Hypersensitive to lights, odors, and sounds. Fear of being alone. Thirsty for large cold drinks. Worse in the open air (opposite Pulsatilla). Often left sided. Pain in the face and jaw that is associated with dental problems. Bleeds bright red blood from the slightest cut.

Verbascum thapsus: Often left sided. Worse from movement, clenching the teeth, or even touching them with the tongue.

Operations: See "Surgery"

Pain

See also under individual ailments, for example "Kidney Stones," "Heart Problems," "Eyes," "Earaches," and "Injuries." Many of the remedies for various pain symptoms will also relieve the pain of those specific ailments.

Unbearable Pain

Note: The following remedies are effective with "unbearable pain." The patient may express this as "I can't stand it any longer," or some similar comment. There are many remedies for pain, but this reaches a level that feels unendurable.

Aconite: *Pain with an intense fear of death.* The patient predicts the time of his death. Restless, has great thirst for cold water, skin is hot and dry. Pain in delicate areas like the eyes or urethra. Pain from a heart attack.

Chamomilla: *Pain with great anger.* Uncivil to anyone who approaches. Unwilling to be touched or spoken to. Worse from heat. Better from applying cold to the affected area. Pain with numbness. Hot, thirsty, hot sweat. One cheek red, the other pale. Children needing this remedy want to be carried or rocked. Green diarrhea.

Coffea: Tossing about in anguish. Worse from touch, noise, open air, strong odors, and cold. Better from lying down, warmth, or holding ice in the mouth during tooth pain. Headache pain feels like a nail driven into the head. Despairing and weeps from pain.

Hepar: Especially for pain with infected areas. *Painful part is extremely sensitive to cold, draft, or the slightest touch.* The patient is extremely chilly and can't get warm. Splinterlike pains. Inflammations smell like old cheese. Very irritable and angry when in pain.

Arsenicum album: Burning pains paradoxically relieved by heat. Great anxiety with fear of death. Chilly, restless, hopeless, and exhausted. Thirsty for small sips. Suspicious. Worse from midnight to 3 a.m.

Hypericum: *Damage to nerves from injuries*, operations, etc. Pain radiates from injury. Often accompanied by tingling and numbness. Worse from cold, dampness, or touch. Neuritis with tingling burning pain.

Phytolacca: *Pain radiates from one point and flies about. Pains like electric shocks.* Pains appear and disappear suddenly. Soreness all over. Restless but worse from motion. Worse from dampness, cold weather, and at night. Better from warmth. Bone pains, rheumatic pains, sore throat, mastitis.

Pain That Radiates from One Point

Hypericum: Injuries to parts rich in nerves, such as fingers, toes, and nails. Extreme pain after wounds. Neuritis. Injuries to the head or spine. Pain radiates up a limb from injury. Worse from cold and touch.

Berberis: Kidney or gallbladder pain that radiates from one point. Symptoms that change and alternate in location and nature. Worse from motion. Bubbling or boiling water sensation. Burning pain at the end of urination, which extends to the hip and legs.

Argentum nitricum: Pain of stomach ulcers. Worse in a warm room or lying on the right side. Better from cold air and pressure. Abdomen distended with gas. Very anxious.

Magnesia phosphorica: Painful cramps or spasms that are better from warmth and better bending forward or doubling over.

Dioscorea: Painful spasms that are better from bending backward or stretching out. Worse from doubling up (opposite Magnesia phosphorica).

Phytolacca: Pain radiates from one point and flies about. Pains like electric shocks. Restless, but worse from motion. Worse from moving, rising from a bed, and from hot drinks. Better from warmth, cold drinks, and lying on the abdomen.

Pain That Moves from Place to Place—Wandering Pain

Pulsatilla: Pain moves from place to place. Patient is worse from warmth, craves fresh air, desires sympathy, and weeps easily. Thirstless. Yellowish-green secretions.

Lac caninum: Pain moves from one side to the other and then back again (e.g., from left to right, and then to the left again). Worse from touch, at night, and during rest. Better from fresh air, cold drinks, and lying on the right side.

Kali bichromicum: Pain felt in small spots that could be covered with a thumb. Pains move from one place to another and occur every day at the same time. Worse from 2 to 5 a.m. and on waking. Very chilly. Thick, stringy, yellow discharges. Ulcerations.

Ledum: The painful area feels cool to touch but is worse from heat and better from cold. Chilly but can't bear a warm bed. Perspires at night and pulls off the covers. Worse at night and from motion. Puncture wounds, bruises, black eye, etc.

Kali sulphuricum: Ailments with yellow discharges. Dreads hot drinks. Worse in a warm room. Neck, back, and limb pain. Arthritic pains.

Pain—Throbbing

Aconite: With restlessness and fear of death. Sudden intense onset (also Belladonna). Face red. Skin hot and dry. Great thirst. Worse from cold and at night.

Antimonium tart: With thick mucus rattling in lungs. Worse from heat. Waves of nausea. Tongue coated white. Great drowsiness.

Belladonna: Face hot and red. Sudden intense onset (also Aconite). Pupils dilated. Worse from noise, light, drafts, becoming cold (especially the head), or being jarred. Mentally agitated or angry.

Hepar: Pain with great sensitivity to draft, cold, or the slightest touch. Irritable.

Ledum: The painful part feels cool to the touch, but is better from applying cold and worse from warmth. Puncture wounds, bruises, or black eyes.

Phosphorus: Pain with fear of being alone and desire for company. Sensitivity to light, noise, and odors. Great thirst for cold drinks. Burning pains. Tendency to bleeding of bright red blood. Worse lying on the left side. Worse from warm food. Better after napping.

Some Conditions and Causes of Pain

Representative remedies for some conditions and causes of pain.

Anxiety from the pain: Aconite, Arsenicum, Phosphorus, Natrum carb, Kali arsenicum.

Band (feels like there is a band around some part of the body): Cactus.

Bearing down pain (uterus, abdomen): Sepia.

Bending backward feels better: Dioscorea.

Bending over double (doubling over) feels better: Colocynth.

Bones, pain in: Ruta, Eupatorium, Aurum.

Bruising pain; fear of being approached: Arnica.

Burning pain with fear of death, restlessness, thirst: Arsenicum.

Cold and dampness, worse from; thirsty and restless: Rhus tox.

Despair from pain: Aurum, Arsenicum, Chamomilla, Cinchona.

Left side (pain on the left side, which comes on after sleep): Lachesis.

Motion (pain worse from the slightest motion): Bryonia.

Nerves (pain from injured nerves): Hypericum.

Puncture wounds, pain from: Ledum, Hypericum.

Right side (pain on the right side, from 4 to 8 p.m., worse from being covered): Lycopodium.

Spasms of muscles (better from warmth, pressure): Magnesia phosphorica, colocynth.

Splinterlike sensation: Nitric acid, Hepar sulph, Argentum nitricum, Silica.

Spots (pain in small spots): Kali bichromicum, Lachesis.

Sudden onset: Aconite, Belladonna, Nitric acid, Arsenicum, Colocynth, Pulsatilla, Nux vomica.

Throbbing pain (sudden onset, heat, redness, worse from touch or being jarred): Belladonna.

Ulcerative pain (internally): Lachesis, Pulsatilla, Silica, Ranunculus bul, Argentum nitricum, Rhus tox, Bryonia, Nux vomica, Causticum, Colocynth.

Violent behavior from pain: Chamomilla, Hepar sulph, Aurum.

Weakness from pain: Arsenicum, Phosphoric acid, Rhus tox, Silica.

Panic Attack: See "Fears"

Peritonitis

Peritonitis is an acute inflammation of the membrane that lines the abdominal cavity. It can be triggered by perforation of the gastrointestinal tract or female genital tract, allowing bacteria into the area. It can also be caused by wounds that penetrate the abdomen (including surgery). Symptoms include severe, constant abdominal pain and tenderness. The pain is worse from the slightest movement, even deep breathing. Symptoms include fever, chills, rapid pulse, abdominal bloating, nausea, vomiting, and diarrhea. The patient may lie on her back with her knees drawn up. Sometimes surgery is necessary.

*__Aconite:__ When it first comes on. Sudden onset with fever, chill, abdominal pain, restlessness, and fear of death. Skin is hot and dry. Very thirsty. Worse from any motion, pressure, or lying on the right side.

***Bryonia:** The patient is worse from the slightest movement and lies perfectly still. Deep breathing causes pain, so he takes short, quick breaths. Thirsts for large cold drinks. High fever and violent, sharp pain. Irritable.

***Mercurius corrosivus:** Foul breath, excess salivation and may drool. Intense perspiration and feels worse afterward. Bloody stools. Abdomen swollen and tender. Cutting pains.

***Colocynth:** Painful internal spasms, which cause the patient to double over. Better from warmth. Sharp knifelike pains.

***Belladonna:** Sudden, intense onset. Abdomen bloated, hot, and extremely tender. Worse from the slightest jar or touch. Face red and hot, but hands and feet cold. Pupils dilated. May be drowsy or delirious. Worse from noise and light. Bloody diarrhea. Sensation as if someone is gripping his abdomen with their nails.

***Carbo veg:** Head hot but breath and body cold. Craves air and wants to be fanned. Abdomen bloated with belching. Foul-smelling stools.

***Arsenicum:** Burning pains, but better from warmth. Fearful, restless, great thirst for small frequent sips. Abdomen is so bloated, it feels like it will explode. Very weak. Worse alone and after midnight.

Lachesis: Very talkative and frequently changes subjects. Lies on his back with his knees drawn up. Abdomen is very tender. Stops breathing when he falls asleep. Worse after sleep, from warmth, from the pressure of clothes, and from light touch. Tongue trembles so much he can't stick it out. Wounds look purple.

Rhus tox: Restless, constantly changing position in spite of the pain. Muttering delirium. Worse from cold, dampness. Very thirsty. Dreams of great exertion.

Baptisia: Slurs speech and looks intoxicated. Falls asleep while being spoken to. Body feels stiff and sore. Bodily discharges have a putrid odor. His face is dark red. Delusion that he is broken and tosses around the bed trying to get the pieces together. Fears to sleep because he might suffocate.

Apis: Thirstless, or just drinks tiny sips. Urine dark and scanty. Swelling of the face. Sudden knifelike pain through the abdomen. Burning, stinging pain, which is better from cold. Worse in a warm room and from touch or pressure. Better from cold air, uncovering.

Arnica: Especially when due to injuries. Worse from touch, and averse to being approached. Head hot and body cold. Offensive-smelling discharges.

Veratrum album: Cold sweat, especially on the forehead. Very chilly. Watery diarrhea, vomiting. Anxious, restless, thirsty. Craves cold drinks.

Pinkeye: See "Conjunctivitis"

Plague, Bubonic

Bubonic plague is a bacterial disease transmitted by the bite of the rat flea, or by ingestion of feces of the flea. There are two forms of this disease, the *bubonic* and the *pneumonic*. The pneumonic form can be transmitted from person to person from coughing (airborne).

Bubonic Form

Incubation is two to five days. Comes on suddenly. Chills, high fever, and headache. Pulse is fast but weak. Swollen and tender lymph nodes at the groin, under the arm, and below the jaw. Restless, delirious, confused, and uncoordinated. If untreated, death is usually from heart failure after three to five days.

Pneumonic Form

Comes on in similar manner with chills, high fever, headache, fast but weak pulse. Then a cough develops and patient coughs up specks of blood. Subsequently coughs up pink to bright red foamy mucus. Pneumonia develops with difficult, rapid breathing. Death may occur in one and a half to two days if untreated.

A third form, septicemic plague, can result in death before the lymph nodes enlarge. There is also a benign form of plague characterized by a single enlarged lymph node. It is a self-limiting condition.

Prevention

Yersinia pestis (nosode 30c) once a week, or **Baptisia**, or **Tarentula cubensis. Ignatia** tincture in 1-drop doses may also act preventively.

Remedies for Plague

Hepar sulph: Inflamed areas are extremely sensitive to touch, cold, and draft. The patient feels like a wind is blowing on him. Chilly and wants to be covered. Irritable.

Baptisia: Offensive discharges. Face is dark red, and the patient looks intoxicated. Sore muscles. Delusional. Tongue feels burned, gags on solid food but can drink fluids, falls asleep while answering a question.

Pyrogenium: Offensive discharges, restlessness, extreme pain, violent burning sensations, high temperature with low pulse or vice versa, perspiration that does not relieve fever. Muscles sore and better from motion.

Lachesis: Restless and exhausted, feels sore and bruised, yellow eyes, gags on fluids but can eat solids (opposite Baptisia). Worse after sleep, from heat, or from tight clothing. Hemorrhage of dark blood.

Belladonna: Face bright red, hot. In early stages with delirium, fever, dry heat, shooting pains, and dilated pupils. Worse from noise, light, and being jarred.

Arsenicum album: Diarrhea, restlessness, exhaustion, burning sensations relieved by heat. Very fearful. Better from warmth and company.

Tarentula cubensis: Hard swelling with burning, stinging pain, and purple discoloration. Anxious and very restless.

Nitric acid: Sticking pains as if from splinters, tendency to bleeding. Irritable. Very sensitive to noise. Strong odor to urine, like a horse's urine. Urine feels cold when it passes. Chilly and worse from cold.

Carbo animalis: Glands swollen, hard, and painful. Very weak. Digestion weak. Sensation of cold in the stomach and chest Sensation as if his eyes were loose in their sockets. Easily frightened, sad, weeps when he eats, avoids conversation. Better from warmth.

Mercurius: Profuse sweating—patient feels worse afterward. Foul odor to breath and perspiration. Skin moist. Tongue flabby, with the imprint of teeth. Has excess saliva and may drool, but also has great thirst for cold drinks. Trembling, especially of the hands and tongue. Creeping chilliness. Worse during the night, after sweating, from lying on the right side, the warmth of the bed, drafts, and hot or cold temperatures.

Phosphorus: If there is difficulty breathing or other signs of pneumonia. Craves ice-cold drinks. Desires company and fears being alone. Buboes ulcerate with a colorless discharge.

Yersinia pestis (nosode 30c)**:** Give an occasional dose in between other remedies.

Pneumonia

Pneumonia is an inflammation of the lungs. It may be caused by a bacterial, viral, or fungal infection, or result from inhaling chemical fumes or aspirating certain liquids. Symptoms include difficulty breathing with pain in the chest or side, fever, painful cough, chill, headache, pale or blue face, rapid pulse (100–130 beats per minute), and fluid in the lungs. In the early stages, the patient coughs up pink sputum, which then goes to rust-colored and finally yellow.

***Aconite:** Sudden onset from chill, during cold, dry weather. In the beginning with high fever, hard dry painful cough, and thin, blood-streaked mucus. Great anxiety, restlessness, fear of death. Skin hot and dry. Extreme thirst.

***Ferrum phos:** Early stages have few clear symptoms. The patient has difficulty breathing and coughs up blood. Face is alternately red and pale. Slow onset with low fever. Sweaty. Better from lying down and from cold applications. Worse from 4 to 6 a.m., at night, and from cold drinks, being jarred, or motion.

***Phosphorus:** Coughs up rust-colored sputum or bright red blood, burning sensation in the chest, feeling of weight on the chest, or the chest feels tight. Can't lie on the left side and is better lying on the right. Hard, dry cough that makes him tremble. Afraid to be alone, thirsty for ice-cold drinks, startles easily, sensitive to light, noise, and odors. Better after short sleep.

***Arsenicum:** Extreme anxiety and restlessness, wants company, worse from midnight to 3 a.m. Thirsty but for small sips, exhausted, has burning sensations that are better from heat.

***Antimonium tartaricum:** Rattling mucus in the chest that is too thick to cough up. Feels like she's suffocating and has to sit up. Burning in the chest and throat. Pulse is rapid and weak. Better lying on the right side. Cold sweat on the face. Worse lying down and from warmth.

***Bryonia:** Sharp pains with each breath or from the slightest movement. Better lying still on the painful side. Dry cough, rust-colored mucus, thirsty for large cold drinks. Great urge to take a deep breath, which is painful. Worse from warmth and motion. Irritable.

***Lycopodium:** Worse between 4 and 8 p.m. and sometimes between 4 and 8 a.m. Nostrils flare when struggling to breathe. Face pale with a frown. Short, dry cough. Salty or bitter-tasting mucus. Flatulence. Satisfied by a small amount of food. Wakes irritable or angry.

Hepar sulph: If pneumonia fails to resolve and keeps producing yellow sputum. Very chilly, worse from any draft. Irritable. Discharges smell like old cheese. Better from heat, damp weather. Worse from cold, cold food, drafts, and touch.

Sulphur: Chest feels heavy. There are burning sensations anywhere in the body. The patient wants windows open, and is worse from the warmth of the bed and lying on his back. Irritable. Discharges smell foul and irritate the skin. Redness, itching of the anus, lips, nose, and eyes. Sudden diarrhea in the morning. When other remedies fail to act, it rouses the "Vital Force." Better from fresh air, moving, and lying on the right side. Worse from bathing, being in a warm room or bed, at 11 a.m., standing, or drinking milk.

Mercurius: Foul odor to breath and perspiration, excess saliva, great thirst, tongue flabby with the imprint of teeth, copious perspiration after which he feels worse, blood-streaked thick green mucus, stabbing pain at bottom of the right lung. Worse at night and from the warmth of the bed.

Pulsatilla: Can't stand a closed room, and craves cool, fresh air even when chilly. Gentle, yielding, better from sympathy and company. Coughs every time he breathes. Cough worse lying down and in the evening. Thick, bland yellowish-green mucus. Dry mouth but no thirst.

Ipecac: Nausea and vomiting accompany other symptoms. Coughs with every breath. Coughs up blood. Tendency to bleeding. Clean tongue with excess saliva. Better from open air. Worse from the slightest motion and from warmth, especially damp warmth.

Poisoning

See "Food Poisoning," "Drug Overdose," and poisoning from specific substances, such as "Lead," "Arsenic," or "Mushrooms." If there is a homeopathic version of the poison, you may try that also.

If there is a local "poison information center" in your area, call them immediately. It is often necessary to remove gross amounts of the poison. Sometimes vomiting is recommended, but for caustic substances it can make the patient worse. Consult the poison information center.

To help neutralize acidic poisons: milk of magnesia, milk, or egg white.

To help neutralize alkaline poisons: equal parts of vinegar and water.

Poison Ivy, Oak, Sumac

Contact with the toxin from these plants produces an itching, burning rash and sometimes small blisters. Symptoms develop anywhere from a few hours to a week after exposure. The reaction can be prevented or reduced by washing the area with soap and water within an hour of exposure. Contaminated clothes should also be washed.

***Rhus tox** (30–200c)**:** Better from hot water. Very restless.

Ledum: Better from cold application.

Anacardium: Large blisters filled with yellow fluid. Itching is better from hot water (also Rhus tox).

Graphites: Honey-colored fluid, which oozes out and dries to yellow crystals. Worse at night and from heat.

Polio

Polio is a communicable viral disease. Symptoms include fever, headache, stiff neck and back, deep muscle pain, extreme sensitivity or numbness in body parts, muscle weakness, and loss of reflexes. Also, paralysis of the face and throat with difficulty in swallowing, and paralysis of limbs.

Prevention

These two remedies have been used effectively for prevention. See below for distinguishing characteristics.

***Lathyrus sativa**

Gelsemium

Remedies for Polio

Aconite: Symptoms come on quickly. Numbness of the hands and feet, tingling as if from an electric current, hands and feet icy cold, or hot hands and cold feet. Restless, thirsty, very frightened. Legs weak. Red patch on the palms of both hands.

Lathyrus sativa: The patient's legs feel rigid and he walks stiffly and uncertainly. His knees knock when walking. Extreme reaction to knee-jerk reflex. Weakness of legs. Sudden paralysis of lower limbs. Trembling in upper body. Incontinence of bladder.

Gelsemium: Much trembling and weakness. Can't control his legs and he totters. Dull drowsy look on face, eyelids droop, double vision, paralysis of the tongue, can't move his muscles. Thirstless. Chill up the back.

Rhus tox: Legs feel stiff, as if made of wood. Better from moving and worse after rest. Worse from cold or dampness and at night. Restless in spite of weakness. Trembling after exertion. Thirsty. Tongue coated but with red triangular tip.

Plumbum: Loss of knee-jerk reflex. Trembling of arms. Extreme sensitivity of the skin so it can't be touched, or numbness. Symptoms appear slowly. Paralysis of single parts. Wrists hang down. Extreme constipation. Better from hard pressure and rubbing. Worse from light touch. Worse lying on the right side.

Prostatitis

This is an inflammation of the prostate gland. The acute form, which comes on rapidly, is usually due to a bacterial infection. There is also a nonbacterial variety. Acute prostatitis can also result from surgical procedures such as catheterization or cystoscope. Symptoms include pain in the area between the anus and the scrotum, frequent urination, retention of urine, burning upon urination, constipation, weakness, chills, fever, and low back pain.

***Sabal serrulata:** Urinary retention due to inflamed prostate. Cystitis may accompany an enlarged prostate. Semen feels hot when ejaculated. Loss of sexual power. Aversion to sympathy.

***Chimaphila:** Feels like he's sitting on a ball. Must stand to urinate. Pain and itching extending from the bladder to the penis. Bloody mucus in urine.

Pulsatilla: For people who are emotional, who desire company and sympathy, who are uncomfortable in a warm room, who crave fresh air, who feel worse from eating fat, pastries or pork, and who have very little thirst.

Apis: For people who are usually warm and worse from heat. Very little thirst. Worse from touch or pressure. Burning or stinging pain relieved by cold. Frequent urging with painful urination.

Staphysagria: Pain extending from anus to urethra. For people who suppress anger and other emotions. Worse after sex and from tobacco.

Thuja: Offensive odor to semen and genitals. Worse from cold or dampness. Often has numerous warts. For prostatitis that started after vaccination.

Nitric acid: With sticking pains as from splinters. Strong-smelling urine. Profuse perspiration on hands and feet. Highly irritable.

Silica: For people who are chilly, easily exhausted, fastidious, who fear failure and hate being tested. Worse from drafts. Ridged fingernails, offensive foot sweats. For prostatitis after vaccination.

Copaiva: Prostate feels hard. Burning pain while passing urine. Urine passed by drops.

Belladonna: Comes on rapidly, throbbing sensations, worse from touch, craves lemonade.

Hepar sulph: Chilly and worse from cold and drafts. Inflamed parts very sensitive to touch. Irritable.

Rabies

Rabies is a virus, usually transmitted by saliva during an animal bite. It can also be contracted from contact with mucous membranes or an open wound. After being infected, symptoms may occur in anywhere from ten days to over a year. Symptoms begin with mental depression, weakness, restlessness, and fever. Extreme excitement, salivation, and painful spasm of the larynx follow. The spasms make it difficult to drink, and the patient will refuse liquids in spite of great thirst. Death can occur in three to five days due to asphyxia, paralysis, or exhaustion.

> **Note:** If possible, observe the animal that did the biting. If it does not develop symptoms within ten days, then it probably didn't have rabies.

Prevention of Rabies

This is only to be used if the bite is from a rabid animal or if there is high probability of it: **Hydrophobinum** (30c) three times a day for one week followed by **Belladonna** (3c) twice a day for six months.

> **Note:** When using a remedy for extended periods, it is best to dissolve it in a bottle of water and take half-teaspoon doses. Tap the bottle ten times against a book or table before each use. If you should develop a reaction to the remedy, stop for a week and try it again.

Remedies for Rabies

***Hydrophobinum:** Treatment may be started with this nosode of hydrophobia. Follow with appropriate remedies.

***Belladonna:** Face red, hot, and sweaty. Neck veins bulging. Thirsty but can't swallow water. Delirium, convulsions, striking, biting, and spitting. Worse from noise, light, or being jarred.

***Stramonium:** Can't bear the sight of water or any glistening object. Unable to drink. Delirium, convulsions. Fears darkness and being alone. Better from light. Awakes screaming.

***Hyoscyamus:** Twitching, jerking muscles. Insomnia. Extreme thirst but can't swallow. Much perspiration. Talkative (or very quiet), jealous, and suspicious. Fumbles with his hands and picks at things. Worse from touch.

Cantharis: Itching and burning sensations. Anger and convulsions. Worse from the sight of water or bright objects.

Lachesis: Face red, delirious, very talkative, worse from heat, worse after sleep, difficulty swallowing especially liquids, sensitive to light touch, can't bear anything tight around his neck or waist. His tongue trembles so much, he can't stick it out.

Radiation, Exposure to

Exposure to radiation: Cadmium sulph or homeopathic X-ray.

Radiation burns: Homeopathic X-ray, Phosphorus, Fluoric acid, or Radium bromide.

Radiation Sickness

Radiation sickness is characterized by nausea, vomiting, bloody diarrhea, exhaustion, blistering of the skin, ulceration of mucous membranes, bleeding from the nose, mouth, and rectum, bruising, sloughing of skin, open sores on the skin, and hair loss.

***Cadmium sulph:** Terrible nausea. Black vomit. Also vomits green mucus, blood, or a substance looking like coffee grounds. Freezing cold and can't get warm. Blue circles around his eyes. Bloody-black, offensive stools. Extreme exhaustion.

***Ipecacuanha:** Constant nausea not relieved by vomiting. Bloody, slimy stools. Bleeding from lungs with nausea. Tongue clear. Blue rings around eyes. Profuse salivation. Thirstless. Better from open air, rest, pressure, and closing the eyes. Worse from the slightest motion and from warmth.

***Phosphorus:** Bleeding bright red blood from any orifice. Craves ice-cold drinks but vomits them after they become warm in the stomach. Heightened sensitivity to noise, odors, and lights. Startles easily. Fears being alone. Exhausting diarrhea. Feels he is about to die. Worse lying on his left side.

Arsenicum: Anxious, chilly, restless, exhausted, and thirsty for small sips. Burning pains relieved by heat, fear of being alone. Worse after midnight.

Scarlet Fever

Scarlet fever is a contagious disease caused by a streptococcus infection of the throat. It usually begins with sore throat, high fever, and vomiting. A pink rash—which starts on the neck and chest—follows a day later. The rash has a "sandpaper" quality. Sometimes the rash comes out only partially, or not at all. The tongue goes from bright red to a deep red color. The rash may last two to three weeks. Other symptoms are a bright red color in the folds of the underarm and groin, "strawberry tongue," and muscle aches.

Prevention of Scarlet Fever

Scarlatinum (nosode 30c) or **Belladonna**.

Remedies for Scarlet Fever

***Belladonna:** Red hot face, eyes red, pupils dilated. Throat hot, red, and dry. High fever. Worse from light, noise, or being jarred. Sometimes delirium.

***Rhus tox:** Drowsy but very restless. Constantly moving about to find a comfortable position. Worse after rest. Coarse rash. Very thirsty. Stiff muscles. Worse from cold. Better from warm drinks. Worse at night. Throat puffy and dark red.

***Apis:** Burning and stinging pain in the throat and on the skin. Throat swollen. Dry mouth but no thirst. Worse from heat and better from cold. May be drowsy and sleep much, or suffer from insomnia. Delirium with shrieking. Urine scanty and dark. Edema (swelling of tissues).

***Lachesis:** Face and rash are a purplish color. The patient feels worse after sleep. Can't bear anything around his neck. Left-sided sore throat, which feels worse from dry swallowing or drinking liquids. Bleeding of dark blood from the nose, mouth, or bowels. Worse from warmth. Sometimes very talkative.

***Mercurius:** Foul breath, excess salivation, spongy tongue with the imprint of teeth, great thirst. Much sweating and always worse after it. Ulcers in throat. Worse at night and from the heat of the bed.

***Ammonium carbonicum:** Bursting headache in the forehead. Face is puffy and dark. Very drowsy. Rash not fully developed. Chilly and worse from open air. Worse at 3 a.m.

***Ailanthus:** Dark, swollen throat with feeble pulse. Secretions that burn the nose. Foul odor of breath. Half-conscious and doesn't understand what's going on. Delirium with muttering. Pupils dilated. Tongue dry and cracked.

Aconite: Extremely anxious, high fever, hot dry skin, great thirst, and sore throat. Pulse strong and fast.

Bryonia: Worse from any movement. Swollen joints. Thirst for large drinks. Constipated, pulse weak.

Ipecacuanha: Nausea and vomiting, excess salivation, and difficulty breathing. Tongue clear. Thirstless. Worse from heat.

Lycopodium: Worse between 4 and 8 p.m. Right-sided throat pain. Face pale and bloated. Swollen hands, feet, and abdomen. Red, sandy deposit in urine.

Phosphorus: The rash suddenly disappears and breathing becomes difficult. Burning sensations. Thirst for cold drinks. Fear of being alone.

Nitric acid: Discharge that burns the nostrils and lips. Ulcers in the mouth. Vomits all food. Very chilly. Splinterlike pains. Foul-smelling discharges. Worse from touch, moving, or cold.

Chamomilla: Ulceration and cough after recovery. Highly irritable. Great sensitivity to pain.

Sciatica

Symptoms of sciatica include sharp, shooting pain that begins in the buttocks and extends down the back of the thigh and leg to the ankle. Sometimes numbness and tingling or sensitivity to touch occur. The pain and numbness may be worse from walking or standing.

***Colocynth:** Worse from moving and from cold. Must lie perfectly still. Often left sided. Lightninglike pain from the lower back down to the heel. Worse from touch, cold, or anger. Sometimes numbness (also Gnaphalium, Rhus tox, and Chamomilla).

***Magnesia phosphorica:** Worse from moving and from cold. Worse from uncovering. Right-sided. Better standing.

***Rhus tox:** Better from moving or walking. Walks with stiffness. Worse from cold and dampness. Better from warmth. Very restless. Thirsty. Worse at night. Worse when first beginning to move, but improves with further motion. Sometimes numbness (also Gnaphalium) and burning.

***Bryonia:** Worse from the slightest movement. Worse sitting up. Thirst for large, cold drinks. Better lying on the painful side and from pressure. Better from cold water. Irritable.

***Nux vomica:** Chilly, irritable, sensitive to noise, odors, and criticism. Better from warmth. Worse in the morning. Can't lie on the painful side. Constipation with straining, which increases the pain.

***Kali iodatum:** Better from moving and fresh air. Worse from heat and lying down.

***Gnaphalium:** Numbness with pain (also Rhus tox, Colocynth, and Chamomilla). Sometimes burning. Worse lying down and moving. Better sitting in a chair.

Chamomilla: Unendurable pain, especially at night in bed. Very angry. Worse from motion. Left-sided. Sometimes with numbness (also Gnaphalium, Rhus tox, and Colocynth).

Arsenicum: Chilly, anxious, restless, and thirsty for small sips. Burning pain relieved by heat. Temporary relief from moving. Better from warmth. Exhausted from the least effort.

Plumbum: Accompanied by extreme constipation. Worse from heat, motion, light pressure, and at night. Better from massage.

Seizures: See "Convulsions"

Septicemia: See "Blood Poisoning"

Shingles: See "Herpes Zoster"

Shock

Shock is a life-threatening condition that occurs when blood flow to the body is dramatically reduced. Such a situation may come about from a heart problem (cardiogenic shock), bleeding or dehydration (hypovolemic shock), an allergic reaction (anaphylactic shock), an infection (septic shock), or a problem with the nervous system (neurogenic shock). Symptoms of shock include pale, cold, clammy skin; rapid, weak pulse; and shallow, rapid breathing. Also weakness, restlessness, and anxiety. Keep the person lying down with his head lower than his body. Keep him warm but not overheated.

In the unconscious patient, place the remedy between his lips and teeth so it won't be inhaled. Repeat the remedy as often as needed, even every ten minutes.

***Arnica:** First choice. Especially after an injury.

***Aconite:** Where fear predominates. Pale on rising.

Carbo veg: Head hot with hot sweat, but cold breath. Hands and feet icy cold. Hungry for air and wants to be fanned. Belching.

Veratrum Album: Skin blue, cold sweat on forehead, freezing cold and wants to be covered. Vomiting and diarrhea. Postoperative shock.

Camphora: Icy coldness of the whole body, but refuses covers. Pulse weak.

Cantharis: Shock due to burns.

Sinusitis

Inflammation of the lining of the sinuses (hollow spaces) in the head. Symptoms include headache (often on waking), swelling of the eyelids, pain between the eyes, runny or stuffy nose, pain in the jaw, teeth, or cheeks, swelling around the eyes, postnasal drip (causing sore throat), earache, fever, or weakness. Causes include bacteria, viruses, fungi, and allergies (to airborne substances, medicines, chemicals, etc.).

Acute sinusitis is often triggered by a cold and lasts about three weeks. Chronic sinusitis can last for months or years and requires treatment by a professional homeopath. The following remedies can provide relief from acute sinusitis.

***Kali bichromicum:** Greenish-yellow mucus, which is thick, sticky, and stringy. Postnasal drip. Inability to breathe through the nose and loss of sense of smell. Shooting pain from the root of the nose to the eye. Migraine headache, especially over the eyes. Worse from cold, dampness, after sleep, after eating, and from 2 to 5 a.m.

***Hydrastis:** Sinusitis often after a cold. Thick, sticky, yellow mucus (sometimes white). Air feels cold in the nose. Sensation of a hair in the right nostril. Constipation. Worse inhaling cold, dry air and eating bread. Worse at night.

***Mercurius vivus:** Greenish-yellow mucus, sometimes blood streaked. Nostrils become raw. The patient perspires a lot and feels worse afterward. Headache with the feeling of a tight band around the head. Pain at the root of the nose. Craves cold drinks. Worse at night, from heat or cold (better from moderate temperature), lying on the right side, and from drafts.

***Pulsatilla:** Nonirritating greenish-yellow mucus, especially in the morning. Headache, which is better from walking in fresh air. No thirst. Weepy. Craves peanut butter. Worse from warmth, warm food or drink, lying down, and from eating rich or fatty food. Better from cold, cold food and drinks, fresh air, sitting up, company, and sympathy.

Thuja: Thick, yellow-green mucus with blood or pus. Worse after breakfast. Often in patients with asthma or warts. No appetite. Dislikes onions and garlic, and gets sick from onions. Worse from cold, damp weather. Worse at night and at 3 a.m. and 3 p.m. Worse from coffee, tea, fatty food, and sweets.

Silica: Chilly, always wrapping up, worse from drafts. Constipated with stools that recede after effort. Night sweats on the upper part of the body. Sweats on the head and feet. Dry, hard crusts in the nose that bleed when plucked. Timid, yet stubborn. Lacks confidence and fears failure. Better from warmth and covering the head. Worse from cold air, drafts, mental stress, and lying on the left side.

Arsenicum: Thin, watery, burning discharge, which irritates the nostrils. Very anxious about health, restless, chilly, fatigued by the least effort, thirsty for small sips of water. Affects patients with asthma. Worse from midnight to 3 a.m. Burning pains relieved by heat. Worse from cold, cold drinks or food, dampness, exertion, or being alone. Better from warmth, fresh air, company, walking, or sitting up.

Kali iodatum: Worse from heat and feels better walking around in cool, fresh air. Eyes swollen with burning in the eyes and sinuses. Worse from warmth, dampness, at night, from cold food, and changes of weather. Worse from evening to early morning. Mucus is usually watery and burning, but it can be thick and green with a bad odor. Pressure at the root of the nose.

Hepar sulph: Very chilly and worse from cold and draft. Wants to be covered. Any painful part is also worse from cold, draft, and the slightest touch. Sinusitis after colds. Mucus drips down the throat. Thick, yellowish mucus, which smells like old cheese. Coughs or sneezes from cold air.

Nux vomica: Chilly, chilly from moving, irritable, angry, impatient, and constipated (must strain to pass stool). Oversensitive to light, odors, sounds, or criticism. Worse in the morning, from cold dry air, uncovering, mental strain, or the pressure of clothes. Worse from coffee, stimulants, and overeating. Nose congested with the odor of old cheese (also Hepar) or sulphur. Mucus from the nose irritates the nostrils.

Slipped Disk: See "Spine Injuries"

Smallpox

Smallpox is a highly contagious disease caused by the variola virus. Symptoms usually begin within seven to fourteen days after exposure. At first there is high fever, chills, weakness, and head- and backaches. Vomiting and convulsions may occur in young children. About the third day, the fever goes down and a rash develops on the face, arms, and legs. The rash begins as flat, circular red spots, which eventually become pus-filled and later begin to crust. This is followed by development of scabs. Sometimes the "pox" merge into each other, rather than remaining separate.

Smallpox is spread by contact with the saliva of ill persons. The disease is infectious until all of the scabs have fallen off. However, it is most infectious during the first week of illness.

> **Note:** Chickenpox versus smallpox—in chickenpox the rash develops from day one. Lesions may be oval-shaped instead of circular. The spots come out in successive stages rather than all at once as in smallpox.

Prevention

Variolinum (nosode 200c) once a week or **Malandrinum** (30c) once a day.

Kali muriaticum (6c) three times a day or **Sarracenia** (3c) three times a day.

If the above remedies are not available, then Aconite, Belladonna, or Antimonium tartaricum may be tried.

Remedies for Smallpox

*__Variolinum__ (200c): In addition to prevention, it may be given at the onset and then once a week by itself, to reduce the severity of the disease.

***Aconite:** First stage of illness with fear of death, high fever, thirst, and restlessness. Skin hot and dry.

***Bryonia:** Early stage with high fever and extreme thirst for cold drinks. Lies perfectly still and is always worse from any movement. Dryness of mucous membranes. Worse from heat. Irritable.

***Belladonna:** First stage with high fever, intense inflammation of skin and mucous membranes. Much heat and redness, especially about the head. Throbbing sensations. Spasms of the bladder, insomnia, delirium, convulsions, extreme sensitivity to light, sound, and jarring. Worse from cold or drafts. Craves lemonade.

***Antimonium tart:** Top remedy for smallpox. After lesions become pus filled. Difficult breathing, blue face, drowsiness, and twitching muscles. Coated tongue, weakness, back pain, and nausea. Also, thick mucus in airways causes choking with rattling in the lungs. Worse in a warm room. Better from cold open air. Can't stand being looked at. Wants to be left alone.

Arsenicum: Restlessness in spite of great weakness, extreme anxiety, fear of being alone, burning pains relieved by warmth, thirst for small sips. Lesions may form on the mouth and throat.

Mercurius: Swollen glands, especially under the jaw, excess saliva with drooling, greenish mucus-laden stools. Worse at night, from the warmth of the bed and after perspiring. Great thirst.

Kali muriaticum: Gray coating at the back of the tongue, swollen lymph glands, thick white discharges from mucous membranes, eczema, blisters on the skin filled with thick, white fluid.

Thuja: In middle or later stages, a dark red outline forms around the painful pustules. Pain in the arms and hands. Worse from cold and dampness, and sometimes from the heat of the bed. Worse at 3 a.m. Green discharges. The patient imagines that his body is brittle and fragile, as if made of glass.

Rhus tox: Extremely restless in spite of exhaustion (also Arsenicum), dry tongue with much thirst, blood in pustules and in stool. Foul brown crusts form on the lips and teeth (from stomach secretions).

Pustules become dark. Worse at night and after being still. Worse from cold or dampness. Better from warmth and changing position. Fears to sleep.

Phosphorus: When pneumonia or hemorrhage appear. Bright red blood coughed up from lungs. Back feels broken. Hard, dry cough. Blood appears in pustules. Craves ice-cold drinks. Fears to be alone. Worse lying on the left side. Worse in the evening, when alone, and from warm food or drink.

Apis: Stinging, burning pain of the skin and throat. No thirst. Passes very little urine. Better from cold air or cold applications. Worse from heat, touch, or pressure. Drowsy. Wants to be left alone.

Muriatic acid: End stage of the disease with the patient in a state of collapse. There is a great deal of perspiration. Incontinence of the bladder and bowels. Diarrhea, fever, and weakness. Slides down in the bed. Worse from touch, cold drinks, or talking. Better lying on the left side.

Lachesis: The patient is worse after sleep, and fears going to sleep. Extreme sensitivity to light touch, and intolerance of tight clothing, especially around the neck. Left-sided symptoms. Worse swallowing liquids (solids are better), worse from heat or hot drinks. May be very talkative. Hemorrhages of dark blood. Skin appears purple.

Snakebite

Bandage the limb with a *wide* bandage (not a tourniquet) to slow the spread of venom. Don't cut or suck out the wound. Bites by poisonous snakes are more likely to produce swelling and discoloration of the tissue. Get professional help as soon as possible.

Unless you have the remedy for the specific snake, then use:

Aconite: Every fifteen minutes.

Ledum: A dose of Ledum after the first dose of Aconite should help restrict dispersion of the venom.

Note: Specific remedies are available for each type of snakebite. If all you have is Lachesis, try that. If collapse occurs (pale, cold, clammy skin; rapid, weak pulse; shallow breathing) give Carbo veg every ten minutes, between the lips and teeth.

Snake	**Remedy**
Rattlesnake	Crotalus horridus
Water Mocassin	Toxicophis
Copperhead	Cenchris contortrix
Coral Snake	Elaps corallinus
Cobra	Naja
German Viper	Vipera torva
Bushmaster	Lachesis

The above remedies are available from some of the homeopathic pharmacies.

Herbs Reported to Antidote Snakebite

Golondrina (Euphorbia polycarpa) is an herb that can be used both prophylactically and for treating snakebite. It is supposed to render the body immune to snake poisons. It is used in drop doses of the tincture.

Euphorbia prostata is also reported to be effective against snakebite, especially of the rattlesnake.

Sore Throat

Most sore throats are minor, but some serious ailments start that way. If you can cure an ailment at that stage, it may not go any further. At the end of this list see "Some Distinguishing Features of Sore Throat" to help make the selection.

***Aconite:** *Comes on suddenly, from exposure to cold.* High fever, anxiety, restlessness. Throat red, hot, dry, and burning. Great thirst for cold water. Used at first sign of a sore throat, it will often abort it.

***Belladonna:** *Sudden onset. Face red and hot.* Throat and tongue bright red, dry, and burning. Throat feels constricted, making it difficult to swallow. Coughs food through the nose. Most often right sided. The patient feels worse from noise, lights, or being jarred.

***Lachesis:** *Left-sided sore throat or moving from left to right.* Comes on after sleeping, worse from warmth, worse swallowing liquids (eating solid food doesn't hurt). Throat looks bluish red. External throat is sensitive to touch. Sensation of a lump in throat, making him swallow.

***Phytolacca:** *Dark red throat, pain radiates to ears when trying to swallow,* glands swollen. Burning pain. Lump-in-throat sensation (also Lachesis, Hepar, and Nitric acid).

***Mercurius:** *Raw, burning throat. Foul breath, much saliva,* great thirst. Sweats profusely and feels worse afterward. Tongue coated yellow. Worse at night and from the warmth of the bed.

***Hepar sulph:** *Very chilly and worse from cold or drafts.* Just putting the hand out of the covers worsens the pain or cough. Pus in the throat, splinterlike pains, pain extends to the ear when swallowing. Throat is sensitive to touch. Highly irritable.

***Lycopodium:** *Starts on right side and may move to left.* Better from warm drinks. Worse from 4 to 8 p.m.

Arsenicum: *Burning in the throat, which is relieved by hot drinks.* Thirst for frequent small sips. Chilly and better from warmth. Very anxious, restless, and exhausted. Worse at midnight. Doesn't want to be alone.

Apis: *Burning, stinging pain, like a bee.* Worse from heat and better from cold. No thirst. Throat looks swollen.

Pulsatilla: *Patient is worse in a warm room and craves fresh air. No thirst* (also Apis). Desires sympathy and company. Weeps easily. Worse from empty swallowing.

Gelsemium: *Comes on slowly over a period of days.* Chill up the back. Wants to be left alone. Limbs feel heavy and eyelids droop. Body hot with cold hands and feet.

Baptisia: *Throat dark red and swollen. Sometimes painless.* The throat is constricted, and the patient can only swallow water. Drowsiness, heavy eyelids, falls asleep while being spoken to.

Lac caninum: *Pain moves from one side to the other and back again.* Choking feeling, like the throat is closing. Unable to swallow. External throat is sensitive to touch. Worse from empty swallowing.

Nitric acid: *Feels like there are splinters or sharp bones in the throat.* Pain extends to the ear when swallowing. Swallowing is very difficult. Ulcers in the throat. Patient is very chilly.

Capsicum: Pain is worse when not swallowing (also Apis). Burning pain like hot pepper. Throat swelled, and red or purple (also Lachesis). Chilly after drinking. Face is red but cold.

Some Distinguishing Features of Sore Throat

Warm drinks, better from: Arsenicum, Hepar sulph, Lycopodium (better or worse).

Warm drinks, worse from: Lachesis, Apis, Phytolacca, Lycopodium (better or worse)

Left-sided sore throat (or moving from left to right): Lachesis, Lac caninum.

Right-sided: Lycopodium, Belladonna, Phytolacca, Mercurius, Lac caninum.

Right-sided and moving to the left: Lycopodium.

Alternating sides (left to right and back to left or vice versa): Lac caninum.

Waking, worse upon: Lachesis.

Cold air, worse from: Hepar sulph, Belladonna.

Drafts, worse from: Hepar.

Liquids, difficulty swallowing: Lachesis, Mercurius, Nitric acid.

Sensation as if a splinter or bone is in the throat: Hepar sulph, Nitric acid.

Stinging pain: Apis, Gelsemium.

Empty swallowing, worse from: Lachesis, Arsenicum, Belladonna, Lac caninum, Pulsatilla.

Not swallowing (pain even when not swallowing): Apis, Capsicum.

Swallowing impossible: Belladonna, Gelsemium, Lac caninum, Lachesis, Nitric acid.

Suffocating (feels like he is suffocating): Lachesis, Apis.

Touch (worse when external throat is touched): Lachesis.

Spine Injuries

(See also "Slipped or Ruptured Disk" in this Section)

Symptoms depend on the severity of the injury and what part of the spine is injured. Symptoms may include loss of muscle control, loss of bladder or bowel control, numbness, breathing difficulties, and paralysis.

***Arnica:** After any injury. The patient may say he is okay and refuse to let anyone touch him.

***Hypericum:** Top remedy for injuries to the spine. Follows Arnica. Patient feels intense pain and is unable to walk. Crawls on hands and knees. Worse from being touched or bumped.

***Natrum sulph:** After Arnica and Hypericum. Pains in the lower back as if from a blow. Terrible pain in the neck at the base of the brain. Worse from damp weather, lying on the left side, and lying for long in one position. Very chilly, but profuse sweat at night.

Bryonia: *Pain is worse from the slightest motion*. Wants to lie perfectly still. Better from lying on the painful side. Irritable. Worse from warmth.

Rhus tox: Back feels stiff and is painful when first starting to move, but *continued movement makes it feel better*. Worse in damp or cold weather. Better from warmth. Restless.

Kali carb: Worse from 3 to 5 a.m. Pain extends from the buttocks to the thighs. The back feels weak. Worse from cold and better from warmth. Irritable but doesn't want to be alone.

Slipped or Ruptured Disk

The cartilage disks which separate the vertebrae and cushion the spine can slip out of place or rupture, due to injury or strain. This may put pressure on nerves. When this occurs in the lower back, the individual may experience severe pain that extends to the buttocks, legs or feet. The pain may be aggravated by the least motion. Other symptoms include tingling or numbness, spasms, and weakness of the limbs. When the injury occurs in the neck region, the symptoms include pain in the neck, shoulder, arm, or even the hand. The pain will often be worse when moving the head. Spasms in the neck may also occur.

Bryonia: *Pain is worse from the slightest motion.* Wants to be perfectly still. Better lying on the painful side. Very thirsty. Irritable.

Hypericum: Top remedy for injuries to the spine. Intense pain and inability to walk. Crawling on the hands and knees. Worse from being touched or bumped.

Agaricus: Spine sensitive to touch. Worse from cold air, pressure, and touch. Twitching of muscles. Constantly yawning from pain.

Aesculus: Worse from walking or stooping. Back feels weak. Sticking pains, hot pains, or pains that move around. Hands and feet swell after washing. Especially in the lower back.

Splinters

(And other embedded objects, such as shards of glass)

A sterilized needle (passed through a flame) can be used to gently remove the skin over a splinter. It may then be possible to remove the splinter with the needle or a sterilized pair of tweezers. However, in spite of the best efforts, some splinters may defy removal. Homeopathic Silica stimulates the body's natural tendency to expel things that don't belong there.

Silica (6c)**:** Twice a day for a few weeks or until object is expelled.

> **Note:** Do not use Silica if you have a medical implant such as a pacemaker. The remedy may stimulate the body to expel it.

Sprains

A sprain is an injury to the ligament around a joint. Symptoms include pain, swelling, and sometimes bruising.

***Arnica:** Immediately after the injury.

***Rhus tox:** Stiffness and pain, which is worse after rest and better from continued motion. Must keep shifting position.

Bryonia: Worse from any motion, better from pressure, better from lying on the affected part.

Ruta: Tendons, especially ankle, heel, and wrist. Repetitive motion syndrome. Worse after rest.

Hypericum: When nerves are damaged and there is much pain.

Staphylococcus Infection

These infections are now resistant to many antibiotics. They may exhibit in numerous ways, including local abscesses, tonsillitis, mastitis, cellulitis, cystitis, osteomyeletis, pneumonia, endocarditis, and meningitis. Local infections can enter the bloodstream and become more serious.

Most at risk are newborns, nursing mothers, people with lung disorders, diabetics, burn patients, anyone with an open wound (e.g., surgical wound), or individuals with indwelling catheters.

Antimonium crudum: Tongue has a thick white coating. Irritable and can't bear to be touched or looked at. Worse from heat, but also from cold bathing. Nostrils chapped and covered with crusts. Cracks in the corners of the mouth. Eyes dull, sunken, and red. Constant belching and bloating after eating.

Arsenicum: Very anxious and restless, chilly, thirsty for small frequent sips, exhausted from the least exertion. Burning pains, which are better from warmth. Foul-smelling diarrhea. Afraid to be alone. Worse from midnight to 3 a.m. Better from warmth and sitting up.

Dulcamara: Ailments come on after exposure to cold, wet weather. Chilly and worse from cold or dampness. Excessive discharges of thick, yellow mucus. Dry, burning heat during fever. Burning thirst for cold drinks. Coughs after exertion. Chill triggers an urge to urinate. Green, slimy, bloody, or mucus-laden stools. Better from moving. Worse at night.

Hepar sulph: Extremely chilly. Coughs when uncovered. Choking cough. Painful pus-filled wounds. Infected part is extremely sensitive to touch, cold, draft. Sensation as of a splinter in inflamed parts (e.g., the throat). Putrid ulcers surrounded by little pimples. The patient feels like wind is blowing on him. Very irritable, especially at night. Better from warmth, wrapping up the head. Worse from cold, draft, and touch.

Iris versicolor: Anguished look on face. Terrible burning sensation on the tongue and in the throat, esophagus, and stomach. Profuse saliva. Sour, burning vomit. Watery stools, which burn like fire. Perspiration smells like vinegar. Intense right-sided headache. Ringing in the ears. Worse at night and after rest.

Kali bichromicum: Tough, thick, yellow, stringy mucus. Pains occur in small spots. Pains fly from one place to another. Sensation as if there is a hair on the back of the tongue or in the nostril. Punched-out ulcers with overhanging edges or crusts. Ulcers with dark dots in them. Cutting pains in the thighs. Sensation as if a drop remains after urinating. Tongue is shiny, cracked, dry, and red (or yellow). Better from heat, motion, or pressure. Worse from cold, dampness, from 2 to 3 a.m., and after sleep.

Nitric acid: Splinterlike pains anywhere in body. Very chilly. Discharges are thin, brown, have a foul odor, and abrade the skin. Pains come and go suddenly. Urine smells strong, like a horse's urine. Deep, bleeding cracks in the skin. Foul-smelling foot sweats. Bloody saliva with green-coated tongue. Intense pain in the anus after stool. Profuse sweat on the hands and feet. Fear of disease and death. Better from warmth and hot applications. Worse from cold, light touch, being jarred, motion, and at night.

Phosphoric acid: Very weak, apathetic, and listless. Seems "burned out," gives one word answers. Blue rings around the eyes. Weak feeling in the chest from talking. Feels like his eyeballs are pressed into his head. Crushing headache on top of his head. Nightly pains as if his "bones were scraped." His face feels as if egg whites had dried on it. Painless diarrhea containing undigested food. Profuse sweat during the night and morning. Sensitive to odors, which "take away his breath." Better after a short nap, from warmth, and after stool. Worse from cold or drafts and loss of fluids.

Rhus toxicodendron: Symptoms worse after rest and better from continued movement. Extremely restless and must keep moving. Stiffness and pain in the joints and muscles. Worse from cold and at night. Coughs when putting his hands out of the covers. Hot, painful swollen joints. Skin red, burning, and itching, and better from warm water. Unquenchable thirst. Dreams of great exertion. Better from heat, warm drinks, changing position, and stretching. Worse from lying still, being in a cold, damp environment, from draft, and after midnight.

Silica: Very chilly, worse from drafts. Easily exhausted, thirsty, and hypersensitive to touch and noise. Perspires easily, especially on the head and feet, offensive sweat. Painful parts feel cold. Pus fills inflamed areas. Hard crusts form in the nose, which bleed when detached. Sensation of a hair on the tongue. Sticking pain in the tonsils. Better from warmth, covering the head. Worse from cold, drafts, dampness, light, noise, excitement, or after vaccination.

Pyrogenium: Foul-smelling discharges (breath, stool, sweat, or vomit). Exhausted, but extremely restless. Feels bruised all over. High fever with a slow pulse, or low fever with a fast pulse. Aware of his heart beating. Fevers that begin with pain in the legs. Better from moving about and from warmth. Worse from becoming cold.

Stings: See "Bites and Stings"

Streptococcus Infection

Streptococcal infections can occur anywhere in the body. The symptoms, which include pain, fever, headache, weakness, nausea, and vomiting, cannot be distinguished from other types of bacterial or viral infections. (See also "Necrotizing Fasciitis.")

Arsenicum: Very anxious and restless, chilly, thirsty for small frequent sips, exhausted from the least exertion, burning pains that are better from warmth. Foul-smelling diarrhea. Afraid to be alone. Worse from midnight to 3 a.m., from cold, and when alone. Better from warmth and sitting up.

Belladonna: Sudden intense onset of symptoms. Burning, heat, throbbing pain, and redness. In systemic infections, the face is red and hot, the pupils dilated, and the hands and feet cold. Delirium with biting, spitting, or kicking. Worse from light, noise, being jarred, being in the sun, drafts on the head, or seeing bright objects. Better from quiet, being in a dark room, standing or sitting up, or bending the head backward.

Arnica: For infections occurring after injuries. Much bruising. The head is hot and the body cold. Foul odor of bodily secretions. Taste of rotten eggs in the mouth. Says there is nothing the matter with him. Won't let anyone approach or touch him. His body feels bruised, and the bed feels too hard. Offensive bloody diarrhea. Feels like his stomach is pressed against his spine. Worse from touch, at night, or from becoming heated.

Streptococcinum: Sensitive to noise, light, and drafts, but better from fresh air. Can't bear pressure on the abdomen while lying down. Sensation as if his spine is vibrating. Infected, pus-filled tonsils. Swelling of glands in the neck. Tongue coated white with a red tip. Migraine with vomiting of bile.

Sulfuric acid: Chilly, great weakness (both mentally and physically), trembling, with much perspiration and bruising. Bodily secretions smell sour. Heartburn. Sour belching, which sets teeth on edge. Water feels cold in the stomach. Hot flushes followed by cold perspiration and trembling. Pains come on gradually but end suddenly. Brain feels like it is loose inside his forehead. He feels hurried. Mental fatigue. Worse from fresh air, from cold, and in the evening. Better from hot drinks, warmth, and lying on the affected side.

Stroke

Stroke is characterized by the death of brain cells, from either a burst or blocked blood vessel. The stroke may be preceded by dizziness, nausea, or vomiting. Stroke symptoms include headache, nausea, vomiting, numbness or tingling, weakness or paralysis on one side of the body, speech disturbance, difficulty swallowing, mood changes, vertigo, convulsions, or coma.

Homeopathic remedies administered immediately may prevent further tissue damage and make a positive outcome much more likely. Remedies have been effective even after prolonged coma.

*__Arnica:__ Given immediately, it can dramatically alter the outcome. Stimulates the absorption of blood clots. Left- or right-sided paralysis, but more often left. The head and face are hot, but the body is cool. Afraid to be touched. Pulse strong. If conscious, the patient says the bed feels too hard.

*__Aconite:__ Extreme fear. Strong pulse, face red, skin hot and dry. One cheek red, the other pale. Burning headache.

*__Lachesis:__ Left-sided paralysis. Face may be pale, or purple and puffy. Convulsive movements. Sense of suffocation. Cannot stand to have anything tight around the neck. Worse after sleep and from heat.

*__Opium:__ Coma with constricted pupils. Face bloated and dark with hot sweat. Eyes bloodshot. Labored breathing, deep snoring, pulse full but slow, body rigid. Unresponsive to pain, light, and noise. If conscious, the patient says the bed feels too hot.

*__Belladonna:__ Right-sided symptoms, face bright red and bloated, pupils dilated, eyes red and bulging, mouth drawn to one side. Strokes caused by high blood pressure and/or emotional excitement.

Phosphorus: Suddenly becomes unconscious, pulse and respiration almost gone. Face red but cool to the touch. Mouth drawn to left. Totally unresponsive. One-sided paralysis (right or left). If conscious, the patient has great thirst for cold drinks. Fear of being alone and of the dark. Worse lying on the left side.

Gelsemium: Nausea, headache, limbs feel heavy, eyes droop, stupor, coma, or general paralysis (not one-sided).

Nux vomica: Left-sided paralysis (Lachesis, Arnica). Sensitive to light and noise. Worse in the morning. When mental symptoms or speech impairment occur after a stroke. Strokes caused by the abuse of alcohol, coffee, drugs, or food.

Cocculus: With vertigo, nausea, or vomiting. Can't bear the thought or odor of food.

Nux moschata: Long-standing coma. Totally unresponsive. Cold extremities, mucous membranes dry. Tongue sticks to the roof of the mouth.

Baryta carbonica: In the elderly with loss of speech, trembling limbs, high blood pressure, and foul foot sweats.

Zincum: When there are no reflexes.

Stye
(See also "Eyes")

A stye is an inflammation of a sebaceous gland at the edge of the eyelid, with formation of pus. Swelling of the lid with pain. Hot compresses are often helpful.

Pulsatilla: For the beginning stage.

Staphysagria: If Pulsatilla fails or if the stye leaves a hard nodule after healing.

Hepar sulph: With extreme sensitivity to cold, touch, or draft.

Sunburn

*__Belladonna:__ Administer every two hours as needed. Face and head red, hot, and throbbing. Worse from light, noise, being jarred, lying down, or from drafts on the head. If thirsty, the individual craves lemonade.

***Cantharis:** Severe sunburn with smarting pain relieved by cold. Much blistering of the skin. Restless, thirsty. Pupils dilated. Objects appear yellow. Burning pain on urinating.

Urtica urens: Burning, stinging, and itching pain. Worse after sleep, from touch, or from applying water. Better from lying down.

Pulsatilla: Much itching, which is worse from warmth. Better from cold application. Thirstless. Craves fresh air. Emotional and weeps easily.

Apis: Edema (swelling of tissues) with stinging pain. Urination difficult, reduced urine output. Better from cold application. Thirstless. Restless or drowsy. Worse from heat, hot drinks, and touch.

Externally: Apply the diluted tincture of either **Urtica Urens** or **Hypericum**, four drops in five ounces of water. Another option is to apply cold tea or plain yogurt.

Sunstroke/Heat Stroke

When someone who has been exposed to the sun or high temperature develops a high fever and the following symptoms, sunstroke (heat stroke) must be considered—face flushed; red, hot, dry, or burning skin; high fever; vomiting; weakness; chest pain; cramps and twitching muscles; convulsions; vomiting; delirium; or coma. Rapid heartbeat and respiration. The temperature can rise rapidly to 105 or 106 degrees. This is a serious condition, which can be fatal if not treated.

If the temperature is 106 degrees or higher, an ice-water tub bath should be used. If that is not available, then cover the victim in a blanket soaked in water and massage the skin. Take his rectal temperature every ten minutes. Bring the temperature down to 102. DO NOT let the temperature fall below 101, as hypothermia may set in.

***Belladonna:** First choice. Use as soon as heat stroke is suspected. Face bright red, eyes bloodshot, fever, throbbing in the head. Worse from light, noise, being jarred, or lying down. Easily startled. Repeat every fifteen minutes for the first several doses.

***Glonoine:** Staring, jaws clenched. Throbbing in the whole body. Sees black spots in front of his eyes, and has a deathly feeling in the pit of his stomach.

***Aconite:** Fear of death, hot dry burning skin, restlessness, and great thirst.

***Lachesis:** Delirious and talkative, can't stand anything around his neck, his nose bleeds, and his tongue trembles when he sticks it out. Chronic problems after sunstroke (also Natrum carbonicum).

Carbo veg: Alternate with Belladonna if collapse occurs. Hot head but cold breath and cold extremities. Craves air and wants to be fanned. Belching.

Camphora: A state of collapse with icy-cold skin. Severe headache, delirium, and convulsions.

Gelsemium: Confused, looks intoxicated, eyelids droop, no thirst, pupils dilated.

Opium: Coma, face pale, eyes half open, pupils constricted, involuntary passing of urine and stool, muscles rigid.

Cactus grandiflora: The patient feels like there is an iron band around his chest and he can't breathe. Worse lying on the left side.

Natrum carbonicum: For chronic effects after sunstroke. Weakness from heat, exertion, and drafts.

Surgery

Preparing for Surgery

Arnica: Use on the day of the operation, to help the body deal with the trauma. A few doses of Arnica 30c may be given the day before the operation.

Aconite: For terror.

Phosphorus: If much bleeding is expected.

After Surgery

Arnica (30c or 200c)**:** To help the body recover. Helps reduce pain and bleeding, and speeds healing.

Phosphorus: For excessive bleeding of bright red blood. Can be used before the operation if bleeding may become a problem.

Cinchona: If the patient suffers from loss of blood or other body fluids.

Pain after Surgery

(See also "Pain")

Hypericum: First choice for pain.

Bellis perennis: For pain from deep injury to breasts or pelvic organs.

Hamamelis: Pain, soreness, and bruised feeling. Dark red blood oozes from the wound.

Calendula (30c or 200c)**:** For extreme pain and wounds that fail to heal.

Aconite: Unbearable pain with hot dry skin, thirst, and constant fear of death.

Staphysagria: For surgical wounds that heal poorly after they have drained. Also for operations that involved stretching of sphincters.

Symphytum: If bones were worked on.

Postoperative Shock

***Veratrum Album:** Cold sweat on the forehead, face pale to blue and cold, pulse rapid and feeble. Preceded by much vomiting.

***Strontium carbonicum:** With constant oozing of dark blood from mucous membranes. The patient sees bright colors before his eyes. Trembling from cold and worse from drafts.

Opium: The face is swollen and dark, the pupils constricted. Eyelids droop. Lower jaw hangs down. Labored breathing with deep snoring. Coma.

Carbo veg: The head is warm but the breath and body cold. The abdomen is distended with belching. Craves fresh air and wants to be fanned.

Anesthesia, Bad or Lingering Effects of

***Phosphorus:** First choice. Antidotes the effects of modern anesthetics as well as chloroform and ether.

Acetic acid: Antidotes all anesthetic gases; use one dose.

Antimonium tart: Effects of ether. Thick mucus in chest that can't be coughed out.

Hepar sulph: Weakness from ether. Sensitive to the least draft or cold.

Chloroformum: Liver problems after chloroform.

> **Caution:** If the patient is not fully conscious, dissolve the remedy in a tablespoon of spring water and place just a few drops of this on his tongue.

Infection

Pyrogenium: If infection threatens after an operation.

Tapeworm: See "Worm Infestations"

Teething

Most children begin teething between six and eight months of age, although some take longer. Symptoms include insomnia, extreme irritability, inflammation of the gums, refusal to eat, a desire to bite things, diarrhea, and low-grade fevers.

***Chamomilla:** First choice. Child is irritable, angry, restless, impossible to placate, and wants to be carried. One cheek is red, the other pale. Hot and thirsty. Green diarrhea. Convulsions.

***Belladonna:** Face red and hot, eyes red. Moaning. Worse from light, noise, and touch. Sometimes there are convulsions.

***Coffea:** Wide awake and can't sleep. Better from cold water in the mouth.

***Kreosotum:** Pain becomes worse during the night. Gums swollen and filled with dark fluid. Teeth decay soon after they appear. Restless. Constipation or diarrhea with undigested food.

Magnesia phosphorica: Convulsions from teething. Diarrhea. Better from warmth.

Aconite: Very fearful, restless, and thirsty. Head hot, gums hot, bites his fingers. Fever.

Silica: Slow dentition in thin children with large heads. Chilly. Offensive foot sweats. Constipation.

Calcarea carbonica: Profuse perspiration on the head especially during sleep. Pudgy children with large heads. Slow dentition.

Calcarea phosphorica: Slow dentition in pale, thin children with thin necks. Intolerance of milk. Diarrhea. Worse from cold and drafts.

Podophyllum: Foul-smelling diarrhea, which gushes out. Worse in the early morning.

Cypripedium: Insomnia from teething. Laughs and plays all night.

Apis: Brain symptoms from teething. Child cries out with a shriek during sleep. Skin itches. Burning, stinging pains, which are better from cold. Little or no thirst.

Rheum: Child smells sour and is also angry and restless.

Mercurius sol (or vivus): Much saliva and may drool. Foul breath. Perspires freely and feels worse afterward. Worse at night and from the warmth of the bed.

Tetanus

Tetanus is caused by a neurotoxin that prevents muscles from relaxing. The muscles go into powerful spasm. The source of the toxin is a bacteria (*Clostridium tetani*), which enters the body through a wound. Muscles near the wound may go into spasm. Subsequently, there is stiffness of the jaw and neck. The jaw becomes rigid and there is difficulty swallowing. Painful muscle spasms of the back, arms, legs, and face occur. There is very high fever, thirst, and a wild, excited expression with a fixed smile and elevated eyebrows. Patients may be sensitive to the slightest jar, noise, or draft, which triggers painful convulsions with much perspiration.

Prevention

Ledum: Use 30c every twelve hours, or Ledum 200c once a day for two days followed by Hypericum.

Hypericum: Use 30–200c as needed.

Magnesia phosphorica is another option.

Remedies for Tetanus

Hypericum: Extreme pain at the site of the wound.

Aconite (30–200c)**:** Great fear with numbness and tingling.

Belladonna: Flushed face, delirious with wild-eyed look. Rapid onset of symptoms. Worse from noise, draft, or the slightest jar.

Passiflora tincture: Use undiluted, ten drops two to three times a day. Stiff neck and shoulders, difficulty swallowing, face twisted into a smile.

Nux vomica: Patient is conscious, with the face distorted and the body bent backward. Spasms triggered by light, noise, or touch. Very chilly.

Stramonium: Convulsions triggered by seeing any shiny object. Grinding of teeth, trembling hands, terror.

Hydrocyanic acid: Difficulty breathing, chest tight, feeling of suffocation. Lips and skin blue. Frothing at the mouth, jaws clenched, body bent backward, and face distorted.

Camphora (tincture to 6x)**:** Freezing coldness of the whole body, but refuses covers. Corners of the mouth drawn up showing teeth.

Note: Keep Camphor tincture well away from other remedies, as its vapor can antidote them if they are exposed to it.

Cuprum metallicum: Hands contracted, thumbs drawn in, frothing at the mouth. Limbs jerking, great nausea. Face and lips blue, jaws contracted, loss of consciousness.

Lachesis: Symptoms come on after sleep. Throat feels like it's closing. Patient can't bear anything touching the throat. Extremely talkative in the early stages. Face blue. The wound looks purple.

Veratrum album: A near-collapse state. Cold sweat on the forehead, hands and feet curled inward, patient can't breathe.

Tick Bite: See "Lyme Disease"

Tonsillectomy

Arnica: A few doses before the operation.

Calendula (12c or 30c)**:** After the operation. If Calendula is not available, use Arnica 30c or 200c. Also, Calendula tincture diluted six drops in a half cup of water as a gargle.

Tonsillitis

The tonsils are actually lymph nodes that normally remove bacteria from the blood. During periods of infection they become overloaded and inflamed. Symptoms of tonsillitis include sore throat, difficulty swallowing, fever and chills, headache, and changes in the voice.

***Aconite:** Use at the first sign of symptoms. Sudden onset of chill, fever, pain in the throat, tonsils swollen, throat dry. Much anxiety and restlessness.

***Mercurius:** Right-sided or starting on the right. Excess salivation but thirsty. Foul breath. Better from cold drinks. Worse at night and from the warmth of the bed. Tongue is heavily coated and shows the imprint of teeth.

***Hepar sulph:** Pus has formed in the tonsils. There are sticking pains like splinters. The patient is very chilly and worse from any draft. Better from warm drinks. Pain extends to the ears when swallowing (also Phytolacca).

***Lachesis:** Left-sided or starting on the left and moving to the right. Worse from warmth. Swallowing liquids is more painful than solids. Can't bear anything to touch the throat. Throat looks dark or bluish.

***Belladonna:** The right side is more painful. Throat is bright red, the face red and hot. Worse swallowing liquids. It is almost impossible for the patient to eat due to the feeling that the throat is closing.

Apis: Burning, stinging pain, which is worse from warmth and better from cold. The whole throat is swollen, but also the tongue, making it difficult to breathe. No thirst.

Lycopodium: Starts on the right side and may go to the left. Better from warm drinks. Worse from 4 to 8 p.m.

Baryta carbonica: Tonsils inflamed, pus has formed, swallowing is very painful and eating impossible. Can only drink liquids. Glands in the neck are swollen. Feels like there is a plug in the throat. Very chilly.

Phytolacca: Throat pain extends to the ears. There are tiny blisters on the throat, which is dark red. Can only swallow cold drinks because heat causes pain. Throat is very dry.

Silica: Very chilly. Swallowing is impossible. Ulcers on the throat. Pricking sensation in the throat.

Lac caninum: Throat looks shiny. Pain goes from right to left and back again, or vice versa.

Toothache and Dental Work

(See also "Teething")

Dental Work

Arnica: 30c before and 30–200c after.

Hypericum: For pain. May be used before and after *if not using a local anesthetic*. If using a local anesthetic, use Hypericum afterward only. Hypericum protects nerves so well that it could prevent the local anesthetic from working.

Phosphorus: If there is much bleeding or if you tend to bleed a lot from dental work.

Hepar sulph (6x or 6c)**:** To prevent infection after dental work.

Tooth Extraction

Arnica: 30c before the extraction. After, 30–200c for a couple days.

Hypericum: Taken after the extraction for pain, every three or four hours in addition to the Arnica.

Hepar sulph (6x or 6c)**:** To prevent infection.

Pyrogenium: If an infection develops and Hepar is not sufficient.

Dental Abscess

A dental abscess is an infection in the nerve of a tooth. It can occur from tooth decay or an injury. There is usually intense pain with throbbing, which is worse from lying down.

Belladonna: In the beginning of an abscess with throbbing and redness.

Hepar sulph (6c)**:** Pus-filled pocket or root canal. Painful to touch and worse from cold.

Mercurius: Foul breath, bad taste in the mouth and excess saliva.

Myristica seb (6c)**:** (Not to be confused with Myrica.) If Hepar and Mercurius fail.

Silica: After abscess has drained a bit, this helps finish the process.

> **Note:** Hepar, Mercurius, and Myristica help bring the abscess to a head and drain by itself. With these remedies it may not be necessary to lance the abscess. Once the abscess is draining, rinse the mouth with warm to hot salt water every two hours.

Toothache—Dry Socket

Inflammation of the bone beneath the extraction. A part of the healing process is formation of a blood clot in the socket where the tooth was. If this fails to occur or the clot is dislodged, there will be a dull, throbbing pain. It may extend to the ear and be accompanied by a bad taste in the mouth. This typically occurs several days after the extraction.

***Ruta graveolens.**

Coffea cruda: If pain is unbearable but feels better from cold water.

Toothache

Plantago (6c every 15 minutes)**:** If there is an open cavity, then Plantago tincture placed in the cavity will help.

Chamomilla: The pain is unbearable, and the patient is angry and feels hot.

Coffea: If the pain is better from ice water. The mind won't shut down and the individual is unable to sleep.

Pulsatilla: Desires sympathy and weeps from pain. Craves fresh air and feels worse in a stuffy, warm room. The pain feels better from cold water.

Hepar sulph (6x or 6c)**:** The pain is worse from the slightest touch, cold, or draft. Inflammation of the root. Gums may be swollen. Hepar sulph is excellent for root canal problems.

Mercurius sol (or Mercurius vivus)**:** Excess saliva and bad breath. Tongue shows the imprint of teeth. The inflammation may be at the root. Pulsating pain, worse at night, worse from hot or cold and when eating.

Kreosotum: Teeth are decayed. Spongy gums. Toothache especially in the upper molars. Better from warmth. Irritable. Children needing this remedy often want to be carried.

Staphysagria: Pain extends to the eyes. Worse from cold, touch, warm drinks, and during menses. Feelings of suppressed anger.

Hypericum: Pain after a tooth extraction.

Cheirianthus: Wisdom teeth coming in.

Travel Sickness: See "Motion Sickness"

Tuberculosis

Tuberculosis is a contagious disease caused by *Mycobacterium tuberculosis*. It is spread by breathing in infected droplets or by eating infected food. It most often affects the lungs, but may also involve other parts of the body.

Many patients with the initial (acute) stage of pulmonary tuberculosis show no symptoms, except fever and weight loss. Others, particularly children, experience symptoms such as fever, drowsiness, fatigue, and loss of both appetite and weight.

Patients with the chronic phase show fever, fatigue, weight loss, night sweats, morning cough with green-yellow mucus, coughing up blood, chest pain, and difficulty breathing.

The treatment of chronic tuberculosis is beyond the scope of this book. The following are some remedies for the acute phase.

Prevention

Drosera: First choice.

Bacillinum: Best given with professional guidance in 1M potency. *One dose only!*

Some Remedies for Acute Tuberculosis

Arsenicum: Exhaustion from the least effort, extreme anxiety, restlessness and constantly changing position. Thirst for frequent small drinks, chills, burning pains relieved by warmth, diarrhea. Worse from midnight to 3 a.m.

Bryonia: Worse from moving, can't breathe deeply without discomfort, white tongue with vomiting after cough, thirsty for large cold drinks, irritable. Better lying still.

Cinchona: Exhausting perspiration especially when asleep. Sweats as soon as he closes his eyes. Worse from touch, noise, cold, drafts, fruit, or at night. Coughs when taking a deep breath, worse from lying on the left side, worse from moving. Hungry at night. Abdomen bloated with no relief from belching. Mind is active at night.

Silica: Extremely chilly and very thirsty. Perspires easily with foul foot sweats. Tickling cough. Coughs after cold drinks. Foul-smelling pus. Worse from cold air, drafts, uncovering, light, and noise. Better from covering, especially the head. *Note: Do not use Silica for tuberculosis that is inactive or in remission.*

Bacillinum: Fever and wasting. Stimulates the body's defenses against tuberculosis.

Baptisia: Fever, drowsiness, heavy eyelids, falls asleep while being spoken to.

Belladonna: Face red and hot, throbbing sensations, delirium, bores head into the pillow. Worse from noise, light, or being jarred.

Dulcamara: Symptoms worse in cold, damp weather. Very chilly. Better from moving.

Ferrum phos: Face alternately flushed and pale. Symptoms come on gradually. Coughs up blood.

Pulsatilla: Thirstless, feels suffocated in a warm room and craves fresh air. Desires sympathy and company, weeps easily. Cough relieved by sitting up, worse lying on the left side, worse from heat.

Sulphur: Sensations of heat and burning. Burning sensation of the hands and feet. Dry cough. The patient has to sit up to catch his breath. Night sweats. Itching skin, which is worse from warmth. Best given in a single 200c dose and not repeated.

Sanguinaria: Very sensitive to odors. Cheeks are red and hot. Burning sensations. Dry throat with thick mucus. Foul-smelling belching triggered by cough. Cough triggered by tickling in the back of the breastbone. The patient feels uncomfortable lying down and must sit up. Worse lying on the right side, from moving, from touch, and between 2 and 4 p.m.

Cimicifuga: Chilly but wants fresh air. Sore muscles, especially in the neck. Sensitive to drafts and better from covering up. Talkative, gloomy. Dry cough, night sweats. Insomnia.

Typhoid Fever

Typhoid is a bacterial disease contracted by consuming contaminated food or water. Symptoms include sustained fever as high as 104 degrees, slow pulse in spite of high fever, weakness, stomach pains, diarrhea, bloody stools, vomiting, severe headache, chills, and confusion. Sometimes a characteristic rash of flat, quarter-inch rose-colored spots appears on the abdomen or chest. The abdomen is bloated and tender. The face is flushed and the pupils dilated. The fever gets higher every day for seven to ten days. After a few weeks, the fever starts to go down for part of the day.

Prevention

Salmonella typhi (nosode 30c): once a week

Baptisia: If Salmonella nosode is not available.

Avoid contaminated food or water. Boil water or cook food thoroughly.

Remedies for Typhoid Fever

***Baptisia:** Early stages. Rapid onset with high temperature. *Face flushed dark red. Restless, mentally confused, or delirious and imagines his limbs are scattered about the bed. Falls asleep while being spoken to.* Chilliness and soreness of body. Pulse fast and full. Offensive odor to the urine, sweat, and stool. Tongue dry with a brown stripe down the center. Lips and teeth are covered in brown crusts.

***Pyrogenium:** *Bed feels too hard.* Restless. *High pulse with low temperature or the reverse.* Foul diarrhea. Better from motion. Profuse perspiration, which does not lower body temperature.

***Rhus tox:** Low fever, *anxious, restless and keeps changing position* (also Arsenicum), *weakness, stiff neck, painful stiffness in the arms and legs.* Dizzy when closing the eyes, coughs up bloody material. Heavily coated tongue, lips covered with brown crusts, tongue is red or has a red triangle at the tip. Refuses all food. Despairing. Fears being approached. Dreams of great exertion. Worse from cold, worse after midnight, when first beginning to move, and from getting wet. Better from warmth and changing position.

***Arsenicum album:** Useful in the second or third week. *Anxious, afraid of death, restless with constant changing of position, thirsty for frequent small sips, and extremely exhausted.* Red tongue, foul diarrhea. Tongue is dry and dark. Very cold with cold sweat, but many burning sensations. Burning inside the veins, stomach, and abdomen, yet the patient craves hot drinks. Inside and outside of the mouth are covered with foul, black crusts. Bleeding ulcers in the mouth. Worse from midnight to 3 a.m., when alone, and from cold. Better from warmth.

***Belladonna:** *Delirium with screaming* and attempts to escape from the bed. *Face red and hot*, pupils dilated. Tongue swollen and red. Heavy snoring with twitching of the limbs. Worse from noise, lights, and jarring

***Bryonia:** Comes on slowly. Low fever. *Worse from any movement.* Sharp pains in the chest. Better from lying on the painful side. The patient lies very still, in delirium asks to go home, talks about business. Irritable if disturbed, and thirsty for large, cold drinks. Tongue white with a bitter taste in the mouth. Faints when sitting up.

Phosphoric acid: *Almost too exhausted to speak. Gives one word answers.* Very chilly. Craves fruit, juicy things, or cold drinks. Passes great quantities of clear urine at night. Profuse perspiration, incontinence of the bowels and bladder. Crushing headache on top of the head.

Gelsemium: Early stage. *Eyelids droop, limbs feel heavy, drowsy, looks intoxicated.* Chill goes up the spine, wants to lie perfectly still, trembles. Weakness and tremors. No thirst.

Lachesis: *Worse after sleep*, tendency to *hemorrhage of dark blood*, worse from touch. *Can't bear tight clothing around the neck or waist.* Pain in the shin bones. Tongue trembles. May be very talkative. Suspicious and thinks he is being poisoned.

Hyoscyamus: *Incoherent muttering.* Aversion to drinks. *Mindless picking at the face, clothes, or sheets.* Thinks he is possessed by a devil.

Stramonium: *Looks frightened and wants company and light.* Pupils dilated, eyes half-closed. Black diarrhea. Delirious with biting, scratching, or lewd language. Convulsions.

Echinacea: Use as a tincture, forty drops per dose. Gums bleed easily, tongue and lips tingle. Foul-smelling discharge from the nose, cracks at corners of the mouth, and aching in the limbs. The throat is dark, and the tongue is like raw beef. Headache with flushing of the head and neck.

Phosphorus: *If pneumonia threatens.* Abdomen bloated and sensitive to touch. Worse lying on the left side. Bloody stools of bright red blood. *Burning thirst for ice-cold water.* Fearful when alone. Better from company and reassurance. Sensitive to odors, sounds, and lights.

Sulphur: When well-indicated remedies are not working. Fever goes up and down. Feet feel hot. Mouth is dry and cracked. Worse from heat and at 11 a.m.

Crotalus horridus: Dark hemorrhages that won't coagulate but exude from any orifice. Skin is yellow, cold, and dry. Patient looks intoxicated. Tongue is fiery red. Symptoms come on fast.

Carbo veg: *In the last stages with collapse. Craves air and wants to be fanned.* Head is warm, but breath is cool. Hands and feet icy cold. Face pale to blue. Cold sweat. Dark hemorrhages.

Ipecacuanha: *With nosebleeds and bloody stools of bright red blood.* Nausea with clean tongue.

Hamamelis: *With nosebleeds and bloody stools of dark blood.*

Muriatic acid: Suffers extreme physical weakness but is mentally alert. *Slides down in bed from weakness.* Passes stool while urinating. Lower jaw drops. Worse lying on the right side.

Cinchona: Administer 30c every six hours for debility after symptoms improve.

Typhus

Typhus is an acute contagious disease, transmitted by body lice and ticks. Symptoms include sudden onset of severe headache, pain in the back and limbs, and extreme weakness. The fever rises to 105 degrees in a few days and stays there. The pulse is rapid and weak. The tongue is coated and rolled up in the back of the mouth. *The patient exhibits bluish spots on his abdomen, which do not disappear with pressure. The pupils are contracted.* Stupor and delirium follow.

Prevention

Baptisia or **Rhus tox**.

Remedies for Typhus

***Rhus tox:** Restless, extremely chilly, thirsty for cold drinks. Muscle or joint pain, which is worse after rest, from cold, and at night. Anxious at night. Cheeks dark red. Tongue red and dry with a red triangle at the tip. During delirium, the patient answers questions slowly. Dreams of great exertion.

***Baptisia:** Appears intoxicated. Great weakness. Face hot and flushed. Falls asleep while being spoken to. Eyelids droop (also Gelsemium). Confused as if drunk. Body feels sore, especially the parts lain on. Offensive stools. Delusion that his body is scattered over the bed. Dull headache, frightful dreams. Tongue is brown in the center, with red edges. Ulcers in the mouth. Thirst for large drinks.

***Arsenicum:** Extreme anxiety, fear of death. Restlessness, thirst for small sips, great exhaustion. Pale face, sunken eyes, diarrhea, burning pains that are better from warmth, dry lips. Tongue is black to brown, the chest feels heavy, and breathing is difficult. Skin burning hot with small red marks. Fear of being alone.

***Phosphorus:** When the ailment goes to the heart or lungs. Difficulty breathing, pain in the lungs, coughs up rust-colored or bright red-streaked mucus. Pneumonia. Worse lying on the left side. Must lie on the right side. Pain in the arms and legs. Profuse night sweats. Burning pains. Flushes of heat to the face. Craves ice-cold drinks, which may be vomited shortly after drinking. Afraid to be alone or in the dark. Do not repeat the remedy too often.

***Mercurius:** Lymph glands swollen, excess saliva, tongue flabby with the imprint of teeth, foul breath. Profuse perspiration (which gives no relief), intense thirst, blood-streaked stools, chilly. Worse from the heat of the bed and at night.

Lachesis: Worse after sleep, tendency to hemorrhage of dark blood. Worse from light touch, can't bear the pressure of clothing around the neck or waist, tongue trembles. May be very talkative. Suspicious and thinks he is being poisoned. Semicomatose.

Bryonia: Worse from any movement, lies very still, in delirium asks to go home, talks about business. Irritable if disturbed, and thirsty for large, cold drinks. Tongue is white with a bitter taste in the mouth. Dry cough with stitching pains in the chest. Faints when sitting up.

Belladonna: Delirious with biting, striking, or spitting. Face red and hot, pupils dilated, dry cough at night, head throbbing. Incontinence of the bowels and bladder.

Ulcers of the Skin

Ulcers have numerous causes, including injury, irritating chemicals, exposure to cold or heat, circulatory problems, and bacterial or fungal infections. The following are some important remedies for ulceration of the skin.

Arsenicum: The patient is anxious, chilly, restless, and thirsty for sips of water. The ulcer has intense, burning pain (like fire), which is better from warmth. There is a foul, thin, greenish-yellow discharge. The ulcer has elevated margins, grows larger, and sometimes feels cold.

Carbo veg: The patient is chilly, yet craves fresh air and wants to be fanned. He may have bloating of the abdomen with belching. The ulcer can be painless or have burning pain. The ulcer may bleed and have a foul odor. Ulcers in folds of the skin.

Hepar sulph: The patient is irritable, very chilly, and can't get warm. The pain of the ulcer is made worse from cold, drafts, or the slightest touch. The pains often feel like splinters (also Nitric acid). The ulcer is surrounded by pus-filled pimples. It bleeds easily if touched and discharges pus, which smells like old cheese.

Lachesis: The patient is worse from heat, and after sleeping. He can't stand the pressure of tight clothing, especially around his neck. The ulcer has a purple discoloration. It is painful, has a dark margin, and is sensitive to touch.

Mercurius corrosivus: Very red and deep ulcers, discharging corrosive watery pus. It grows larger while penetrating and disintegrating tissues. The patient sweats profusely at night. He has cold, clammy skin yet is worse from warmth.

Nitric acid: Brown foul discharge, splinterlike pain (also Hepar), bleeds when touched. Burning, stinging pain, which is worse at night. Flat ulcers with raised, jagged edges. Thin, bloody discharge. The patient is chilly and worse from cold and from touch. He is anxious, complains, and is irritable in the morning.

Silica: Cold feeling in ulcer, or burning, stinging pain. Brownish discharge. Better from warmth. The ulcer takes a long time to heal. The patient is pale and thin with cold, clammy feet and hands. Offensive foot perspiration. Sensitive to noise, drafts, and cold. Better from warmth. Very thirsty.

Anthracinum: Horrible burning pains, and a thin, brownish discharge. The lesion is blue or black. The patient is restless, exhausted, and may sense his own death.

Fluoric acid: Painful, worse from warmth and better from bathing with cold water. Worse at night and better in the daytime. The patient can't stand a warm room, is better from a short nap, and craves spicy food.

Mezereum: Thick, yellowish-white crusts with dense yellow pus underneath. The ulcer itches and has a shiny, glazed look. Pimples around the ulcer itch and burn. Worse at night and when touched. The patient is chilly, but the ulcer is worse from warmth. He is anxious when alone and desires company. Feels anxiety in his stomach. Craves fat.

Pulsatilla: Burning like hot coals in the ulcer. Itching and stinging. Ulcers have hard red borders. Discharge of greenish yellow pus. Better from cool air and cool bathing. The patient craves fresh air. He weeps and desires sympathy. Little or no thirst.

Causticum: Ulcers that bleed and discharge green or gray fluid, which corrodes surrounding tissue. Spreads itself rapidly. Burning pain. The patient feels better from sips of cold water and craves smoked foods.

Some Distinguishing Features of Skin Ulcers

Black ulcers: Arsenicum, Lachesis, Carbo veg, Anthracinum, Silica.

Surrounded by pimples: Arsenicum, Carbo veg, Hepar, Lachesis, Mezereum.

Varicose veins, ulceration of: Pulsatilla, Causticum, Arsenicum, Carbo veg, Lachesis, Silica.

Ulcers of the Stomach

Symptoms of a stomach ulcer include abdominal pain, nausea, vomiting (sometimes blood), bloody or black stools, fatigue, and weight loss.

Argentum nitricum: Vomiting blood. Pain right after eating. For people who desire a cool environment with fresh air and who are worse from heat. Craves sweets, which make him belch. Anxious, hurried, and impulsive. Phobias.

Lachesis: The patient feels worse after sleep and from heat. Can't bear anything tight around the neck. Intense and very talkative. Better right after eating, or everything disagrees. Craves coffee, alcohol, wine, or oysters.

Rhus tox: Anxious, chilly, restless, and thirsty. Craves milk. Worse from cold drinks and at night. Better from warmth and motion. Pain relieved by lying on the abdomen (also Acetic acid). Stomach distended after eating.

Natrum muriaticum: Craves salty food. Sweats while eating. Skin oily. Better from fresh air, fasting, tight clothing (opposite Lachesis), lying on the right side. Mouth and lips are dry with a deep crack in the middle of the lower lip. Worse from company and consolation.

Acetic acid: Gnawing pain, bloating of the stomach, vomiting food and blood. Burning pain better from lying on the stomach. The patient may be thin, weak, and wasting. Bloody diarrhea. Excess salivation. Cold sweat on the forehead. Food ferments in the stomach.

Magnesia carbonica: Bitter vomiting. Thin green stools. Can't digest milk and vomits it. Better walking about. Worse from rest, milk, drafts, night, or a change of weather. Can't stand quarreling.

Magnesium muriatica: Worse lying on the right side, in a warm room, or from milk (also Magnesia carbonica). Chilly but craves fresh air. Anxiety at bedtime. Worse from fat and salt. Can't stand quarreling (also Mag carb).

Uremia

Uremia is a condition due to buildup in the blood of waste products from renal insufficiency. Any condition that reduces blood flow to the kidneys may result in uremia. Symptoms include weakness, loss of alertness, loss of appetite, nausea, vomiting, bad taste in the mouth, foul breath, and yellowish-brown discoloration of the skin. See also "Nephritis," "Urine Retention," and "Urination—Painful."

Terebinthina oleum: The patient feels very cold with burning sensations. Pain causes him to urinate. Urine has the odor of violets. Burning pain in the kidneys extending to the bladder. Urine is smoke-colored, thick, and slimy. Bloody urine. Coughs up mucus. Worse from cold, pressure, while urinating, and at night.

Belladonna: Sudden and violent onset. Dark and cloudy urine. Pain extending from the kidney to the bladder. Sensation of burning and heat. Worse from touch, noise, light, being jarred, and cold drafts. Pains come and go quickly. Craves lemonade. Convulsions.

Cantharis: Flushed face. Violent, sharp, burning pains in kidney area. Kidney area is sensitive to touch. Pain before, during, and after urination. Worse after drinking cold water or coffee. Better from warmth, rubbing, and cold. Restless and excitable, with furious delirium. Worse from being approached or touched. Shreddy burning stools.

Helleborus niger: Slow in answering questions. Unconscious. Sighs involuntarily. Picks at his lips and clothes. Abdomen distended. Moaning and rolling the head from side to side. Bores his head into the pillow. Horrible smell from the mouth. Lower jaw falls. Muscles twitch, and the patient cries out in his sleep. Better from warmth and lying down.

Urtica urens: Body smells like urine. Itching skin. Uremia occurring after burns or from eating shellfish. Better lying down. Worse from touch.

Plumbum: Coma, pale face, cheeks sunken, respiration slow. The patient feels like his abdomen is drawn to his spine by a string. Pupils contracted. Chilly and worse from cold.

Urine, Retention of

There are numerous causes of an inability to urinate, including inflamed prostate, spasms, paralysis of the bladder, infections, and growths.

*__Arnica:__ After injuries or overexertion. Also associated with dysentery. Painful retention.

*__Apis:__ Associated with edema, total lack of thirst, drowsiness or coma, and burning, stinging pains relieved by cold. Brightly colored urine. Kidney problems, enlarged prostate. Worse from heat, touch, or after sleeping.

*__Arsenicum:__ Anxious, restless, chilly, exhausted, and thirsty for small sips. Burning pains paradoxically relieved by heat. May occur without any urging to pass urine. Better from warmth.

*__Cantharis:__ Urine (sometimes bloody) is passed by drops with a painful burning sensation. Painful urging to urinate with spasms. Scalding pain on urination. Worse from touch, and from drinking cold water or coffee. Burning thirst but aversion to fluids.

***Terebinthina:** Bright-colored or bloody urine passed in drops with sharp pain. Due to spasm of the urethra or bladder. Better from motion. Urine smells like violets.

***Belladonna:** Sudden intense onset. Throbbing or cutting pains and sensation of heat. Dark, cloudy, or bloody urine. From paralysis of the bladder or acute infections. Mentally agitated. Worse from light, noise, being jarred, drafts, cold, or company.

***Aconite:** After exposure to cold or from fevers, especially in children. Sudden violent onset.

***Nux vomica:** Painful urging without effect. Chilly, irritable, angry, hypersensitive to noise, lights, and odors. Constipated with urging. Craves spicy food, stimulants, or fats. Worse in the morning, from cold, uncovering, or the pressure of clothes.

Opium: After a fright. Also helpful in nursing children and after operations. Drowsy, hot perspiration, burning thirst but no appetite.

Causticum: Retention of urine after labor or surgical operations. Also after burns to the skin or tissue. Easier to pass urine when sitting. Burning pain during urination.

Conium: Hot urine, which stops and starts. Must stand to pass urine. Perspires during sleep. After injuries to the spine. Inflamed prostate. Craves salt, sour foods, or coffee. Aversion to company.

Gelsemium: After fright. Slow onset. Little or no thirst. Faced flushed. Limbs feel heavy. Drowsy, eyelids droop. Trembling.

Lycopodium: Right-sided pains. Sediment in urine looks like red sand. Must strain, cries out before passing urine. Worse from 4 to 8 p.m. Better from moving, warm food or drink, being uncovered, or cold application. Worse from being in a warm room or the pressure of clothes.

Pareira brav: Constant urging and straining with pain going down the thighs. Must get on hands and knees and press head to floor to pass urine. Urination painful. Urine smells of ammonia.

Rhus tox: After exertion or exposure to damp, cold weather. Restless and thirsty.

Plumbum: Sense of a string pulling the spine to the abdomen. Abdomen drawn in. Constipation with hard black stools. Better from hard pressure and rubbing. Foul belching. Vomits brown liquid or fecal matter. Very chilly and better from warmth.

Hyoscyamus: Very talkative or silent, fumbling with the hands and picking at the face and clothes. Twitching muscles. Worse from touch, cold, or lying down.

Veratrum album: During cholera. Exhaustion, freezing cold, diarrhea, cold sweat on forehead.

Vaccination, Treating the Effects of

(See also chapter 7, "Preventing Illness with Homeopathy," to learn about the use of homeopathic remedies as a safe, effective alternative to vaccination)

Thousands of people have reported adverse reactions to vaccination, including liver damage, encephalitis, immune suppression, mental retardation, paralysis, epilepsy, asthma, seizures, autism, sudden infant death syndrome, learning disabilities, brain damage, and death.

The United States government's National Vaccine Injury Compensation Program has paid out over $724.4 million for people injured or killed by vaccines. However, the problem is much larger than even that figure suggests. The FDA estimates that only 10% of vaccine adverse reactions are reported. Further, these reports only represent the immediate effects. Delayed and long-term effects are not even considered. Insurance companies know which side of this controversy to bet on—they refuse to cover vaccine adverse reactions.

A physician friend of mine vaccinated his own healthy infant some years ago. The child became severely retarded shortly thereafter. For him and for thousands of other people, the debate about the safety of vaccines has been settled.

In the midst of all this, there are still no long-term studies on the safety of vaccines. There is evidence, however, which shows that vaccines have limited effectiveness. Whole populations have come down with the very illness for which they were vaccinated.

In the United States, hepatitis B vaccine is being given to infants a day or two after birth. Considering that this disease is spread by intravenous drug use and promiscuous sex, one wonders about the fervor to vaccinate infants.

In France, fifteen thousand people have sued the government over adverse effects from hepatitis B vaccine, including neonatal deaths, neurological damage, and autoimmune disease. Hepatitis B vaccination for school children has been discontinued.

To vaccinate or not is a personal decision. In making that decision, one should realize that vaccination is not without risk. Nor does it offer absolute protection. There are, however, alternatives.

The Role of Homeopathy in Immunization

Homeopathy has two roles here. First, remedies given just before vaccination may reduce the risk of side effects. Remedies administered after vaccination can help prevent and sometimes cure illnesses resulting from vaccination.

Secondly, homeopathic remedies can be used in place of vaccines as a safe and effective alternative. Over the last two hundred years, homeopathy has proven itself effective in preventing illness during epidemics.

Prior to Vaccination

Ledum: A dose or two followed by a dose of **Hypericum** may prevent side effects.

Thuja: One dose is another option.

Immediate, Delayed, and Long-Term Side Effects of Vaccination

***Thuja:** Top remedy for effects of vaccination and allergy shots. Usually one or two doses will be sufficient. Thuja should not be repeated frequently. Stomach pain, cough, eye inflammation, paralysis of lower limbs, asthma, mental changes, warts, and insomnia. Thuja may help virtually any ailment that develops after vaccination.

***Silica:** Convulsions, backache, diarrhea, nausea, weakness, listlessness, chilliness, abscesses, asthma, swelling at site of injection.

Antimonium tartaricum: Asthma attack with thick mucus and rattling in the chest.

Kali muriaticum: Gray coating at the back of the tongue, swollen lymph glands, thick white discharge from mucous membranes, eczema, or blisters on the skin filled with thick white fluid. Silica follows well.

Homeopath Dr. Tinus Smits recommends using homeopathic doses of the offending vaccine. He states that this has helped patients even years after the vaccination. He recommends using a 200c potency prior to vaccination. For effects after vaccination, he suggests that a 30c be tried first. A succession of higher potencies is also used.

For instance, if the offending vaccine was hepatitis B, then a homeopathic remedy "hepatitis B vaccine 30c" would be used. Because it is made from the vaccine, the remedy will be homeopathic to the disease portion of the vaccine as well as the additives (e.g., formaldehyde, aluminum). Remedies made from vaccines are available from some homeopathic pharmacies.

Dogs and Cats—Vaccination Effects

Dogs and cats are also subject to side effects from vaccination. The remedies are equally effective for them.

Silica: If there is listlessness and loss of appetite immediately after the vaccination.

Thuja: For any other symptoms and to prevent any long-term adverse effects of the vaccination. Just one or two doses.

Vomiting

(See also "Motion Sickness," as well as "Morning Sickness" in chapter 6)

Note: For weakness from loss of fluids, use **Cinchona**.

***Ipecacuanha:** Nausea not relieved by vomiting. Clean tongue (not coated). Patient has excess saliva and may drool. Cough with nausea. Worse from motion. Sometimes with diarrhea. Vomits food, mucus, bile, or blood. Very anxious.

***Antimonium crudum:** Heavy white coating on the tongue. Nausea right after eating or drinking. Worse from eating fats, pastries. Worse from being touched or looked at. Better from lying down and from warmth.

***Antimonium tartaricum:** Nausea, retching, vomiting, and deathly faintness. Thick, white coating on the tongue. Craves small, frequent sips of cold water. Fear from nausea. Fear of being alone. Must lie on the right side to avoid vomiting. Thick mucus rattling in the chest.

***Nux vomica:** Tongue coated in back. Feels like a stone is inside the stomach. Constipated and strains at stool. Very chilly and better from warmth. Hypersensitive to noise, odors, lights, or criticism. Anxious, irritable, and angry. Worse from overeating, spices, coffee, alcohol, or drugs. Worse in the morning in bed. Sometimes unable to vomit.

***Iris versicolor:** Vomiting very sour material that burns the throat. Feeling of heat inside. Vomits bile. Nausea with headache or alternating with headache. Worse after exertion. Lots of thick, stringy saliva. Worse from sweets and milk.

***Tabacum:** Constant nausea, which is worse from moving and opening the eyes. Wants to uncover his abdomen, which decreases the symptoms. Better from fresh air. Watery diarrhea, weakness, and cold sweat accompany the nausea and vomiting. Worse from the odor of tobacco.

Phosphorus: Craves cold drinks, which are vomited when they become warm in the stomach. Vomits food by the mouthful. Worse from warm food and lying on the left side. Sensitive to light, odors, and sounds. Desires company. Burning in the stomach extending to the throat and bowels. Better from a short nap.

Cadmium sulphuricum: Intense nausea and retching with black vomit. Everything eaten is vomited. If anything touches the lips, it triggers vomiting. Burning pain in stomach. Desires sips of cold water, which also stimulate vomiting. Includes vomiting from cancer, chemotherapy, and radiation poisoning.

Argentum nitricum: Vomits sticky mucus. Much belching with bloating of the stomach. Burning pain. Pain that radiates from a point in the stomach. Green diarrhea like chopped spinach. Worse from warmth, sweets, at night. Better from cold. Very anxious.

Colchicum: Nausea on looking at, smelling, or even thinking about food. Worse from motion, cold, strong odors, bright light, and touch. Wants to lie perfectly still. Chilly. Discouraged.

Pulsatilla: Worse from eating fatty or rich food. Worse in a warm room and craves fresh air. Desires sympathy and may weep describing the pain. No thirst. Vomits food long after it was eaten. Sensation as if there is a stone in the stomach.

Bryonia: Worse from the least motion and lies perfectly still. Dry mouth with dry, cracked lips. Thirst for large, cold drinks. Worse from warm drinks. Nausea and faintness when rising up. Stomach sensitive to touch. Sensation as if there is a stone in the stomach.

Crotalus horridus: Abdomen hot and tender. Can't bear clothing around the stomach. Vomits food, bile, and blood. Black or coffee-ground vomit. Can't lie on the right side. Bleeds dark blood from any orifice. Bloody sweat. Worse after sleep. Hypersensitive to light. Eyes yellow.

Arsenicum album: Burning pains, sometimes like hot coals, which are oddly relieved by heat. Chilly, terribly anxious, and exhausted. Wants frequent sips of water. Fears death or serious illness. Foul-smelling vomit and diarrhea. Can't stand the sight or smell of food. Vomits blood, bile, or green mucus. Exhausted by the least effort. Worse after midnight.

Veratrum album: Violent retching and forcible vomiting. Freezing cold with cold sweat on the forehead. Thirst for cold water, which is vomited immediately after drinking. Copious, painful, watery diarrhea. Worse from drinking or moving.

Cocculus: Nausea from riding in cars or boats, or from watching moving objects. Most patients will be averse to food or drink, but some may crave cold drinks. Worse when cold. Profuse salivation. Worse from loss of sleep and the odor of food. Aversion to fresh air (opposite Tabacum).

Cinchona: Weakness after vomiting, diarrhea, and other loss of fluids. Yellow, painless diarrhea. Vomits undigested food. Worse from the slightest touch, or after eating. Abdomen bloated. Cold feeling in abdomen after drinking. Profuse perspiration at night. Chilly and worse from cold.

West Nile Virus

West Nile virus is spread to both people and animals by an infected mosquito. Most people exhibit only mild symptoms or none at all. Rarely, West Nile virus can result in a serious and sometimes fatal illness known as West Nile encephalitis.

West Nile virus may present as flu-like symptoms such as fever, chills, and muscle and joint pain. It may also evolve to a more serious stage with incoordination, staggering, convulsions, pneumonia, kidney failure, heart failure, rapid loss of weight, and death. There is no specific conventional therapy and treatment is symptomatic.

Prevention

Prevention may be attempted with the **West Nile virus** nosode (30c). If that is not available, then:

Ledum: As soon as possible after any suspect mosquito bite. Every four hours for three or four doses.

If the Ailment Develops

If it presents as flu-like symptoms, see the remedies under "Flu." If it presents as the more serious encephalitis, see the remedies under "Encephalitis."

Whooping Cough—Pertussis

Pertussis is a very contagious bacterial disease characterized by a spasmodic cough ending in a high pitched "whoop." It starts out very much like a cold. In the next stage (after ten to twelve days), the patient coughs five to fifteen times in rapid succession, followed by a deep inspiration sounding like "whoop." This pattern is repeated over and over. Large amounts of sticky mucus are coughed up, sometimes resulting in vomiting. There is usually a low-grade fever. The infection normally lasts about six weeks, although coughing may continue for months.

Prevention

Pertussin (nosode 30c).

Drosera: Use 6c twice per day if Pertussin is not available.

Remedies for Whooping Cough

***Pertussin** (nosode 30c)**:** Give this initially, one dose. It may prevent the disease from progressing further.

***Drosera:** This is almost a specific for whooping cough. Give in 30c potency every fourth day. Barking cough, vomiting, bleeding (nose, throat, etc.).

Antimonium tart: Rattling in the chest. Sticky mucus that can't be coughed up. Feels like he's choking. Vomits mucus and food.

Carbo veg: Greenish-yellow mucus. Short of breath, wants to be fanned. The head is warm but hands and feet are freezing cold. Face is pale. Belching.

Cuprum: Cough with convulsions. Lips blue, frothing at the mouth, vomiting bile. Spasms that begin in the fingers and toes. Body becomes rigid. Cough worse after eating solid food.

Phosphorus: Tickling in the chest incites hacking cough. Mucus is white or rust-colored to bright red. Hoarseness and sometimes loss of voice. Burning in the chest. Cold sweat at night. Desires cold drinks. Wants company.

Sanguinaria: Dry, tickling cough, which is relieved by sitting up. Thick, yellow, sweet-tasting mucus. Pain in the chest relieved by passing gas or burping. Diarrhea in the night.

Ipecac: Vomits mucus mixed with blood. Repeated hollow cough leaves the patient out of breath. The body becomes stiff during a coughing spell and the patient turns blue. Tendency to nausea and bleeding. Tongue is clean, with much saliva.

Kali carbonicum: Puffy eyelids. Cough is worse after midnight, especially from 3 to 5 a.m. Worse from cold.

Worm Infestations

Tapeworm

A tapeworm is a flat, parasitic worm that is acquired from eating infected and undercooked beef, pork, or fish. In the beginning of the infestation, symptoms may include diarrhea, abdominal discomfort, gas, vomiting, and weakness. Chronic infestations produce more vague symptoms, such as bloating, water retention, weight loss, and constant hunger. Segments of the worm or its eggs may be found in the stool.

Calcarea carbonica (200c, one dose): If 200c is not available, use Calcarea carb 30c every seven days for three to four weeks.

Natrum muriaticum (200c, one dose): If Calcarea carbonica fails.

Another method of relieving tapeworm: Scald two ounces of pumpkin seeds with boiling water to remove the skin. Crush the green seeds to a paste and give it to your patient. This works best after a one-day fast. Follow this a few hours later with a standard dose of castor oil.

Pork Tapeworm

A more serious infestation giving rise to trichinosis. The larval form of the worm forms cysts.

Silica (6c): Three times a day. This may prevent the formation of cysts.

Bryonia: If cysts form in the muscles, this may relieve the pain.

Hookworm

A type of roundworm that enters the body through the skin, migrates to the lungs (producing a cough), and then to the intestines. Often there are no symptoms, but those that occur may include a raised, itchy red rash, fever, coughing, and abdominal pain. Anemia may develop, which in children can result in slower growth, tissue swelling, and heart failure. The worm's eggs appear in the stool. The condition is usually contracted from walking barefoot in larvae-infected soil.

Cardus marianus (3x)**:** Three times a day for one month.

Calcarea carbonica (200c, one dose)**:** If Cardus marianus fails. If 200c is not available, use Calcarea carbonica 30c every seven days for three to four weeks.

Ascarid (Long Roundworms)

A parasitic worm that grows to fourteen inches. It is acquired from eating infected food.

Abrotanum (3c or 6c)**:** Three times a day for one month. Follow with a few doses of Calcarea carbonica.

Calcarea carbonica: If Abrotanum fails.

Natrum muriaticum: If Abrotanum and Calcarea fail.

Sabadilla: Thirstless. Craves sweets and hot foods.

Threadworms (Pinworms)

Cina: Twice a day for five days.

Spigella: If Cina fails.

Wounds

See also "Wounds—Infected," in this section. The following remedies are useful in reducing pain, preventing tissue damage, preventing infection, and speeding healing.

*__Arnica:__ *Ragged wounds*, cuts and tears with jagged surfaces. *Also bruises.* Blows from blunt objects. After any trauma to the body.

***Staphysagria:** *Wounds made by a sharp object*, leaving a clean cut. Wounds from knives, razors, glass, etc.

***Ledum:** *Puncture wounds*. This includes wounds from needles, nails, and similar objects as well as insect stings. Ledum may help prevent tetanus after puncture wounds. Follow with Hypericum if the wound is very painful.

***Hypericum:** *Wounds that are very painful*, or where the pain shoots up the limb from the injury. For injury to parts rich in nerves, such as fingertips and teeth. Important for injuries to the spine. *May help prevent tetanus in puncture wounds*, which become very painful. It follows Ledum in these cases.

Belladonna: Wounds that are hot, red, and throbbing. Before pus forms. (See "Wounds—Infected.")

Ruta: Sprains, tears, and other *injuries to tendons and bones.*

Symphytum: *Injuries to bones and tendons.* Also, *injuries to the eye* from a blunt object.

Bellis perennis: *Injuries to the breast* and to deeper tissues.

Calendula: Used in 30c potency to speed healing and reduce pain.

Calendula: For external use. The tincture is diluted, one part to eight parts of water and the wound is bathed in this. *Note: This should not be used for very deep wounds that need to drain. It may heal the surface tissue before the deeper layers.*

Phosphorus: Minor wounds that bleed excessively.

Silica: Wounds that are slow to heal, especially in the person who is chilly.

Wounds—Infected

Note: If there is a red line extending up the limb from the wound, see "Lymphangitis." If the skin becomes cold and black or blue, and gives off a foul odor, see "Gangrene."

***Hepar sulph:** *Wound is extremely sensitive to touch, cold, and the slightest draft.* Filled with pus. Sometimes there are splinterlike pains. Odor like old cheese. The patient is better from warmth.

***Lachesis:** *Wounds look purplish, and may have black edges.* The patient is worse from warmth, touch, pressure, and after sleeping. Can't bear tight clothing, especially around the throat. Tendency to bleed dark blood. Sometimes very talkative.

***Apis:** *Stinging, burning pain, which is better from applying cold.* Skin rosy red or bluish and sensitive to touch. The patient has little or no thirst and is worse in a hot room and better from cool air.

***Arsenicum:** *Burning pain, which is better from heat.* The skin is dry and may be have blue or black spots. The patient is very anxious, chilly, restless, and thirsty for frequent small sips. Worse from cold, after midnight, and when alone.

***Anthracinum:** *Terrible burning pains and great weakness.* Foul-smelling discharges. Black or blue blisters. Bleeding of black blood. Anxious with fear of death. Great thirst but difficulty swallowing.

***Pyrogenium:** *With fever. Foul odor to the wound and foul-smelling discharges (breath, stool, sweat, or vomit).* Exhausted but extremely restless. Feels bruised all over. High fever with a slow pulse or low fever with a fast pulse. Patient is better from moving about and warmth. Worse from becoming cold.

Crotalus horridus: Wound may look purplish (also Lachesis). Tendency to bleed thin, dark blood. Patient can't stand tight clothing around the waist. Very sensitive to light, especially from a lamp. Face is yellow. Skin is sensitive on the right side of the body. Tongue scarlet red. Breath smells moldy. Worse after sleep and lying on the right side. Despairing, weeping.

Echinacea angustifolia (tincture, 30- to 40-drop doses)**:** May be used in addition to other remedies. Helps trigger the immune function. Wait a half hour after administering other remedies.

Silica: Pus continues to drain but the infection doesn't end. Patient is chilly.

Yellow Fever

Yellow fever is a viral disease transmitted by a mosquito. It is characterized by sudden onset, fever, slow pulse, vomiting black blood, jaundice, and hemorrhage from the nose and gums. The pulse is initially raised, but is later slower than expected, with a fever. Other symptoms may include flushed face, red tongue, nausea, vomiting, and extreme exhaustion with restlessness. Jaundice occurs after the third day, when the temperature rises to 103–104 degrees. The pulse will be abnormally slow in spite of the high temperature. As the condition proceeds, the patient becomes dull, confused, and may experience delirium, convulsions, and eventually coma. No specific conventional treatment exists.

Prevention

Yellow fever (nosode 30c)**:** once a week, or

Crotalus horridus, or

Arsenicum album: if the other remedies are not available.

Remedies for Yellow Fever—Earlier Stages

Aconite: Earliest stage. Fear of death, high fever, restlessness, and thirst for large drinks. Face is hot and red, pulse is strong.

Belladonna: Face red and hot, pupils dilated, pulse strong, body hot but with cold hands and feet. Frontal headache, delirium.

Bryonia: Worse from the least movement, headache in the back of the head, neck pain. Thirst for large drinks, delirium.

Eupatorium perfoliatum: Deep aching in bones. Restless due to a sore feeling. Thirsty for cold drinks. Chill beginning in the lower back. Very little perspiration.

Ipecacuanha: Nausea and vomiting, nausea after drinking water, nausea not relieved by vomiting. Much salivation with a clear tongue, thirstless, worse from heat.

Lachesis: Worse after sleep, difficulty speaking. Can't stand anything touching his throat, worse lying on the left side, left-sided symptoms.

Dark hemorrhages that don't coagulate, yellow skin. *Also useful in latter stages.*

Remedies for Yellow Fever—Latter Stages

***Carbo veg:** Short of breath, collapses with cold breath, body icy cold, faint pulse. Burning pain in the throat, stomach, and abdomen. Vomits with burning pain after eating.

***Arsenicum album:** Black vomit, great anxiety and restlessness, fear of being alone. Thirst for small sips, chills, burning pains relieved by heat.

***Crotalus:** Face red and swollen, skin yellow, pulse faint, hemorrhages from every orifice. Bloody sweat, black vomit, right-sided symptoms.

***Cadmium sulph:** The patient feels freezing cold. Black vomit with horrible nausea, which is worse from moving. He feels extreme exhaustion and wants to keep quiet. Worse after sleep. Afraid to be alone. Severe insomnia, or sleeps with his eyes open. Awakens suffocating.

***Lachesis:** Worse after sleep and lying on the left side. Difficulty speaking, can't stand anything touching the throat. Left-sided symptoms, dark hemorrhages that don't coagulate. Yellow skin. *Also useful in latter stages.*

***Cantharis:** Suppression of urine, burning pains, slow pulse, and cold sweat on the hands and feet. Burning thirst but aversion to drinking. Fears mirrors, the sound of water, and bright objects.

Cuprum: Convulsions beginning with spasms of the hands and feet. Face cold and blue. Better after perspiring and from drinking cold water. Worse from touch. Craves cold drinks.

Phosphorus: Bright red hemorrhages, great thirst for large drinks, hypersensitivity to light, sound, and odors. Can't bear to be alone. Worse lying on the left side, from warm food, and in the evening. Better from cold food and drink, and lying on the right side. Use Phosphorus if pneumonia threatens.

Cinchona: To regain strength while recovering. Weak, chilly, bloated abdomen, perspires day and night.

4
Organ Remedies

Homeopathic remedies often have an affinity for particular organs. Here are some remedies that strongly affect the heart, lungs, liver, and kidneys.

Heart

Digitalis: *Sensation as if the heart suddenly stopped beating. Palpitation from the least movement.* The patient feels like he must keep very still. Worse from being raised up in bed or lying on the left side.

Convallaria: *The patient feels as if the heart stopped beating and then started suddenly.* Palpitation and irregular heart movements, difficulty breathing while lying down, must sit or stand. Diminished urinary secretion, liver feels "full," edema. Worse lying on the back and in a warm room.

Crataegus: Use in low potency (3x) or tincture every three to four hours for several weeks. Use when the heart is failing steadily, with rapid pulse and difficulty breathing, which is worse from exertion. Blue tinge to the face, swelling of ankles. Almost every case can benefit from the tincture, which acts as a nutrient for the heart.

Aconite: *Intense fear of death, skin hot and dry. Restless, thirsty.* Sudden and intense onset of symptoms.

Cactus grand: *Sensation as if an iron band is around the chest, being drawn tighter.* Pulse fast, but feeble. Worse lying on the left side. Swelling of left hand. Worse at 11 p.m. Dreams of falling.

Spigella: Violent audible palpitation, sharp sticking pains, pressing pains, pain radiates to throat, left arm and shoulder blade. Pain followed by numbness. Pain is worse from the slightest movement. Craves hot water. Foul odor from the mouth.

Naja: *Constricted feeling in the throat and chest. Worse lying on the left side.* Very chilly. Palpitations cause choking and keep the patient from talking. Pain in the heart extending to the nape of the neck and the left shoulder.

Lachesis: Vertigo or palpitation with fainting. The heart feels as if it is too large for the chest, or as if it is constricted by cords. Feeling of pressure in the heart with red face and cold feet. Worse after sleep, and from tight clothing, light touch, and hot drinks. Better from lying on the right side, cold drinks, and fresh air.

Arsenicum: *Tightness in the chest with a burning sensation. Fear of death and being left alone.* Very chilly, restless, and exhausted from the least effort. Better from warmth and covers. Thirsty for frequent small sips. Face pale.

Latrodectus mactans: *Pain extends down the left arm to the fingers* with numbness. The patient screams with pain. Gasps for breath. Skin cold. Constriction in the chest. Worse during and after sleep.

Iodum: *Sensation as if there is a tight band around the heart itself,* as opposed to the whole chest. Face flushed, worse from heat. Patient is usually very thin. Restless and anxious.

Spongia: *Heart feels as if it is getting bigger* and bigger, too large for chest, as if it might burst out. Worse lying down. Chilly and worse from any draft. Numbness in the arm or hand.

Lycopus: *Horrible pounding feeling in the heart with a throbbing feeling in the head and neck.* Worse lying on the right side (opposite Naja / Lachesis). Can't stand the smell of food.

Laurocerasus: *Face looks purple, lips blue, gasping for air. Worse if totally sitting up or lying down.* Best when just reclining. Very cold. Worse from motion.

Lungs

Carbo veg: Patient is hungry for air and wants to be fanned. Skin pale or blue. The head is hot but the body is icy cold. Coughs with burning in the chest. Pulse feeble, fingertips blue. Feet icy cold up to the knees. Abdomen bloated with gas and better from belching.

Antimonium tartaricum: Suffocating from thick mucus, which can be heard rattling in the chest. Unable to cough it up. The patient feels like she must sit up. Burning in the chest and throat. Pulse rapid and weak. Better lying on the right side. Cold sweat on the face. Worse lying down and from warmth. Drowsy. Paralysis of the lungs.

Phosphorus: Afraid to be alone, thirsty for ice-cold drinks, startles easily, sensitive to light, noise, and odors. Can't lie on the left side and is better lying on the right. Coughs up rust-colored sputum or bright red blood, has a burning sensation in the chest, a feeling of weight on the chest, or the chest feels tight. Hard, dry cough that makes the patient tremble. Better after short sleep.

Bryonia: Sharp pains with each breath or from the slightest movement, better lying still on the painful side. Dry cough, rust-colored mucus, thirst for large cold drinks. Great urge to take a deep breath, which is painful. Worse from warmth and motion. Irritable.

Lycopodium: Worse between 4 and 8 p.m. (sometimes 4 and 8 a.m.). Nostrils flare when struggling to breathe. Face pale with a frown. Short dry cough. Salty or bitter-tasting mucus. Much flatulence. Satisfied by a small amount of food. Wakes up irritable or angry. Better from moving, warm food or drink, and belching. Worse from the pressure of clothes and being in a warm room.

Mercurius: Foul odor to breath and perspiration. Excess saliva, great thirst, tongue flabby with the imprint of teeth. Copious perspiration after which the patient feels worse. Blood-streaked, thick green mucus, stabbing pain in the bottom of the right lung. Worse at night and from the warmth of the bed.

Sulphur: When other remedies fail to act, it rouses the "Vital Force." The chest feels heavy, with burning sensations. The patient wants windows open. Worse from the warmth of the bed and from lying on the back. Irritable. Discharges smell foul and irritate the skin. Redness and itching of anus, lips, nose, and eyes. Sudden diarrhea in the morning. Better from fresh air, moving, and lying on the right side. Worse from bathing, being in a warm room or bed, at 11 a.m., standing, and drinking milk.

Arsenicum: Extreme anxiety and restlessness, wants company, worse between midnight and 3 a.m. Thirsty for frequent small sips, exhausted, with burning sensations that are better from heat.

Pulsatilla: Can't stand a closed room, craves cool fresh air even when chilly. The patient is gentle, yielding, and better from sympathy and company. Coughs every time he breathes. The cough is worse when lying down and in the evening. Thick, bland, yellowish-green mucus. Dry mouth but no thirst.

Ipecac: Nausea and vomiting accompany other symptoms. Coughs with every breath. Coughs up blood. Tendency to bleeding. Clean tongue with excess saliva. Better from open air. Worse from the slightest motion and from warmth, especially damp warmth.

Hepar sulph: Very chilly, worse from any draft. Irritable. Discharges are yellow and smell like old cheese. Worse lying on the left side. Coughs when any part of the body is uncovered. Choking cough; has to rise and bend his head backward. Better from heat, and damp weather. Worse from cold, cold food, drafts, or touch.

Kidneys

Apis: No thirst. Pain in the kidneys. Edema of the face and limbs. Passes urine but in small amounts. Worse from heat and better from cold. Puffy under the eyes. Skin is sensitive to touch. Difficulty breathing, which is better from sitting up. Worse from heat, touch, or lying down.

Berberis: Kidneys are sensitive to touch, and worse from moving. Pain with numbness. Burning pain, and a bubbling sensation in the area of the kidneys. Pains that radiate from one point to the back, hips, and legs. Pain and stiffness in the lower back. Frequent, strong urge to urinate. Worse from moving. Dry mouth with sticky saliva.

Phosphorus: Blood in urine. Great thirst for cold drinks. Desires company and fears being alone. Worse lying on the left or painful side. Better after short sleep. Very sensitive to odors, light, or noise. May urinate pure blood.

Natrum sulph: Urination frequent but scanty and dark. Brown, bitter coating on the tongue. Sour vomiting. Very chilly with profuse sweats at night. Loose stools in the morning. Very large stools. Very sensitive to light. Worse in the morning and in damp weather. Skin itches while undressing.

Lycopodium: Abdomen full of gas with much flatulence. Symptoms worse between 4 and 8 p.m. Excessive secretion of urine at night, with red sediment like brick dust. Pain in the back before urinating. Chilly, yet craves open air. Desires warm food or drink. Nostrils flare when trying to get air. Craves sweets.

Equisetum: Kidney pain, especially on the right side, extending to the lower back. Frequent urging with severe pain at the end of urination. Constant urge, passes large volumes of light-colored urine. Urinary retention. Worse on the right side, at end of urination, from pressure, or sitting down. Better from continued motion or lying down.

Terebinthina oleum: Very cold with burning sensations. Pain causes the patient to urinate. Urine has the odor of violets. Burning pain in the kidneys extending to the bladder. Urine is smoke-colored, thick, or slimy. Bloody urine. Coughs up mucus. Worse from cold, at night, from pressure, and when urinating.

Arsenicum: Anxious with a fear of death or being alone, restless. Thirsty for small frequent sips of water, chilly, and exhausted. Craves warmth. Watery diarrhea, and edema of the face. Urine scanty, burning. Urine is sometimes black.

Cantharis: Violent, sharp, burning pains in the kidney area. Kidney area is sensitive to touch. Pain before, during, and after urination. Intense urging to pass urine, which feels hot, scalding. Worse after drinking cold water or coffee. Better from warmth, rubbing, and cold. Restless and excitable, with furious delirium. Worse from being approached or touched.

Solidago: When urine is obstructed or when kidneys malfunction, this may act as the homeopathic "catheter." Kidneys are sensitive to touch and pressure. Pain in the kidneys extending to the abdomen and thighs. Stinking dark urine passed with difficulty.

Liver

Lycopodium: Dull, aching pain in the liver. Worse after eating. Much gas. Feels full after a few bites of food. Desires sweets. Worse between 4 and 8 p.m. Can't stand tight clothes. One foot is cold, the other warm. Fluid in the abdomen from liver ailments.

Natrum sulphuricum: Sharp pains in the liver. Worse lying on the left side, from moving, and in the morning. Vomits bile. Stools are dark green. Diarrhea when first standing. Depressed and dislikes to be spoken to, especially in the morning. Suicidal thoughts.

Nux vomica: Angry, irritable, oversensitive to noise, odors, and light. Very chilly. Dislikes the pressure of clothing. Liver enlarged and hard. Wakes between 3 and 4 a.m. Constipation with straining.

Phosphorus: Unquenchable thirst for cold drinks, a tendency to hemorrhage of bright red blood, perspiration during sleep. Fear of being alone, worse lying on the left side, burning sensations. Desires company. Very sensitive to odors, lights, or noises. Startles easily.

Bryonia: Lies very still and is worse from any motion. Mouth is dry with great thirst for large, cold drinks. Liver sore and swollen. Feels better lying on the painful side. Constipation. Better from pressure. Bursting headache. Irritable and wants to be left alone.

Hydrastis: Pain in the liver extending to the right shoulder blade. Worse from lying on the back or the right side. Thick, yellow, stringy mucus. Weak digestion, constipation. Pains from liver cancer.

Magnesia muriatica: Exhausted and unrefreshed after sleep. Chilly, but craves fresh air. Worse from milk, fat, or salt. Tenderness and pain in the liver extending to the spine. Better from hard pressure. Worse lying on the right side. Liver enlarged with bloated abdomen. Heart palpitations while sitting, but improved from moving.

Taraxacum: Liver enlarged and hard. Tongue white with clear patches, bitter or sour taste in the mouth. Cold fingertips. Great quantities of urine voided often. Feels like bubbles are bursting in his abdomen. Perspires heavily at night. Pain in the back of the head after lying down. Headache from liver problems. Impatient and irritable.

Leptandra: Black tarlike stool, vomits bile, tongue yellow, shooting pains around the liver. Burning pain in the liver.

Belladonna: Pain in the liver is worse from pressure, breathing, coughing, or lying on the right side. The patient's face is red with hot perspiration. Pupils dilated. Can't bear light, noise, being jarred, or cold air. For ailments that come on quickly.

Cardus marianus: Face yellow, headache, nausea and vomiting, urine and stool golden yellow. Hard, difficult stools alternating with diarrhea. Worse from eating (opposite Chelidonium). Worse when moving. Lower potencies are best, but give what you have.

Chelidonium: Pain in the upper right side of the back, face yellow, liver area feels painful when touched. Much nausea and sometimes vomiting. Temporarily better from eating. Better from hot drinks. Lower potencies best (6c–12c), but give what you have.

Cinchona: Abdomen bloated with much belching, which gives no relief. Liver is enlarged, hard, and sensitive to the slightest touch. Face yellow, bitter taste in the mouth, constipation or painless diarrhea. Circles under the eyes, ringing in the ears.

5
Remedy Descriptions

Here you will find the main symptoms associated with each remedy. Included are conditions that make the person feel *better* or *worse* (e.g., worse lying down, better after eating). Also listed are causes of illness associated with that remedy (e.g., ailments from damp weather, from loss of fluids). Finally, there are examples of ailments that have been treated with that remedy. Each remedy covers many more ailments than are listed under it.

The remedy you choose should look, feel, or sound like what your patient is going through. If the remedy description matches the patient, that remedy should cure, regardless of the name of the ailment. Note: The patient doesn't need to have *all* the symptoms listed for the remedy to work.

Aconite

Sudden intense onset, especially after exposure to dry, cold weather or after fright. Fear, restlessness, unquenchable thirst, and red, hot, dry skin. Use Aconite for the first stages of ailments that come on fast after exposure to cold. If given in the first twenty-four hours, it can prevent an illness from taking hold. A few pellets at the first sign of a sore throat, earache, or cold can stop it in its tracks. *Top remedy for panic.* Short acting remedy. Repeat it several times. **Worse:** from cold air, between 12 and 2 a.m. **Better:** from sweating, sleep.

Antimonium tartaricum

Leading remedy for thick, suffocating mucus in the lungs. The secretions become so thick that they block the airways and can't be coughed up. You can hear the *rattling of mucus* in the chest. Choking, very drowsy, perspiring, and nauseous. Asphyxia of newborns, asthma, croup, pneumonia, whooping cough, apparent death from drowning, etc. **Worse:** from lying down, during the nighttime, or from being in a warm room. **Better:** from sitting up, lying on the right side, moving, or vomiting.

Antimonium crudum

Tongue has thick, white coating. Irritable and can't bear to be touched or looked at. Worse from heat, but also from cold bathing. Nostrils chapped and covered with crusts. Cracks in the corners of the mouth. Eyes are dull, sunken, and red. Constant belching and bloating after eating. Callouses, constipation, prolapsed rectum, disordered stomach, eczema, sunstroke, etc. **Better:** from fresh air, lying down. **Worse:** from cold bathing, sweets, the heat of sun, and overeating.

Apis mellifica

Burning, stinging pain relieved by cold. Edema (swelling) of tissues. No thirst. Right-sided complaints, or complaints that move from right to left. Top remedy for bee stings and anaphylaxis (life-threatening allergic reactions). Also meningitis, inflammation of ovaries, kidney disease, etc. *Whenever you have stinging pain relieved by cold, along with edema, think of Apis.* **Better:** from cold, motion, sitting up, fresh air, and cold water. **Worse:** from heat, touch, pressure, lying down, being in a warm room, after sleeping.

Argentum nitricum

Feels anxious and hurried. Craves sweets, which disagree. Can't stand a hot room and craves fresh air. Anticipatory anxiety, panic attacks, trembling hands, claustrophobia, agoraphobia, or fear of heights. Eyes feel painful with a discharge of pus. Palpitation, which is worse lying on the right side. Sensation of a splinter in the throat when swallowing. The patient feels as if parts of his body are expanding. Feels as if he is being squeezed. Migraine with the feeling that the head is enlarged. Green stool like spinach. Anxiety, prostate enlargement, ophthalmia, etc. **Better:** from fresh air, cold, and belching. **Worse:** from any kind of warmth, sweets, at night, or from strong emotions.

Arnica

First remedy for injuries. Everything from bumps, bruises, and broken bones to shock and heart attack. Also for dental work and surgery—both before and after. Will speed healing, reduce pain and bruising, and minimize bleeding. Also for exhaustion from overwork. *After an injury, the individual says he is "okay," but doesn't want to be approached or touched.* Infections occurring after injuries. Much bruising. Head hot and body cold. Foul odor of bodily secretions. Taste of rotten eggs in the mouth. **Worse:** from touch, at night, or becoming heated.

Arsenicum album

Anxious, restless, chilly, thirsty for small frequent sips, burning pains relieved by heat, extreme weakness from any exertion, pale face, and putrid discharges. Diarrhea, flu, food poisoning, asthma, blood poisoning, anxiety attacks, heart attacks, etc. **Better:** from heat and warm drinks, and from elevating the head. **Worse:** between midnight and 3 a.m., when alone, and from cold.

Baptisia

Muscular soreness and putrid secretions. Drowsy, falls asleep while being spoken to, eyelids droop (also Gelsemium), confused as if drunk, body feels sore, especially the parts lain on. Tongue feels burned. Putrid secretions.

Delusion that his body is scattered all over the bed. Toxic states due to infections in the blood. Typhoid fever, diphtheria, influenza, dysentery, etc. **Worse:** from damp heat, pressure, walking, and on awaking.

Belladonna

Sudden, intense onset of symptoms. Heat, burning, throbbing pain, redness, inflammation, spasms. Delirium with biting, spitting, or kicking. Face is red and feels hot. Hands and feet are cold. Pupils dilated. Often right-sided complaints. Scarlet fever, ear infections, abscesses, rabies, whooping cough, mania, delirium, etc. **Better:** from quiet, being in a dark room, standing or sitting up, bending the head backward. **Worse:** from light, noise, being jarred, being in the sun, drafts on the head, or from seeing bright objects.

Bryonia

Worse from the slightest motion. The patient lays perfectly still. Irritable if disturbed. *Great thirst for large drinks*, mucous membranes dry. Dry mouth and throat, dry cough. *Stitching pains.* Bursting headache, with pressure from within. Red, hot, swollen joints. Constipation or hard, dry stools. Sprains, rheumatic pain, pneumonia, bronchitis, appendicitis, flu, etc. **Better:** from pressure, lying on the painful side, and from cold air. **Worse:** from any motion, deep breathing, coughing, or being overheated.

Calcarea carbonica

Extremely fearful (of heights, rats, mice, fire, contagious diseases, being observed by others, or violence). Tires easily from exertion. Very chilly with cold, damp hands. Head sweats during sleep, sour-smelling perspiration. The patient craves sweets, eggs, or salt. Can't digest milk. Often—but not always—needed by heavyset people, including children. Tapeworm, delayed development in children, bone diseases, epilepsy, nightmares, rheumatism, etc. **Worse:** from cold, exertion, the pressure of clothes, drinking milk, and during dentition.

Calcarea phosphorica

Weakness (especially after acute illness), headache from mental exertion, craving for smoked meat or fish and salt, intolerance of milk. Fear of bad news. Slow healing of broken bones, delayed dentition, osteomyeletis, osteoporosis, rickets, etc. **Worse:** from drafts, cold, weather changes, and loss of body fluids.

Calendula

Most often used as a diluted tincture to cleanse wounds. Speeds healing and helps prevent infection and scarring. Used in potency for corneal abrasions and painful burns.

Cantharis

Top remedy for burns and bladder infections. Burning, cutting pain (skin, bladder, mouth, throat, stomach, ovaries, etc.). Burning pains with an intolerable urge to urinate. Burning pains with excitement, even rage, and making barking noises. Burning thirst, but with an aversion to drinks. Burns, cystitis, shingles, kidney infections, rabies, mania, etc. **Better:** from cold application and rubbing. **Worse:** from urinating (burning), cold drinks, seeing bright objects (fearful), the sound of water, coffee, and at night.

Carbo vegetabilis

Top remedy for collapse. Hungry for air and wants to be fanned. Much belching. Head hot but breath and body cold. Hot sweat on the head. Pulse feeble, fingertips blue. Feet icy cold up to the knees. Upper part of the abdomen bloated with gas. All food disagrees. Slow oozing of dark blood from small wounds or natural orifices. States of collapse, debility, asthmatic attacks, passive hemorrhage, whooping cough, gangrene, food poisoning, etc. **Better:** from belching, being fanned. **Worse:** from fatty food, from warm wet weather, from wine, and in the evening.

Caulophyllum

Important birthing remedy. Helps to strengthen contractions. Patient feels exhausted. *More weepy than fearful. Emotionally soft, tearful,* and chilly. False labor. Labor pains are ineffective or very painful. *Pains move from place to place.* Drooping of eyelids. Birthing difficulties, premature labor, miscarriages, painful periods, etc. **Better:** from warmth. **Worse:** from cold, open air, motion, and in the evening.

Causticum

Gradual paralysis, contraction of muscles and tendons, raw burning pain, very chilly, craves smoked food. Restless legs at night. Ailments after long-standing grief or fright. Ailments after burns. Very sympathetic and deeply affected by injustice. Passes urine while sneezing or laughing. Gradual paralysis, rheumatism, deep or painful burns that don't heal, Bell's palsy, etc. **Better:** from cold drinks, damp weather, and the warmth of the bed. **Worse:** from cold dry air, stooping, and in the evening.

Chamomilla

Unendurable pain coupled with extreme anger. The patient exclaims, "I can't bear this pain. Do something!" Will not answer civilly. Impatient when being spoken to. Thirsty and hot. One cheek is red and hot, the other pale and cold. Pain with numbness. Headache, earache, teething, toothache, pain in pregnancy, etc. **Better:** from being carried and warm, humid weather. **Worse:** from heat, anger, and at night.

Cimicifuga

Important birthing remedy. Helps regulate contractions and relieve anxiety. *Extremely fearful. Excitable, hysterical, pessimistic, chilly, and talkative.* Sighs a lot. Stiff neck. Pain across the pelvis from hip to hip. *Labor pains felt in the thighs, back, or hips.* Patient feels as if a "black cloud was over everything." Dreams of "impending evil." Fear of death, insanity, or rats. Birthing difficulties, menstrual problems, back pains, etc. **Better:** from warm wraps, gentle motion, open air, and eating. **Worse:** from drafts, damp cold air, strong emotions, and at night.

Cinchona (sometimes called "China")

Ailments from loss of fluids (from bleeding, vomiting, diarrhea, lactation, or perspiration). Fatigue following exhausting illnesses. Very chilly. *Bloating of the abdomen not relieved by belching. Painless diarrhea.* Mentally apathetic or sad. Extreme sensitivity of all senses. Sensitive to cold, drafts, noise, light touch, and odors. Headache with throbbing pain and red face (also Belladonna). Extreme hunger, especially at night. *Ailments that occur periodically, especially every other day (e.g., intermittent fevers).* Loss of fluids, dehydration, anemia, diarrhea, food poisoning, exhaustion after acute ailments, intermittent fevers. **Better**: from hard pressure and lying down. **Worse**: from drafts, cold, motion, loss of fluids, and light touch.

Cocculus indicus

Ailments from loss of sleep or extended caregiving. Motion sickness. Aversion to fresh air. Hunger but aversion to food. Nausea from the odor of food. **Worse:** from motion, loss of sleep, cold, fresh air, and the smell of food.

Coffea crudum

Patient has an overactive mind and can't shut it off. Extreme sensitivity to pain. Aversion to fresh air. Very talkative. Toothache (better from cold water), insomnia after excitement or from drinking coffee, unendurable pain. **Better:** from cold drinks, rest. **Worse:** from noise, odors, or touch.

Colocynth

Violent cramping pains, which make the patient double over to get relief. Crying out with pain. Left-sided pains. Kidney and gallstone pain. Pain with diarrhea, nausea and vomiting. Ailments from anger and anger during ailments. Colic pains, spasms, peritonitis, sciatica, dysentery, etc. **Better:** from bending double, hard pressure, and lying on the abdomen. **Worse:** from anger, drafts, or rest.

Dulcamara

Ailments that come on after exposure to cold, wet weather. Chilly and worse from cold or dampness. Excessive discharges of thick, yellow mucus. Dry burning heat during fever. Burning thirst for cold drinks. Cough after exertion. Chill triggers urge to urinate. Green, slimy, bloody, or mucus-laden stools. Adenitis, colds, herpes, stiff neck, meningitis, scarlatina, etc. **Better**: from moving. **Worse**: from cold, dampness, and nighttime.

Eupatorium perfoliatum

Deep aching in bones, or bones may feel broken. Restlessness. Thirst for cold drinks. Chill in the back. Body feels bruised. Painful eyeballs. Influenza, rheumatism, broken bones, etc. **Better:** from being on hands and knees, and from conversation. **Worse:** periodically (every third or fourth day), between 7 and 9 a.m., from cold air, and from the smell or sight of food.

Euphrasia

Profuse, burning tears with a mild discharge from nose. Burning sensation in the eyes with sensitivity to light. Keeps blinking the eyes. Swollen eyelids. Frequent yawning when walking in open air. Intense cough only during the day. Cough stops at night and is better from lying down. Cough in the morning with much mucus. Stiffness of the upper lip. Absence of menstruation with inflammation of the eye. Irritation of and injuries to the eye. Conjunctivitis, allergies, hay fever, corneal opacities, prostatitis, etc. **Better:** from fresh air, darkness, and lying down. **Worse:** from sunlight, wind, smoke, warmth, and in the evening (except for the cough).

Ferrum phosphoricum

Early stages of inflammatory ailments. Slow onset with low fever. The patient feels ill, but there are no clear symptoms yet. Face alternates red and pale. Tendency to bleeding. Sweaty. Anemia, colds, sore throat, flu, nosebleeds, and other hemorrhages, etc. Right-sided complaints. **Better:** from lying down and from cold applications. **Worse:** between 4 and 6 a.m., at night, from cold drinks, being jarred, and motion.

Gelsemium

Drowsy, sluggish, limbs feel too heavy to move, the eyelids droop, swallowing is difficult, paralysis of body parts. Chill up the back, no thirst. Wants to be left alone. Slow onset. Trembling. Anticipatory anxiety. Gelsemium has been used for influenza, drug overdose, paralysis, hysterical paralysis, bad effects of fear, meningitis, etc. **Better:** from sweating, passing urine, drinking alcohol, or from open air. **Worse:** from heat, hot weather, excitement, bad news, or fright.

Hepar sulphuris calcareum

Infections. The infected part is extremely sensitive to touch, drafts, and cold air. Every little injury starts to form pus. Whether the infection is in the ear or the finger, the patient won't let you touch it because of the pain. Sneezes or coughs when uncovered. *Extremely chilly and can't get warm. Discharges smell like old cheese. Infections with pus* (ear, gums, roots of teeth, wounds, etc.). Most often used in the lower potencies (6x to 6c), which increases pus formation, allowing it to drain. **Better:** from heat, damp weather. **Worse:** from cold, cold food, drafts, and touch.

Hypericum

Injuries to nerves. Any injury where there is excessive pain. Injuries to the head or spine. *Puncture wounds that become very painful.* Also used to prevent tetanus, along with Ledum. Gunshot wounds, dental work, neuralgia, tetanus, etc. **Better:** from lying on the face, bending the head backward. **Worse:** from being jarred, changes of weather, and fog.

Ignatia

Number one remedy for the ill effects of grief, disappointed love, worry, and fright. Ailments triggered by strong emotions. *Much sighing and silent brooding.* Changeable mood—laughter alternates with tears. Hysteria. Feeling of a lump in the throat. *Aversion to tobacco smoke.* Insomnia from grief. **Better:** from changing position, being alone, and from warmth. **Worse:** from consolation, strong emotions, odors, coffee, and tobacco smoke.

Ipecacuanha

Constant nausea and vomiting. Nausea is not relieved by vomiting. Any ailment in which nausea is an added symptom may yield to this remedy (e.g., headache with nausea, hemorrhage with nausea, asthma with nausea, etc.). Clean tongue, profuse salivation, thirstlessness, tendency to hemorrhage, convulsive cough. Asthma, hemorrhage, bronchitis, yellow fever, etc. **Better:** from open air, rest, pressure, and closing the eyes. **Worse:** from the slightest motion and from warmth, especially damp warmth.

Kali bichromicum

Thick, yellow, stringy mucus. Thick mucus plugs in the nose. Chilly and worse from getting cold. Pains appear and disappear suddenly. They often appear in small spots. Pains move from one place to another and appear at regular times. Sensation of a hair on the back of the tongue. Sinusitis, migraine in small spots, postnasal discharge, ulcers of the skin with punched-out edges, etc. **Worse:** from cold damp weather, in the morning, from 2 to 5 a.m., after sleep, from hot weather, from drinking beer.

Lachesis

Left-sided symptoms, or symptoms that start on the left and move to the right. Symptoms come on or get worse after sleep. Hemorrhaging of dark blood. *Purple color of lesions* (boils, wounds, etc.). Extremely talkative and intense. The patient can't stick her tongue out because it trembles so much. Sore throat, which is worse from swallowing liquids, but okay with solids. Infected wounds, appendicitis, gangrene, heart problems, or left-sided paralysis from stroke. **Better:** from cold drinks, open air, hard pressure, and discharges (menses, runny nose, perspiration). **Worse:** After sleep, from heat, empty swallowing or drinking liquids, light touch, and tight clothing, especially around the neck.

Ledum

Any puncture wound (e.g., a nail, bullet, insect sting, animal bite, etc.). *Used to prevent tetanus.* Hypericum follows when the wound is very painful. The injured part feels cold to the touch but is better from cold application. Also, black eye from a blow and bruises that fade to green. Pain in the joints that is worse from motion (e.g., arthritis of the knee, wrist, hand, finger joints, etc.), and rheumatism. Useful before or after vaccinations. **Better:** from cold applications, rest. **Worse:** from the heat of a bed, the motion of joints, evening and night, and wine.

Lycopodium

Right-sided symptoms or symptoms that start on the right and move to the left. Abdomen full of gas with much flatulence. Symptoms worse between 4 and 8 p.m. and 3 and 4 a.m. Craves sweets. Chilly, yet craves open air. Desires warm food or drink. *Nostrils flare when trying to get air.* Can't stand strong smells or noise. Anticipatory anxiety, lack of confidence, fear of being alone, weak digestion. Constipation, sore throat, liver problems, diphtheria, rheumatism, pneumonia, cancer of the lip, etc. **Better:** from uncovering (especially the head), from motion, warm food or drink, cold applications, and burping. **Worse:** between 4 and 8 p.m., from heat except on the throat or stomach, from cold food, oysters, onions, or cabbage.

Magnesia phosphorica

Cramping, spasms of muscles, better from warmth and doubling over. Shooting pains, right-sided complaints, better from pressure. Pains appear and disappear suddenly. Cramps, colic, sciatica, toothache, neuralgia, etc. **Better:** from applying warmth, pressure, doubling up, hot baths. **Worse:** from cold, cold bathing, uncovering, drafts, night, moving, and touch.

Mercurius (Merc vivis or Merc solubilis)

The patient sweats profusely and feels worse afterward. Foul odor to breath and perspiration. Skin moist. Tongue flabby, with the imprint of teeth. Patient has excess saliva and may drool, but has great thirst for cold drinks. Tremors of the hands and tongue. Creeping chilliness. Abscesses, infections with pus (especially blood-streaked pus), infections in the gums or roots of teeth, sore throat, bronchitis, typhus fever, diseases of bone, dysentery, etc. **Better:** from rest, moderate temperature. **Worse:** at night, after sweating, lying on the right side, from the warmth of the bed, drafts, and hot or cold temperatures.

Mercurius cyanatus

Number one remedy to treat diphtheria and also to prevent it. Profound exhaustion, icy coldness, and cyanosis (turning blue). Diphtheritic membrane forms in the mouth, throat, and at anus. The throat is very painful when talking or swallowing. Ulcers in the mouth. Intense thirst, but vomits drinks. Diarrhea or hot, bloody stools. Painful spasms of the rectum or bladder. Mumps, peritonitis, intestinal fever, etc. **Better:** at rest. **Worse:** at night, from swallowing, from cold, and after urination or stool.

Nux vomica

Extremely chilly, chill from uncovering or just moving. Even during fever with hot body temperature, the patient cannot be uncovered. *Irritable, angry, oversensitive to noise, lights, odors, and criticism. Constipation with ineffectual urging for stool accompanies many complaints.* Insomnia between 3 and 5 a.m. Indigestion, asthma in the morning or after eating, backache, convulsions, cramps, gallstones, strangulated hernia, inefficient labor pains with the desire for stool, etc. **Better:** from warmth, covering, wet weather, and napping. **Worse:** from cold, early morning, uncovering, drafts, noise, odors, the pressure of clothes, or after anger.

Phosphorus

Craves cold drinks. Burning sensations (anywhere). Worse lying on the left side. Afraid to be alone and desires company and reassurance. Easily startled and afraid of thunderstorms. Hypersensitive to odors, sounds, or lights. *Tendency to hemorrhage of bright red blood.* Small wounds bleed too much. Craves salt, spices, or ice cream. When a common cold starts to go into the lungs. Pneumonia with burning in the chest, which is worse lying on the left side. Bloody sputum, bronchitis, hepatitis (also use Phosphorus to prevent it), pernicious anemia, hemorrhage, blood in the urine, jaundice, diseases of the liver, yellow fever, etc. **Better:** from short naps, eating, cold food and drink, company, sitting upright, lying on the right side. **Worse:** from being alone, warm food or drink, morning and dusk, lying on the left side, or from odors.

Phytolacca

Body feels sore, especially the eyeballs, breasts, kidneys, and neck. Shooting pains like electric shocks, which come and go suddenly and move about. Throat dark red. Swollen glands. Restless but worse from moving. Hard lumps in the breast. Sinusitis with tough, sticky discharges. Sore throat with pain extending to the ear when swallowing. Swollen breasts, breast abscess, and cancer (burning pains). Diphtheria, mumps, heart problems, etc. **Better:** from cold drinks, warmth, or lying on the stomach. **Worse:** from hot drinks, moving, swallowing, or rising from bed.

Podophyllum

Profuse, offensive-smelling diarrhea, which gushes out forcibly. Cramping pain, nausea, or rumbling before diarrhea. Diarrhea in children when teething. Headaches alternating with diarrhea. Constipation alternating with diarrhea. Rolls head from side to side and groans. Desire to press gums together. Thirst for large, cold drinks. Gastric problems, prolapsed rectum or uterus, vertigo, cholera infantum, etc. **Better:** bending forward and rubbing the right side. **Worse:** from eating, early morning (2–4 a.m.), during hot weather, or during teething.

Pulsatilla

Mild, timid, weeps telling of her problem. Craves company and sympathy. Fearful when alone. Great craving for fresh air, even when chilly. Worse from warmth and closed spaces. Quite thirstless even with dry mouth. Symptoms change in character and from place to place. Bland, yellow-green discharges. No two stools alike. Ailments from fatty foods. Ear infections, bronchitis, measles, mumps, food poisoning, breach birth (Pulsatilla may enable the baby to turn), retained placenta, and other problems of pregnancy. **Better:** from company, sympathy, fresh air, gentle motion, sitting upright, after weeping, or from cold food and drink. **Worse:** from warmth, a closed room, being alone, warm food or drink, fatty food, lying on the left side, or during the evening.

Pyrogenium

Top remedy for septic infections, e.g., blood poisoning, childbed fever, wounds gone bad, never well since an infection. *Foul-smelling discharges (breath, stool, sweat, vomit). High fever with slow pulse or vice versa.* Exhausted but extremely restless. Feels bruised all over. Aware of his heart beating. Fevers that begin with pain in the legs. Typhoid, typhus, ptomaine poisoning, diphtheria, peritonitis, etc. **Better:** from moving about and from warmth. **Worse:** from becoming cold.

Rhus toxicodendron

Symptoms worse from being at rest. Better from continued movement (worse from initial movement). Extreme restlessness and must keep moving. Stiffness and pain in the joints and muscles. Hot, painful swollen joints. *Burning and itching of the skin, which is better from warm water.* Unquenchable thirst. Chilliness. Dreams of doing things requiring great exertion. Craves milk. Influenza, sprains, arthritis, sciatica, poison ivy and any skin inflammation that looks and feels like it, dengue fever, typhus fever, blood poisoning, etc. **Better:** from moving about or changing position, stretching, warmth, dry weather, and warm drinks. **Worse:** from lying still or being at rest, cold damp environments, getting wet, drafts, and at night, especially after midnight.

Ruta graveolens

Bone and tendon pain after injuries or from illness. Bruised, aching feeling with restlessness. Violent unquenchable thirst for ice-cold water. Pain in the eyes as if from strain. Wakes from sleep at the slightest touch. Pain in the rectum after stool. Desires cold drinks. Bruises to bones, eyestrain, injuries, and pain in the wrist. Constipation after injuries. Headache from eyestrain. Lameness after sprains. Easy dislocation of vertebrae, rheumatism, etc.

Better: from warmth and lying on the back. **Worse:** from cold air or temperatures, overexertion, and eyestrain.

Sepia

Bearing-down sensations in the abdomen, very chilly, irritated by company but afraid to be alone. Milky-white discharges, vertigo when kneeling, yellow or brown discoloration on the nose or cheeks. Craves chocolate, pickles, or sour foods. Prolapsed uterus, anus. Aching in the lower back, which is worse from kneeling and better from firm pressure. Painful periods, bladder problems, tendency to miscarriage, problems related to pregnancy, etc. **Better:** from exertion, warmth, loosening clothes, and fresh air. **Worse:** from cold air, in the morning and evening, from birth control pills, and before, during, and after menses.

Silica

Very chilly, worse from drafts, easily exhausted, thirsty, perspires easily (especially on the head and feet), hypersensitive to touch and noise. Malnutrition, constipation, slow-healing wounds, recurrent infections, *ill effects of vaccination*, violent cough when lying down, splinters (Silica causes the body to eject them). **Better:** from warmth and covering the head. **Worse:** from cold, drafts, dampness, light, noise, excitement, and vaccination.

Spongia

Very dry "barking" cough. Palpitation of the heart and difficulty breathing after midnight. Wakes at night with a fear of suffocation. Sensation as if the heart is too big for the chest. Numbness of the left arm. Chilly. Dry cough, croup, goiter, heart failure, whooping cough, etc. **Better:** from lying on the back, warm food, and rest. **Worse:** after sleeping, from cold drinks, exertion, stooping, and lying on the right side.

Staphysagria (also spelled "Staphisagria")

First aid for razorlike cuts from sharp instruments. (For ragged cuts, use Arnica.) *Also for ailments from suppressed anger or humiliation*, including rape and abuse. *Excellent for pain from stretched sphincter muscles.* Cuts, styes, cystitis, painful incision after surgery, sea sickness without vomiting, colitis from anger, etc. **Better:** from warmth, rest, and after a meal. **Worse:** from unexpressed anger, tobacco smoke, touch, or sexual excess.

Sulphur

The patient feels hot, is worse from heat, and craves fresh air. Burning sensations, and red, itching skin, which is worse from heat and bathing. Bodily discharges smell foul and irritate the skin. Redness and itching of the anus, lips, nose, and eyes. Sudden diarrhea in the morning. Craves sweets and spices. Skin ailments, pneumonia, vertigo, lumbago, insomnia, etc. Sulphur is useful when other remedies fail to act in acute diseases; it stimulates the body's resistance. **Better:** from fresh air, moving, lying on the right side. **Worse:** from bathing, being in a warm room or bed, at 11 a.m., standing, or from drinking milk.

Symphytum

Speeds healing and relieves the pain of broken or injured bones. Pricking pains at the site of the injury. (Use Calcarea phosphorica if there is coldness and numbness in the limb.) *Injuries to joints, ligaments, tendons, periosteum. Also for an injury to the eyeball from a blunt instrument (after Arnica).* Ailments resulting from injuries to bone.

Thuja

Top remedy for bad effects from vaccination (see also Silica). *Can be effective even years after the vaccination. Warts.* Yellow-green discharges. Sweats on uncovered parts. Ridges in fingernails. Dreams of falling and of the dead. Feels like his body is fragile or brittle. Gonorrhea, sinusitis, moles, polyps, etc. **Better:** on the left side, from drawing up limbs, warmth, or rubbing. **Worse:** from cold damp weather, at 3 a.m. and 3 p.m., from eating fatty foods or onions, from coffee, after eating, or from bright light.

Urtica urens

Burning, itching of the skin with blistering. Hives and rashes. Pain in the eyes like a blow or a feeling of sand. Bruised feeling in the right deltoid muscle (back). First-degree burns, illness from shellfish, gout pain in the ankles or wrists with itching skin, rheumatism, kidney stones, hives, arthritic nodes in the fingers, diminished breast milk, etc. **Worse:** from cold, damp weather, eating shellfish, at night, or from burns.

Veratrum album

A major remedy for collapse. Patient is freezing cold with profuse cold sweat on the face and forehead. Skin blue. Extreme weakness. Diarrhea with vomiting. Sudden, violent onset of symptoms. Wants to be covered. Craves sour fruit, salt, or cold drinks. Cholera, pneumonia, typhoid, asthma, post-operative shock, angina, dehydration, heatstroke, meningitis, head injury, effects of fright, etc. **Better:** from hot drinks, warmth, walking about, or lying down. **Worse:** from drinking (especially cold drinks), exertion, night, cold weather, and touch.

Important Exotic Remedies

Most of these remedies are nosodes, which are remedies made from a diseased substance. Some are used for prevention and some for both prevention and treatment. A friendly doctor can write a prescription for these.

Anthracinum: Anthrax, boils that spread, gangrene, and ulcers.

Crotalus horridus: Ailments with hemorrhaging from every orifice, blood poisoning, carbuncles, peritonitis, yellow fever.

Diphtherinum: Diphtheria, severe sore throat, myelitis.

Influenzinum: Influenza.

Lathyrus: Polio (no prescription needed).

Malaria officinalis: Malaria.

Pertussin: Whooping cough.

Pestinum or **Plaginum** (Yersinia pestis nosode)**:** Bubonic plague.

Salmonella typhi nosode: Typhoid.

Variolinum: Smallpox.

Vibrio cholerae nosode: Cholera.

Yellow fever nosode: Yellow fever.

6
Pregnancy and Birth

The following topics are listed below in chronological order:

Morning sickness, Threatened Miscarriage, Breech Birth, Inducing Labor, Prolonged or Difficult Labor, Labor Pains—Excessive, Postpartum Hemorrhage, Retained Placenta, Perineal Tears and Episiotomies, Asphyxia of the Newborn, Childbed Fever, Postpartum Fatigue, Remedies for the Baby, Depression After Delivery, Mastitis, Breast Abscess, Colic.

> **Warning**: Do not use Silica during pregnancy. Pulsatilla should only be used in the third trimester and as a 30c or higher.

Morning Sickness

From the fourth week through the third month of pregnancy, mild to severe nausea and vomiting often occurs. Aversion to the smell of food is a common symptom. Balancing the blood sugar with frequent small meals or snacks may help. The remedies below are best taken fifteen minutes before eating.

***Sepia:** *Empty feeling in the stomach not relieved by eating.* Sickened by the thought or odor of food. Craves acidic foods (vinegar, pickles, etc.)

and chocolate. Everything tastes salty. *Irritable around others, but dreads to be alone. Indifferent to loved ones.* Better from vigorous exercise, warmth, and sleep.

***Colchicum:** *Can't bear the smell or even thought of food.* Riding in a car brings on nausea. Vomits from standing up or lying down flat. Must flex knees or crouch.

***Ipecacuanha:** *Continuous nausea not relieved by vomiting. Excess salivation and often drooling. Tongue is clear (not coated).* No thirst. Vomits undigested food, mucus, or bile. Worse from warmth, humidity, stooping, or motion. Better from open air.

***Tabacum:** *Worse from any motion, such as riding in a car* (also Petroleum, Cocculus). *Much cold sweat.* Face looks very pale. Nausea without vomiting. Tendency to spit. *Worse from heat. Better from fresh air.*

***Symphoricarpus racemosa** (200c)**:** *Deathly nausea, continuous retching and vomiting.* More comfortable lying on her back. Worse from any motion. Constipated.

***Antimonium crudum:** *Tongue coated thick white.* Vomiting with convulsions. Craves acids (also Sepia). Better lying down and from warm baths. Aversion to being looked at.

***Nux vomica:** *Nausea in the morning, with cramping pains and constipation.* Vomiting after eating. Irritable. Wakes at 3 a.m. and can't sleep. Chilly and worse from cold, coffee, and spices.

Veratrum album: Vomiting with diarrhea. Freezing cold with cold sweat. Craves cold drinks but is worse afterward. Craves salty and sour foods. Worse from exertion.

Petroleum: *Worse from motion, such as riding in a car* (also Tabacum, Cocculus). Chilly and avoids open air. Strong odor to perspiration. Skin dry and cracking. Hunger during nausea. *Worse from cold* (opposite Tabacum).

Cocculus: *Worse from motion* (also Petroleum, Tabacum). *Chilly and avoids open air.* Worse from loss of sleep. Much saliva, but considerable thirst for cold drinks.

Kreosotum: Nauseous but has to work hard to vomit. Water tastes bitter. Vomiting undigested food, sour fluids, or mucus. Chilly and worse in open air (opposite Pulsatilla). Better from warmth. Better from motion (opposite Tabacum). Weeps from music.

Lactic acid: *Hot, sour vomiting, heartburn, excess salivation.* Better from eating breakfast.

Threatened Miscarriage

Miscarriage refers to the spontaneous termination of a pregnancy before twenty weeks. Signs include vaginal bleeding, which may be accompanied by cramps or backache.

***Viburnum opulus:** First choice. From the first to the eight month. Especially in women with a history of miscarriage. Severe cramping with bearing-down pains that start in the back and go down the thighs. Very restless. Chilly, but wants fresh air. Sick feeling, which is worse from moving. Pains come and go suddenly.

***Arnica:** From physical exertion or injury. Pelvic area feels bruised, and sometimes hemorrhages. Aversion to being touched.

***Belladonna:** Pains are intense and come on suddenly. Feels as if her insides will be pushed out. Face is red and hot. Bright red, hot blood. Worse from noise, light, being jarred, or from cold air. Throbbing sensations. Hands and feet cold.

***Pulsatilla:** *Note: Never use Pulsatilla in less than a 30c potency during pregnancy. The patient must have fresh air. A closed or warm room feels unbearable.* Desires company and sympathy. Weeps easily. No thirst. Discharge of black blood. For the threat of late-term miscarriage.

***Sepia:** From the fifth to the seventh month. *Bearing down sensations in the uterus, bladder, and rectum.* Chilly and either irritable or depressed and weepy. Worse from cold. Worse kneeling. Better from warmth and cold drinks. Yellow discoloration on the face. Craves chocolate, cold drinks, and pickles.

***Caulophyllum:** *Pains that fly about from one place to another.* Worse from open air and better from warmth (opposite Pulsatilla). Chilly. Highly irritable. Eyelids droop.

***Cimicifuga:** Often in the third month. *Pains that fly across the abdomen from side to side.* The patient is doubled up with the pain. The condition may begin after being frightened. Chilly but better from open air (also Pulsatilla). Worse from drafts and cold. Better from warm wraps. Talkative. *Feels like she's enveloped in a black cloud.* Fear of insanity.

Ignatia: *From grief or fright. Much sighing.* Sense of a lump in her throat. Sensitive to strong odors, especially tobacco.

Chamomilla: *After anger.* Pain starts in the back and moves down the inner thighs. The patient is angry, uncivil, and complains of unbearable pain. Discharge of dark blood. One cheek is red or hot, the other pale. Worse from heat or touch.

Sabina: In the second to the third month. Pains go from back to front—from the lower back to the pelvic area. *Worse every time she moves.* Worse from heat, motion, and taking a deep breath. Better from fresh air. Weepy, nervous, and sensitive to noise.

Secale: Often during the third month, with discharges of thin, black blood. Extremely restless with fear of death. *She feels hot inside, but her skin is cold to the touch. Even when icy-cold, she can't bear to be covered.* Worse from warmth. Feels like ants are crawling on her, especially her hands (and so she holds her fingers apart).

Apis: In the first to the fourth month. Stinging, burning pain in the abdomen. Thirstless. Worse from heat or a warm room. Better from cold application. Edema. Desires company and is worse alone. Restlessness alternating with sadness.

Rhus tox: From overexertion. Back and muscles ache, great restlessness. Worse from rest and better when moving. Chilly and better from warmth.

Kali carbonicum: In the second to the third month. Pain extends from the back to the buttocks and thighs. Despondent, fearful, worse alone.

Symptoms come on, or are worse at 3 a.m. Very chilly and sensitive to drafts. Perspires from the least exertion. Upper eyelids are swollen.

Gelsemium: *From sudden bad news*, excitement, strong emotions (also Ignatia, Aconite). Eyelids droop, limbs feel heavy, pain goes upward and into the back. Trembling. Passes large quantities of clear urine. Much anticipatory anxiety.

Remedies Related to the Time of Miscarriage

First month: *Apis, Viburnum.

Second month: *Kali carb, *Cimicifuga, Apis, Sepia, Viburnum.

Early months: Viburnum, Caulophyllum, Sepia.

Third month: Sabina, Secale, Sepia, Kali carb, Mercurius.

Fourth month: Apis.

Eighth month: Pulsatilla.

Breech Birth—Altering the Baby's Position in the Womb

The optimal position for birth is head first. In a breech position, the buttocks, feet, or knees may present first. Breech births are often done as cesarean, but also vaginally. Breeches may turn spontaneously just before labor, but it is best to try turning them at about thirty-two weeks. This can sometimes be accomplished by lying on the back with knees flexed and hips elevated by pillows. The exercise is done for twenty minutes, twice a day. The following homeopathic remedies can sometimes get the baby turned around head first.

***Pulsatilla:** Top remedy. Give 30c every couple hours (up to six doses in one day). Stop the remedy if the baby turns. Another option is Pulsatilla 200c once. If there is no effect, skip a day and repeat the remedy on the third day. This stimulates the muscles of the womb. The mother desires sympathy, company, and craves fresh air. She weeps easily and openly.

Natrum muriaticum: Used when the mother is feeling very private and is worse from company and sympathy (opposite Pulsatilla). She is emotionally withdrawn and only weeps when alone.

Inducing Labor

***Caulophyllum:** *Nervous, restless, excitable, sleepless. Emotionally soft, tearful*, changeable. Chilly, worse from cold, thirsty. Better from warmth. Trembles from weakness. Drooping eyelids. Desires company, but is not talkative.

***Cimicifuga:** Fearful and lacks confidence in her ability to withstand the rigors of birth. Much sighing and trembling. Gloomy and feels like she is under a "black cloud." May feel like she is losing her mind. Very talkative, jumping from subject to subject. Chilly and worse from cold. Better from fresh air, but worse from drafts.

Pulsatilla: She desires company and sympathy. Weeps easily and openly. Wants to please. She craves fresh cool air, even when chilly. Thirstless. Contractions come and go but labor doesn't begin.

Gelsemium: Great anticipatory anxiety. Fear of losing control. She feels drowsy, her limbs feel heavy, her eyelids droop, and her face is flushed. No thirst. Sometimes trembling, with diarrhea, or a chill up the back. Doesn't want to be disturbed.

Prolonged or Difficult Labor

The two top remedies are Caulophyllum and Cimcifuga. If the symptom picture isn't clear, those two remedies may be alternated.

***Caulophyllum:** Strengthens contractions. Prolonged labor with great exhaustion and weak contractions. *Nervous, restless, excitable, sleepless. Emotionally soft, tearful*, and changeable. Chilly, thirsty, and worse from cold. Better from warmth. Trembles from weakness. Drooping eyelids. Desires company, but is not talkative.

***Cimicifuga:** Weak, irregular contractions. Fearful and lacks confidence in her ability to withstand the rigors of birth. Much sighing and trembling. Gloomy and feels like she is under a "black cloud." May feel like she is losing her mind. Fear of losing control. Very talkative, jumping from subject to subject. Chilly and worse from cold. Better from fresh air, but worse from drafts.

***Chamomilla:** *Unendurable pain with extreme anger. She will scream, "I can't stand it anymore!" She is uncivil and abusive from the pain.* Asks for things and pushes them away. She evokes feelings of anger rather than sympathy. Labor pains that press upward. She is thirsty, feels hot, and wants to be uncovered. Very restless. One cheek may be red and the other pale. Sometimes there is pain with numbness.

Aconite: *Sudden and intense fear of death.* Predicts the time of her death. The face is hot, flushed, and may go pale when sitting up. The mouth is dry with extreme thirst for cold drinks. Worse in a warm room. Pains are intense, and frighten her.

Arsenicum: *Very anxious, restless, and keeps changing position.* Exhausted from the least effort. Chilly and wants to be covered. Doesn't want to be left alone. *Thirsty for frequent sips of cold water.*

Belladonna: Angered from the pain (also Chamomilla). *Face red and hot, pupils dilated, throbbing headache. Sometimes delirious, and may hit or bite.* Extremities will be ice cold. Pains come and go quickly and move about. Bearing-down pains as if insides would fall out. Worse from bright light, noise, being jarred, cold air, and drafts. Dry mouth without thirst, or may crave lemonade.

Coffea: *The patient seems as if she drank too much coffee. Super alert, overexcited, thoughts racing, talkative, lively, hypersensitive to pain* and also light, noise, odors, and touch. Hungry. She can also be irritable, despairing, and fearful. Sleepless from an overactive mind. Worse from excitement of any kind.

Gelsemium: *Looks drowsy or intoxicated, eyelids droop, limbs feel heavy.* Trembling. Passes large quantities of clear urine. Much anticipatory anxiety. Creeping chilliness up the back. Thirstless. When Caulophyllum fails to act.

Ignatia: *Sadness. Ailments from grief or other strong emotions. Weeping with much sobbing,* mood swings, or bouts of hysteria. Worse from consolation. Sense of a lump in the throat, loss of appetite, twitching muscles, sensitive to strong odors. Often prescribed based on a history of some recent or unresolved grief. More reserved than the Cimicifuga state.

Natrum muriaticum: *She is depressed, emotionally closed, wants to be alone, doesn't ask for or accept sympathy or help.* This state comes about from long-standing grief. Weeps when alone. Can't urinate when people are nearby. Worse from heat, consolation, and company.

Nux vomica: *With every contraction, there is an urge to move the bowels*, but she passes little or no stool. High strung, irritable, impatient, and oversensitive to noise, odors, lights, and touch. Easily offended and moved to anger and abusiveness (also Chamomilla). Chilly and wants to be covered at all times. So sensitive to pain, she may faint from it.

Opium: *Great sleepiness during labor and lack of pain where it should be expected. A glassy-eyed, drowsy, dreamlike state.* She seems far away and says she is okay. This state can be triggered by great fear, although it looks like euphoria. Contractions are mild or stop altogether. Hot perspiration, red face, worse from heat. Breathing is heavy, labored, and noisy. Babies born of mothers in an Opium state may require the remedy for asphyxia. Opium is also recommended for premature deliveries due to fright.

Phosphorus: *Desires and is better from company, affection, and touch. Great thirst for large, ice-cold drinks.* Sensitive to lights, odors, and sounds. Startles easily and is afraid when left alone. Often tall slender women. Aversion to warm food. Iced drinks may be vomited after becoming warm in the stomach. Burning pains, especially in the palms of the hands.

Platina: *Extreme sensitivity of the genitals*, making her unable to concentrate on labor. Cannot bear to be examined because of the sensitivity. Contractions are weak, painful, and ineffectual. Pains are often felt on the left side. She behaves in a haughty manner, highly displeased with people.

Pulsatilla: *Gentle, yielding, desires company and sympathy. Weeps easily and openly. Craves fresh air and feels oppressed in a closed, warm room.* Dry mouth, but no thirst.

Secale: Extremely restless. She feels very hot, though her skin may be cold to the touch. Pushes away the covers because of the heat. Wants to be fanned. *Sensation as if ants are crawling under the skin. Doesn't like her fingers to touch each other and holds them apart.*

Sepia: Averse to company, yet afraid to be alone. Chilly and sensitive to cold, but with flushes of heat. Weeps for no apparent reason. *Bearing-down sensations in the uterus, vagina, and rectum. Feels better drawing her legs up.* Wants to be covered. Sometimes there are yellow blotches on her face.

Labor Pains—Excessive

***Chamomilla**: *Unendurable pain with extreme anger. She will scream, "I can't stand it anymore!" She is uncivil and abusive from the pain.* Asks for things and pushes them away. She evokes feelings of anger rather than sympathy. Labor pains that press upward. She is thirsty, feels hot, and wants to be uncovered. Very restless. One cheek may be red and the other pale. Sometimes there is pain with numbness.

***Sepia:** Bearing-down pains. Chilly, but with flushes of heat. Worse from cold, but better from cold drinks. Wants to be covered. Irritable from company, but dreads being alone. Worse from consolation. Depressed, irritable, and sarcastic. Weeping spells. Aversion to the thought or odor of food.

***Belladonna:** Angered from the pain (also Chamomilla). *Face red and hot, pupils dilated, throbbing headache. Sometimes delirious, and may hit or bite.* Extremities will be ice cold. Pains come and go quickly and move about. Bearing-down pains as if her insides would fall out (also Sepia). Worse from bright light, noise, being jarred, cold air, and drafts. Dry mouth without thirst, or she may crave lemonade.

***Coffea:** The patient has a fear of death and tosses about in anguish. Angry at sympathy. Mentally hyperactive. Extreme sensitivity to (and worse from) noise, odors, touch, open air, and cold. Better from warmth. Worse from motion. Sleepless.

Aconite: Has a great fear of death and predicts the time of her demise. Pains are sudden, violent, and intolerable. Very restless, with an unquenchable burning thirst. Her face is hot and dry. Worse at night.

Cimicifuga: Fearful and lacks confidence in her ability to withstand the rigors of birth. Much sighing and trembling. Gloomy and feels like she is under a "black cloud." May feel like she is losing her mind. Very talkative, jumping from subject to subject. Chilly and worse from cold. Better from fresh air, but worse from drafts.

Nux vomica: Strong ineffectual urging for stool accompanies the pain. Pain extends to the rectum. Very chilly. Pains better from heat. Oversensitive to sounds, odors, and lights. Highly irritable, angry.

Ignatia: The woman needing this remedy has experienced very strong emotions (fear, grief, etc.) and tried not to express them. The emotional pain comes out as sighing and sobbing, twitching of facial muscles, or a sense of a lump in the throat. Very changeable moods—laughing then crying. Bites the inside of her check. Worse from consolation and touch.

Arsenicum: Fearful, restless, exhausted by the least effort, and thirsty for frequent small sips of cold water. Afraid to be alone. Very chilly and better from warmth. Burning pain relieved by heat.

Kali carbonicum: Intense, sharp lower back pain that extends to the buttocks and thighs. It is partially relieved by pressure and motion. Worse from cold and in the early morning (3–5 a.m.). Swelling of the upper eyelids. Doesn't want to be left alone, but is irritable with company.

Pulsatilla: Mild, yielding, wanting to please. Desires company and sympathy. Highly emotional and weeps easily. Can't bear a warm or stuffy room even when chilly. Craves fresh air. No thirst.

Postpartum Hemorrhage

Postpartum hemorrhage is defined as more than two cups of blood following birth. Do not massage or handle the uterus before the placenta separates on its own.

> **Note:** The remedy Cinchona can help sustain the body after loss of blood.

***Arnica** (200c, or whatever potency you have)**:** First remedy to try. One dose during labor and another immediately after labor may prevent many problems. *She feels bruised, exhausted, doesn't want to be touched, and says she is okay.*

***Belladonna:** *Her face is red and hot*, her neck arteries throbbing, and her pupils dilated. *Hot, bright red blood with clots.* Bleeding stops and starts suddenly. Bearing-down sensation, feels like her insides will fall out. Can't stand noise, light, or being jarred.

***Aconite:** Great fear of death with restlessness. Bright red blood spurts out. Unquenchable thirst. Face hot and dry.

***Chamomilla:** *Angry and uncivil.* She is very sensitive to pain and says it is unbearable. Dark blood. Cold hands and feet, but craves cold air.

***Ipecacuanha:** *Bright red blood often accompanied by nausea.* Pain from the umbilicus to the uterus. Face pale. Gasping for breath, chilly, and shuddering with cold sweat. Much saliva.

***Sabina:** Gushing, bright red, thin blood with dark clots. *Pains that extend from back to front.* Worse from warmth.

***Ferrum metallicum:** *Fiery red face* (also Belladonna). *Cannot bear the slightest noise.* Dark, coagulated blood. Cold hands and feet. Worse at midnight.

Carbo veg: *Dark blood is slowly oozing out. She is very pale and feels breathless; she wants to be fanned.* Much belching, which gives some relief. Her head is hot, but her hands and feet are freezing cold. Pulse is very weak.

Cinchona: *Bloating of abdomen with belching, which gives no relief.* Bleeding with clots of dark blood. Pale face, chilly, and weak, with ringing in ears, thirst, cold sweat, and fainting. Worse from drafts. *Excellent remedy for the effects of loss of blood or other fluids.*

Cimicifuga: Profuse, dark, coagulated blood, accompanied by laborlike pains. Depressed, with much sighing. Feels as if she's in a "black cloud." Stiff neck. Very chilly.

Caulophyllum: Oozing of blood after brief labor or premature delivery. Great weakness. Can't keep her eyes open. Unbearable after-pains. Chilly. *Gentle and weepy, changeable moods, desires company but is not talkative. Craves fresh air.* Chilliness with shivering. Similar to the Pulsatilla state, but more chilly and thirsty and less needy.

Hyoscyamus: *Spasms of the whole body with twitching limbs. Delirium. Bright red blood.* Suspicious, talkative, and quarrelsome. She uses obscene language and laughs at everything. Worse at night.

Hamamelis: *Painless hemorrhage of dark (sometimes bright) unclotted blood, which oozes out.* Accompanied by a hammering headache. Pain in her neck and lower back. Sometimes there is a bruised feeling. Often in women with a history of varicose veins.

Secale: Continuous passive oozing of thin blood. Severe after-pains. Better from cold and uncovering, and worse from warmth or covers. Her skin feels cold to the touch, but she complains of burning heat.

Cinnamonum: *Massive bleeding from premature separation of the placenta. Sudden, profuse, bright red bleeding.* Bleeding during the first few contractions when there is little or no dilation. Also, hemorrhage from overlifting heavy objects prior to going into labor, etc.

Ustilago: Dark (sometimes bright) blood, small clots, with putrid odor. Uterus feels drawn up in a knot. Emotionally depressed.

Retained Placenta

The placenta normally detaches ten to thirty minutes after birth, but sometimes it takes longer. Having the mother nurse the baby assists this process. Never yank on the cord or massage the uterus prior to the placenta detaching. That could trigger hemorrhage.

***Pulsatilla:** Craves fresh air and wants a window open. Gentle, yielding, weepy, and better from sympathy and company. Dry mouth but without thirst.

***Cantharis:** Painful, burning urination. She has a constant desire to urinate, but is only able to pass a few drops with much burning pain. Anxious, restless, or angry.

***Sepia:** Bearing-down sensation, which feels like her uterus will fall out. Extremely chilly, but with flushes of heat. Wants to be covered. Sometimes there are sharp, shooting pains. Averse to company, but afraid to be alone.

Arnica: After a long labor. Feels bruised but says she is okay. Fear of being touched.

Arsenicum: Anxious, chilly, restless, exhausted, keeps changing position, and thirsty for frequent, small sips. Burning pains, which are better from warmth. Afraid of death, afraid to be alone. Looks worried, with a pale face. Better from heat.

Secale: With constant bearing-down sensations (also Sepia). Passive hemorrhage of thin, dark, unclotted blood. She's hot and can't tolerate covers. Worse from heat in spite of cold extremities. Sensation as if ants are crawling on her. Spreads her fingers apart from discomfort.

Belladonna: Face is red, hot, and throbbing. Profuse flow of hot blood that coagulates quickly. Cold extremities. Worse from light, noise, cold air, or being jarred.

Cimicifuga: With rheumatic pains in the back and limbs and much anxiety. *Depressed, with much sighing. Feels like she's in a "black cloud." Stiff neck.* Very chilly.

Caulophyllum: From exhaustion and weakness. Especially if this remedy worked during labor. Chilly. *Gentle and weepy, changeable moods, desires company but is not talkative. Craves fresh air.* Chilliness with shivering. Similar to the Pulsatilla state, but more chilly, thirsty, and less needy.

Gossypium: When the placenta is firmly attached to walls of the uterus and will not budge. Backache, with a sense of weight and dragging in the pelvis. Pains are worse from moving.

Sabina: With bright red bleeding (fluid and clots) and severe after-pains, which are felt from back to front. Desires cool air.

Ipecacuanha: Nausea accompanies all other complaints. Sharp, pinching pain around navel, extending to the abdomen. Hemorrhage of bright red blood. Excess saliva, clear tongue. Worse from motion.

Perineal Tears and Episiotomies

Kegel exercises and perineal massage can help prevent tears and the need for episiotomies. Ice packs lubricated with a diluted Calendula tincture are helpful in the first twenty-four hours.

Externally: Calendula tincture, diluted eight drops to half a cup of water, is used topically to speed healing and prevent infection.

***Arnica** (30–200c)**:** If the area feels bruised and is worse from touch. She complains that the chair or bed feels too hard. Arnica helps to control bleeding, prevent infections, reduce swelling, and speed healing.

***Staphisagria:** Useful for clean, razorlike wounds, such as episiotomies. Speeds healing. Administer 200c once a day for a few days, or 30c three times a day.

***Hypericum:** When there is much pain, especially if it radiates from the wound.

***Calendula:** Use in 30c potency for perineal tears.

Asphyxia of the Newborn

(See also "Remedies for the Baby")

In most cases of asphyxia, the baby's lungs remain in the collapsed state. The airways may also be obstructed by meconium or mucus. The remedies on the next page may be life saving in these critical moments. Aside from remedies, it may be necessary to clear the nose, mouth, and throat with gentle suction.

***Antimonium tartaricum:** Top remedy. The baby's lungs are filled with thick mucus and you can hear rattling sounds. Pale skin. Also, when the baby has aspirated meconium.

***Camphora:** Freezing cold, blue, lifeless. Pulse is small and weak. Use Camphora if the newborn's feces (meconium) have been inhaled. Also, if Antimonium tartaricum fails.

***Opium:** Coma or asphyxia, especially after a fright. The mother may have been frightened. The newborn is pale, limp, or unresponsive. The neck is arched back or the body rigid. The face is purple, blue, or red.

***Laurocerasus:** Gasps for breath or is barely breathing. Face is blue or pale and may twitch. Pulse slow and weak. Worse from sitting up. Better from lying down. Strangulation from wrapped cord.

***Arnica** (200c or whatever you have): After any traumatic birth, especially with bruising or head trauma. Reflexes are diminished.

***Arsenicum album:** For newborns who are limp, pale, make little or no attempt to breathe, and who appear lifeless. Also, when no other remedy is clearly indicated.

***Cinchona:** After great loss of blood by the mother. Baby is pale, rather than blue, and may be unconscious.

Aconite: The baby is hot, purplish, breathless, and pulseless. Often due to fright.

Belladonna: The baby is motionless, with staring bloodshot eyes, hot red face, dilated pupils, twitching muscles, and hot moist skin.

Carbo veg: Near death. Limp, flaccid, cold, doesn't react to stimulation. Pulse weak and intermittent, skin pale. Heartbeat is weak. Respiratory distress and blue skin from a tightly wrapped cord. Also for the moderately depressed and persistently blue baby.

Hypericum: Traumatic injury to the baby's spine. Convulsions after birth related to an injury.

Digitalinum: Babies with congestive heart failure.

Childbed Fever (Puerperal Sepsis)

After the first twenty-four hours, if the mother has a fever of 104 degrees or higher for two successive days, it may indicate childbed fever. Fever may be accompanied by chills, headache, weakness, pale face, and rapid pulse. This is a serious condition resulting from infection.

***Pyrogenium:** *Top remedy for childbed fever. She feels bruised all over and the bed feels too hard. Pulse out of sync with fever. High pulse with low fever or low pulse with high fever. Offensive discharges.* The body parts that are lain on become sore, and she must constantly change position for relief. Tongue shiny and red. Worse from cold. She says she can feel her heart beat. Delusions of having extra limbs. Very talkative during fever.

Rhus tox: *Extremely restless and keeps changing position. Very thirsty.* Her muscles feel stiff and ache, and she wants to stretch. Chilly and worse from cold or dampness. Worse after rest. Anxious at night. Itching skin. Red triangle at the tip of the tongue.

Arsenicum: *Extreme anxiety, fear of being alone, great restlessness, exhaustion from the least effort, and great thirst for small, frequent sips of cold water. Burning pains that are relieved by heat.* Offensive discharges, which may burn. Very chilly. During headache, she wants her body warm but her head cold. Delusion that she is being watched. Worse from midnight to 3 a.m.

Arnica: Fear of being touched or approached. Insists she is okay. Complains of the bed being too hard (also Baptisia, Pyrogenium) and is restless. Bruised feeling. Discharges smell like rotten egg. Her head is hot and her body cold. Given before and after labor, Arnica can help prevent childbed fever.

Pulsatilla: *Craves fresh air and wants a window open, even when chilly. Dry mouth but no thirst. Weeps easily.* Irritable or yielding. Symptoms move from place to place and change in character. The patient is short of breath and better sitting up. Better from sympathy and company.

Lachesis: *Inflamed areas have a purplish hue. She always feels worse after sleep. Sensitive to light touch, even the pressure of bedclothes. Can't bear* *anything to touch her neck.* Left-sided symptoms. Pain temporarily relieved each time she bleeds or discharges other fluid. Difficulty swallowing liquids. Worse from hot drinks. Better from open air. Very talkative.

Sulphur: *She feels hot and wants fresh air* (also Pulsatilla). *Burning pains.* Itching and burning of the skin, which is worse from heat. Offensive odor of secretions (stool, sweat, urine). Redness of orifices (lips, eyes, anus, and vagina). Worse from being in a warm room, after bathing, and when standing. Pushes feet out of the covers at night. *When other remedies fail to initiate a response.*

Secale: *Her skin feels cold to the touch, but she feels burning hot inside. Throws off the covers. Worse from heat and better from cold.* Better from fresh air and being fanned (Carbo veg). Discharge of dark blood and pus. Feels like ants are crawling on her skin.

Echinacea: Used in tincture form: 30-drop doses repeated in addition to other remedies, but not at the same time. Veins look dark and distended. Temperature varies widely from high to low.

Postpartum Fatigue

***Cinchona:** Especially from loss of fluids. Worse from touch, pressure, and drafts. Apathetic. Sometimes there are flu-like symptoms.

***Kali phos:** Exhausted, but with so much nervous energy she can't relax or sleep. Worse at night and from heat.

Sepia: Apathetic and depressed or snappish. Weeps for no reason. Worn out, chilly. Feels dragging-down pains. Yellow discoloration on the face.

Phosphoric acid: Apathetic, forgetful, mentally exhausted. Chilly, craves fruit and juicy things, and feels a sensation of a crushing weight at the top of her head. Blue rings around the eyes.

Pulsatilla: Pessimistic, weeps easily, lacks confidence. Better from company and sympathy. Worse from warm rooms and craves fresh air. Thirstless.

Nux moschata: The patient is very drowsy and can barely keep awake—a dreamlike state. Faints easily. Chilly and worse from cold. Alternating moods. Dry mouth without thirst. Bloating and constipation.

Remedies for the Baby

(See also "Asphyxia of Newborn")

Arnica: For traumatic birth, whatever the cause, especially with bruising or head trauma.

Hypericum: For traumatic injury to the baby's spine, or convulsions after birth.

Aconite: When the baby is very frightened.

Depression After Delivery

Symptoms of postpartum depression generally include weeping, insomnia, feelings of hopelessness, inadequacy, anxiety about the demands of motherhood, mood swings, guilt, and loss of interest in daily activities. Caring, nonjudgmental listening is a powerful tool, along with the remedies below.

*****Sepia:** Chilly and worse in cold air. Better from vigorous exercise such as dancing. Apathetic and takes pleasure in nothing. Emotionally tearful or irritable, critical, or snappish. Wants to be alone. Worse from consolation. Craves chocolate, lemons, pickles, and cold drinks.

*****Natrum mur:** Introverted, solitary, and averse to company. Worse from consolation. Weeps when alone. Worse from heat and sensitive to sunlight. Doesn't express feelings or ask for help. Craves salt.

*****Pulsatilla:** Desires sympathy and company. Gentle, yielding, weeps easily in company. Changeable moods. Craves fresh air and can't stand a warm, closed room. No thirst.

*****Platina:** Disappointed in everyone and seems aloof or contemptuous. Laughs at serious matters. Feels like she's alone in the world. Must have the best of everything. Other people appear smaller to her. Sensation as if parts of her were constricted by bandages. Aversion to meat. Better from fresh air.

Aurum: Takes relief in thoughts of suicide. Talks about suicide. Feels she hasn't fulfilled her duty. Guilt feelings, remorse, self condemnation, disgust for life. Feels hurried and can't do things fast enough. Silent with sudden bursts of anger, especially when contradicted. Sobs in her sleep.

Lachesis: Extremely talkative or intense, jumping from one subject to another (also Cimicifuga). Hot and worse from heat. Can't bear anything tight around her neck. Worse after sleep. Suspicious and jealous.

Cimicifuga: Sadness with much sighing. Feels like she's in a "black cloud." Fears insanity. Very talkative, moving from one subject to another. Chilly and better from warmth, but desires fresh air.

Anacardium: Better while eating, but sad again soon after. Deep loss of confidence. Feels like she has two wills and is torn between them. Easily angered and given to hatred. Cannot bear being contradicted. Failing memory. Things seem unreal to her.

Mastitis

Mastitis is an infection of the breast tissue, which may follow a cracked nipple. The breast may be pink or red, swollen, and tender to the touch. The mother has a high temperature with vague flu-like symptoms. This can develop into a serious infection.

Belladonna: Rapid onset. The breast is hard and swollen with throbbing pain. Red streaks radiate from the nipple. The patient feels worse from light, noise, or being jarred.

Bryonia: The breast is hot, hard, and painful. The patient is worse from the least movement, and wants to lie perfectly still. Very thirsty.

Cimicifuga: The left breast is inflamed and worse from cold and in the morning. Physical symptoms may alternate with a gloomy, dark emotional state.

Mercurius: The breast is very painful and worse from heat. She perspires a great deal and feels worse afterward. Bad breath. She has excess saliva, but is very thirsty. Flabby tongue, which shows the imprint of teeth.

Phytolacca: The breast feels heavy, stony hard, swollen, and tender. Pain radiates outward from one point. Better from heat. Worse from dampness.

Silica: Mastitis with a discharge. The patient is thin, weak, and very chilly. She feels better in a warm room with her head covered. Worse from cold, drafts, dampness, noise, light, and being jarred.

Breast Abscess

***Bryonia:** The breast is hot, hard, and painful, but not very red. Pain, which is worse from the slightest movement.

***Belladonna:** Breast feels heavy, with red streaks radiating from one point and throbbing pains. Worse lying down or from being bumped.

***Phytolacca:** Breasts hard and sensitive. Pain radiates from the nipple to the rest of the body when nursing. Purple discoloration (also Lachesis). Ulcers with pus. Worse from cold.

Hepar sulph (6x or 6c)**:** When pus begins to form. Worse from the slightest touch, or from cold or draft.

Silica: Ulceration with a discharge of pus. The patient is thin, chilly, and exhausted. Worse from cold, drafts, light, noise, or being jarred.

Mercurius sol: Much perspiration, chills, and excess saliva. Worse in a warm room and at night.

Lachesis: Breast inflamed, with a purplish color. Worse after sleep. More often on the left side. The patient feels cold at night but experiences flushes of heat during day.

Colic in Babies

Colocynth: The baby pulls its legs up to its abdomen. Sometimes vomiting. Better from warmth.

Magnesia phosphorica: Similar to Colocynth, but even better from warmth.

7

Preventing Illness with Homeopathy

Homeopathic Immunization

Homeopathic remedies can also help prevent illness. If there were an epidemic and you had no vaccines available, you could use remedies to help prevent the disease or reduce its severity.

At the end of this section is a chart with diseases and the remedies that may help prevent them. Some of the remedies are made from the diseases themselves, such as Variolinum (smallpox) and Lyssin (rabies). Others are regular remedies, whose symptom pictures resemble the disease. Examples are Belladonna for scarlet fever, and Mercurius cyanatus for diphtheria.

How well does it work? Neither homeopathy nor vaccines convey absolute protection. However, the greatest homeopathic physicians, from the early days to the present, have recommended homeopathic prevention. They include Doctors Hahnemann, Boenninghausen, Burnett, Kent, Shepherd, Sankaran, and Eizayaga.

The following are examples of homeopathy's effectiveness in preventing illness.

Polio

In the 1957 polio epidemic in Buenos Aires, the remedy Lathyrus 30c was given to thousands of people. Not one case of polio was reported in these individuals. Between 1956 and 1961, Lathyrus in higher potencies was given to over fifty thousand people worldwide. Only one subject developed nonparalytic polio. Lathyrus is made from the chick pea.

Meningitis

In a 1974 epidemic of meningococcal meningitis in Brazil, 18,640 children were given the homeopathic remedy Meningococcinum 10c, one dose. Only four cases of meningitis occurred in these children. Of the 6,340 children who did not receive the nosode, there were thirty-two cases of meningitis reported.

Smallpox

In the smallpox epidemic of 1902 in Iowa, the homeopathic remedy Variolinum was given as prophylaxis to 2,806 patients of fifteen doctors. Of these, 547 were subsequently known to be exposed to smallpox, but only 14 contracted the disease. The protection rate was 97%.

Scarlet Fever

Dr. Hahnemann used Belladonna to prevent scarlet fever during an epidemic. It worked so well that conventional doctors began using it. Dr. R.E. Dudgeon reported that ten doctors used Belladonna on 1,646 children. Only 123 got the disease, yet the usual infection rate was up to 90%. In 1838, the Prussian government made the use of Belladonna obligatory during epidemics.

Cholera

During the cholera epidemic in Europe in 1849, the death rates were as high as 90%, but only 16% for those receiving homeopathic treatment, including prevention.

Diphtheria

H. C. Allen, MD, (1836–1909) ran the Hering Medical College in Chicago. He reported that the remedy Diphtherinum was used for twenty-five years as a prophylactic and he never saw anyone so inoculated develop the disease. He challenged the conventional doctors to test this assertion and publish their own failures.

In 1941, Patterson and Boyd found that twenty children who had tested Schick-positive (susceptible to diphtheria) became Schick-negative (indicating antibodies to diphtheria) after receiving the remedy Diphtherinum. Similar results were obtained by Dr. Roux in 1946.

The general effectiveness of homeopathic prevention was examined by Isaac Golden, PhD, Homeopathic Coordinator of the Melbourne College of Natural Medicine. He reviewed ten years of records of patients who had received homeopathic remedies to prevent disease. He concluded that homeopathic prevention provided an 89% rate of protection.

Golden stated, "This level of efficacy is more than comparable with the rates of protection for vaccines. Those rates range from 75% to 95%, and may be considered best estimates."

The reported effectiveness of homeopathic prevention appears to vary. Some physicians have reported almost perfect results, while others have found a lower percentage of success. Here is one explanation for this seeming inconsistency.

To state that a particular remedy is the preventive for a particular disease oversimplifies the case. For the remedy to work as a preventive, its symptom picture has to match the symptoms of the disease. In a particular year, the symptoms of influenza might be diarrhea, restlessness, burning pains, great thirst, extreme anxiety, and a desire for company.

Those symptoms fit the remedy Arsenicum. It would be easy to conclude that Arsenicum was *the* remedy for flu.

However, the next year, the flu symptoms might be flushed face, chills up the back, pain in the eyeballs, droopy eyelids, slow pulse, lack of thirst, and a desire to be left alone. Those symptoms fit the remedy Gelsemium. If someone used Arsenicum for that flu, he might conclude that preventive remedies didn't work. Thus, mixed reports of success with preventive remedies are partly due to using the wrong remedy.

With that in mind, take the list below as a guide, not an absolute. The list might suggest Belladonna to prevent scarlet fever, because that has always worked in the past. But if everyone is coming down with symptoms that resemble Rhus tox, then give that remedy.

Remedies for Prevention of Illness

Here is a list of ailments and the homeopathic remedies used for prevention. The asterisk (*) indicates that the remedy is a nosode, which is made from diseased tissue. You can't catch any disease from them because none of the original substance remains. However, some homeopathic pharmaceutical companies require a prescription for them. A dose of 30c potency once or twice a week during the epidemic is most often recommended. If the nosode is available, that should be your first choice. If several remedies are listed, give the one you have, or the one that best matches the symptoms occurring during the epidemic. For characteristics of the remedies, see chapter 5, "Remedy Descriptions."

Amoebic dysentery: *Entamoeba histolytica, Arsenicum album

Anthrax: *Anthracinum

Bubonic plague: *Yersinia pestis nosode, Baptisia

Chickenpox: *Varicella, Antimonium crudum, Pulsatilla, Rhus tox

Cholera: *Vibrio cholerae nosode, Cuprum met, Camphora, Veratrum album

Conjunctivitis: Belladonna

Croup: Phosphorus, Aconite

Diphtheria: *Diphtherinum, Mercurius cyanatus

Hepatitis: *Hepatitis A nosode, hepatitis B nosode, Phosphorus, Chelidonium

Hydrophobia: *Hydrophobinum (Lyssin)

Hypothermia: Aconite

Influenza: *Influenzinum, Oscillococcinum, Gelsemium, Arsenicum, Rhus tox, Eupatorium

Lyme disease: *Borrelia burgdorferi, Ledum

Malaria: *Malaria officinalis, Cinchona, Arsenicum album, Natrum mur

Measles: *Morbillinum, Pulsatilla, Aconite, Arsenicum

Meningococcal meningitis: *Meningococcinum

Mumps: *Parotidinum, Mercurius vivus, Phytolacca

Polio: Lathyrus, Plumbum

Puerperal fever: Pyrogenium

Scarlet fever: *Scarlatinum, Belladonna

Smallpox: *Variolinum, *Malandrinum

Tetanus: *Clostridium tetani, Ledum, Hypericum, Magnesia phos

Typhus: Rhus tox, Baptisia

Tuberculosis: *Bacillinum, Drosera

Typhoid: *Salmonella typhi nosode, Baptisia

Whooping cough: *Pertussinum, Drosera, Carbo vegetabilis

Yellow fever: *Yellow fever nosode, Crotalus horridus, Carbo veg, Arsenicum

Bubonic plague: *Yersinia pestis nosode, Baptisia, Ignatia (tincture)

8

First Aid Remedies for Specific Occupations and Activities

Certain occupations and activities lend themselves to particular injuries or dangers. This section was included because it makes great sense to carry a handful of remedies that might save your life or prevent serious injury. In a critical moment, a remedy administered *immediately* can make all the difference. Take the remedy and then call an ambulance. The remedy could buy you the time you need to survive. Below are the most important remedies for each occupation or activity. If it's an unusual remedy or potency, order it now and keep it handy.

Activists

Arnica: For head injuries and rough lacerations.

Euphrasia: For the effects of tear gas.

Hypericum: For head or spine injuries.

Staphysagria: For sharp cuts as from a knife or razor.

Astronauts

Carbo veg: For asphyxia and the effects of reduced-oxygen environments.

Arnica: Any kind of physical trauma. Microhemorrhages. For takeoff and landing.

Cocculus indicus: To help meliorate the effects of loss of sleep.

Aconite: To help combat the effects of hypothermia. Also for panic.

Coffea: To help sleep when insomnia is due to an overactive mind.

Athletes

Arnica: For sprains, broken bones, and head or back injuries.

Rhus tox: Stiffness and soreness that feels better from moving and worse after rest.

Bryonia: Pain that is worse from the slightest motion. Hot, swollen joints.

Ruta: For bruises in bony areas. Also for injuries to the heel.

Hypericum: Head and spine injuries.

Bartenders

Arnica (200c)**:** For gunshot wounds, stabbings, fists in the face, etc. Just keep this high-potency remedy handy. Use it immediately and then call emergency.

Nux vomica: Top remedy for hangover. It addresses the gastric upset and mental irritability associated with overindulgence.

Bikers

Arnica: Use immediately after any fall, even if you don't think you're hurt. Use especially after scrapes, bruises, ragged cuts, broken bones, and head injuries.

Hypericum: A must for injuries to the head or spine, to be used after Arnica. Especially if there is extreme pain or convulsions, or injuries to parts rich in nerves, such as fingertips.

Calendula gel or cream: Used externally for cuts and scrapes. Helps prevent infection and speeds healing. Wash the area first to remove dirt and debris.

Campers

Arnica: Top remedy for any trauma. For any bruising injury, head injury, or broken bone.

Apis: For bee stings. Use as needed.

Ledum: For any puncture wound, including the stings of insects as well as spider and snake bites. May help prevent tetanus. May be followed by Hypericum if there is much pain.

Calendula gel or cream: Used externally for cuts and scrapes. Speeds healing and helps prevent infection. Wash the injured part first to remove dirt and debris.

Hypericum: For head or spine injuries or any injury that is extremely painful.

Cantharis: For burns.

Carpenters

Arnica: Top remedy for any bruising injury, ragged cut, head injury, or broken bone.

Hypericum: For banged-up fingers and toes that are very painful. Use after Arnica for head or spine injuries.

Ledum: For puncture wounds. May help prevent tetanus. Follow with Hypericum if there is much pain.

Silica: For splinters that are too deep to reach. Causes the body to expel them, even if they've been there for years. Use the 6c potency two to three times a day for ten days. *Note: Do not use Silica if you have any kind of surgical implant.*

Chemists

Cantharis: Top remedy for burns. Can also be used externally by diluting the tincture, eight drops to a pint of water. Dip a clean cloth in this and wrap the wound. Keep it wet with this mixture.

Euphrasia: Top remedy for eye irritation. Can also be used topically by dissolving a couple pellets in spring water and placing a few drops in the eye.

Milk thistle (the herb)**:** To help protect the liver during exposure to solvents and other toxins.

Climbers

Arnica: Top remedy for any bruising injury, ragged cut, head injury, or broken bone.

Hypericum: For banged-up fingers and toes that are very painful. Use after Arnica for head or spine injuries.

Aconite: For hypothermia.

Carbo veg: For the effects of altitude.

Construction

Arnica (30c or 200c)**:** For any bruising injury, broken bone, or head or spine injury.

Hypericum: For any wound with extreme pain. For banged fingers or toes. A must for head or spine injuries. Use after Arnica.

Calendula gel: Externally for cuts and scrapes. Speeds healing and helps prevent infection.

Ledum: For any puncture wound. Follow with Hypericum if there is extreme pain.

Belladonna: Top remedy for sunstroke.

Cooks/Bakers

Cantharis: Top remedy for burns.

Staphysagria: For cuts from knives and other sharp instruments.

Arnica: For ragged cuts.

Calendula gel: Use externally for cuts to speed healing and help prevent infection.

Dancers

Arnica: First treatment for sprains.

Rhus tox: For stiffness and soreness that feels better from moving and worse after rest.

Bryonia: Pain that is worse from the slightest motion.

Ruta: Torn or sprained ligaments. Also for pain in the heel.

Argentum nitricum: Anticipatory anxiety before a performance.

Dentists and Their Patients

Ledum: For puncture wounds. May help prevent infection.

Arnica: Prior to extractions, surgery, or periodontal work. Lessens pain, reduces bleeding, and speeds healing.

Hypericum: For pain after any dental work. Complements Arnica. Best used immediately after the procedure, since it may interfere with local anesthetics.

Hepar sulph (6x or 6c)**:** Three times a day to prevent infection.

Phosphorus: A single dose if there is excessive bleeding.

Doctors

(See also chapter 7, "Preventing Illness with Homeopathy," for remedies to use if you are going to be exposed to contagious diseases)

Ledum: To help prevent infection from puncture wounds. This may be effective regardless of the particular germ or virus. Especially important when there are sharp objects in a contaminated environment.

Calendula (tincture, diluted)**:** To help prevent infection and speed the healing of cuts.

Cocculus: To help dispel the effects of loss of sleep.

Electricians/Electronics

Electric Shock

If the patient is not breathing, begin mouth-to-mouth resuscitation. If there is no heartbeat, begin cardiopulmonary resuscitation. The following remedies may help.

Arnica: For electric shock with or without stoppage of the heart. Give the highest potency you have. Place the remedy between the lips and teeth.

Phosphorus: Pale face, weak pulse. Place the remedy between the lips and teeth.

Cantharis: Burns from electricity.

Farmers

Arnica: For any bruising injury, broken bone, ragged cut, or head or spine injury.

Ledum: For any puncture wound. Follow with Hypericum if there is extreme pain. May help prevent tetanus.

Hypericum: For any wound with extreme pain. Use after Arnica for head and spine injuries.

Calendula gel: Externally for cuts and scrapes. Speeds healing and helps prevent infection.

Apis: Specific for bee stings.

Rhus tox: Top remedy for poison ivy.

Firefighters

Arnica (30 or 200c)**:** For any bruising injury or ragged cut. For head or spine injuries and broken bones.

Hypericum: A must for head or spine injuries to be used after Arnica. Also, any other injury with extreme pain, including burns.

Cantharis: Top remedy for burns. Take a few pellets as needed.

Cantharis externally: A good dressing for burns. Dilute the tincture eight drops to a pint of water. Dip a clean cloth in this and wrap the wound. Keep it wet with this mixture.

Carbo veg: After smoke inhalation. Difficulty breathing, can't seem to get enough air. Also for states of collapse, with shortness of breath, cold breath, and cold hands and feet.

Belladonna (30 or 200c)**:** If you feel overheated, with a flushed face or throbbing head.

Calendula gel or diluted tincture: Used externally for cuts, scrapes, and other open wounds. Speeds healing and helps prevent infection.

Ledum: For any puncture wound. May help prevent tetanus or other complications from a puncture wound. Follow with Hypericum if there is extreme pain.

Cocculus indicus: To help counter the effects of loss of sleep.

Fishermen

Arnica: For any trauma to the body. Broken bones, head or spine injuries, or ragged cuts.

Ledum: For any puncture wound, including insect stings and fish hooks. May help prevent tetanus. Follow with Hypericum if there is extreme pain.

Apis: Specific for bee stings.

Hypericum: For any injury with extreme pain, especially for crushing injuries to fingers and toes. Also for head and spine injuries.

Carbo veg: For use in drowning along with resuscitation. Place the remedy between the lips and teeth.

Calendula gel: Use externally for open wounds. Speeds healing and helps prevent infection.

Forestry/Loggers

Arnica (30c or 200c)**:** For any trauma to the body. Broken bones, head or spine injuries, or ragged cuts.

Ledum: For any puncture wound including insect stings. May help prevent tetanus. Follow with Hypericum if there is extreme pain.

Hypericum: For any injury with extreme pain. Especially for crushing injuries to fingers and toes and for head and spine injuries. For severed digits or limbs.

Calendula gel: Externally for open wounds. Speeds healing and helps prevent infection.

Apis: Specific for bee stings.

Hairstylists

Staphysagria: Cuts from scissors or razors.

Milk thistle (the herb): To protect the liver from chemicals.

Hikers

Arnica: Top remedy for any trauma. For any bruising injury, head injury, or broken bone.

Rhus tox (30 or 200c): For poison ivy. Also useful for sprains with stiffness that is better from movement and worse after rest.

Apis: For bee stings. Use as needed.

Ledum: For any puncture wound including the stings of insects and snake bites. May help prevent tetanus. May be followed by Hypericum if there is much pain.

Calendula gel or cream: Used externally for cuts and scrapes. Speeds healing and helps prevent infection. Wash the injured part first to remove dirt and debris.

Hypericum: For any injury that is extremely painful.

Aconite: For hypothermia.

Joggers

Arnica: First treatment for sprains.

Rhus tox: Stiffness and soreness that feels better from moving and worse after rest.

Bryonia: Pain that is worse from the slightest motion.

Ruta: Torn or sprained ligaments. Also for pain in the heel.

Loggers: See "Forestry"

Machinist/Mechanics

Silica: Helps expel splinters of wood or metal that are too small or deep to be removed. Works even if the splinter has been there for months or years. Silica 6c, three times a day for a couple weeks.

Arnica: For any trauma to the body.

Hypericum: For injuries to parts rich in nerves, such as fingers and toes, injuries to the head or spine, and injuries that are especially painful.

Ledum: For puncture wounds. Follow with Hypericum if there is much pain.

Cantharis: For burns.

Phosphorus: For electric shock (also Arnica).

Miners

Silica: Helps expel foreign objects from the body. May assist the body to expel microscopic particles from the lungs and airways.

Antimonium tartaricum: Thick mucus in lungs that cannot be coughed up. You can hear it rattling.

Arnica: For any trauma to the body. Bruising injuries, broken bones, head or spine injuries, ragged cuts, gunshot wounds, or shock.

Ledum: For any puncture wound. May help prevent tetanus. May be followed by Hypericum if there is much pain.

Staphysagria: Clean, razorlike cuts as from a sharp knife.

Cantharis: A few pellets under the tongue are excellent for burns. The diluted tincture is used externally for burns.

Calendula gel or cream: Used externally for cuts and scrapes. Speeds healing and helps prevent infection. Wash injured part first to remove dirt and debris.

Hypericum: For any injury that is extremely painful. For head and spine injuries.

Hepar sulph: For local infections where pus has begun to form. Use 6x or 6c potency.

Musicians

Argentum nitricum: To help dispel anxiety before a performance.

Cocculus ind: To help recover from loss of sleep.

Nurses

(See also chapter 7, "Preventing Illness with Homeopathy," for remedies to use if you are going to be exposed to contagious diseases)

Ledum: To help prevent infections from puncture wounds. This may be effective regardless of the particular germ or virus. Especially important when there are sharp objects in a contaminated environment.

Calendula (tincture, diluted)**:** To help prevent infection and speed the healing of cuts. Used externally.

Cocculus: To help dispel the effects of loss of sleep.

Painters

Alumina: For the chronic effects of lead poisoning.

Arnica: For traumatic injuries.

Hypericum: For injuries to the head or spine. Use after Arnica.

Milk thistle (the herb)**:** To help protect the liver from the effects of solvents.

Pest Control

For Chronic Poisoning from Arsenic

Arsenicum: For anxiety, chills, restlessness, or burning pains that are better from warmth. Thirst for small sips of water, exhaustion from the slightest exertion, fear of being alone.

Hepar sulph: Chilly, irritable, worse from drafts. Every injury becomes infected. Extreme sensitivity to touch and pain. Splinterlike pains. Craves vinegar.

Carbo veg: For a state of collapse with shortness of breath, distended abdomen with much belching, or burning in the chest, stomach or abdomen. Head hot but hands and feet cold.

Milk thistle (the herb)**:** To help protect the liver from the effects of solvents.

Pilots

Cocculus: Helps the body and mind cope with the effects of loss of sleep. Useful for jet lag. (Melatonin, 3 mg or less, also helps with jet lag. Melatonin for three days before and five days after crossing time zones.)

Arnica (200c)**:** For any kind of trauma, including broken bones and head injuries.

Ruta: For eye strain.

Carbo veg: For the effects of low-oxygen environments, such as a depressurized cabin.

Police

Arnica (200c)**:** For any trauma to the body, including bruising injuries, broken bones, head or spine injuries, ragged cuts, gunshot wounds, and shock.

Ledum: For any puncture wound including the stings of insects. May help prevent tetanus. May be followed by Hypericum if there is much pain.

Staphysagria: Clean razorlike cuts as from a sharp knife.

Cantharis: A few pellets under the tongue are excellent for burns. The diluted tincture is used externally for burns.

Calendula gel or cream: Used externally for cuts and scrapes. Speeds healing and helps prevent infection. Wash the injured part first to remove dirt and debris.

Hypericum: For any injury that is extremely painful. For head and spine injuries.

Postal Carriers

Arnica: For back sprain.

Rhus tox: Back sprain that is worse after rest.

Bryonia: Back sprain that is worse from any movement.

Roofer

Arnica: For any injury—bruises, bumps, falls.

Hypericum: For any injury to the head or spine. Follows Arnica.

Cantharis (30 or 200c)**:** For burns.

Sales

Lycopodium: For loss of confidence.

Staphysagria: Suppressed anger from frustration.

Scuba Divers

Carbo veg: To help revive a drowning victim after CPR.

Tabacum: For seasickness.

Magnesia phosphorica: For cramps.

Kali mur (6c)**:** If the ear feels clogged after swimming.

Secretaries

Ruta graveolens: Carpal tunnel syndrome and other repetitive motion injuries. Also useful for eye strain.

Skiing

Arnica: For any traumatic injury including broken bones and head or spine injuries.

Hypericum: Use after Arnica for head or spine injuries.

Aconite: For hypothermia, both prevention and treatment.

Agaricus: For frostbite.

Carbo veg: Altitude sickness.

Mercurialis perennis: Snow blindness. Pain, burning, watery eyes. Seems like there is a cloud or veil before the eyes. Pupils dilated and eyes very sensitive to light.

Kali mur: Snow blindness. Seems like smoke and mist before the eyes.

Phosphorus: Snow blindness like a veil before the eyes. Letters look red. Green halo around candle light.

Soldiers

Homeopathic remedies are the greatest military secret ever.

Arnica (200c)**:** For bullet wounds, ragged cuts, broken bones, head injuries, shock, or any trauma to the body. Repeat as need in a critical situation.

Hypericum: For any injury that is extremely painful. Use after Arnica for head and spine injuries.

Cantharis (30 or 200c)**:** For burns.

Carbo veg: Homeopaths call this the "corpse reviver." When someone is barely alive, or cold and lifeless, this remedy may pull him back from the abyss.

Cinchona: Loss of blood. This remedy helps the body sustain itself after loss of blood. You still need a transfusion, but it will buy you some time.

Calendula gel: Cuts and scrapes. Speeds healing and helps prevent infection. If a wound can heal in two days instead of four, you're better off.

Aconite: For the sheer terror that can occur in or before battle.

Speakers/Announcers

Argentum metallicum: Total loss of voice from overuse.

Arum triphyllum: Hoarseness from overuse of the voice. Throat may burn.

Telephone Linemen

Arnica (200c)**:** For any trauma including falls, electric shock, ragged cuts, and head and spine injuries.

Hypericum: For any injury that is very painful. Use after Arnica for head and spine injuries.

Phosphorus: Follows Arnica for electric shock.

Tailors

Ledum: Puncture wounds.

Ruta grav: Eyestrain.

Truckers

Cocculus: To help relieve the effects of loss of sleep.

Ruta: Eyestrain.

Arnica: For any injury.

Typists

Ruta grav: Carpal tunnel syndrome. This remedy also helps eyestrain.

Welders

Arnica: For any traumatic injury.

Cantharis: Top remedy for burns.

Phosphorus: Use after Arnica for electric shock.

Carbo veg: For the effects of breathing hot air.

9

Economizing: Making Your Remedies Last Forever

If you ever find yourself running out of a remedy, or if you have to treat many people with a small amount of a remedy, there is a way to extend what you have.

1. Place a few pellets of your remaining remedy in a clean bottle and add 2 to 4 ounces of water (spring, filtered, or distilled). Shake the bottle vigorously for a couple minutes. This conveys the medicinal quality to the water. Each dose of the water (½ tsp.) acts as a dose of the remedy. If you wish to store this for later use, add a bit of pure grain alcohol (NOT rubbing alcohol) or brandy and keep the bottle away from the light.
2. There is a second method of extending a remedy. Purchase some blank pellets. If you have a container of remedy with five or six pellets left, give it several good shakes, then fill that container half full with blank pellets and shake vigorously. The blanks pellets become transformed into remedy by contact with the other pellets and the "dust" from the sides of the container.

A more efficient way to do this is to add a few drops of grain alcohol (the drinkable alcohol) to the few remaining pellets in your bottle. Shake the bottle a few times. Then add the blank pellets and shake again. The alcohol picks up the remedy frequency and transfers it to the blank pellets. *Note that this uses grain alcohol, NOT rubbing alcohol!*

> **Note:** Although the above methods work just fine, I urge people to purchase remedies from homeopathic pharmacies when possible. The pharmacies produce high-quality remedies and they need our support.

Making Remedies from Scratch

Most of the remedies you will ever need are available at health food stores or homeopathic pharmacies. You don't have to make your own remedies. However, there are rare situations where you might want to.

> **Example:** If you've been made ill by some toxin (pesticide, drug, plant, or food) and want to get it out of your system, you can potentize it and use it as a remedy. A remedy made from the offending substance can cause your body to excrete it or defend against it.

You could also make a remedy out of diseased material.

> **Example:** If someone has an infection or a tumor and you've tried everything else, you could make a remedy from the diseased material. A bit of pus, some sputum, or tartar from infected gums can be turned into a remedy. This may act as a specific trigger for the immune system.

Materials

A half-ounce dropper bottle (must be absolutely clean). Water (spring, filtered, or distilled). A clean cup. Disposable plastic is fine. A small quantity of pure grain alcohol (vodka or brandy can substitute).

What You Will Be Doing—Overview

Start with a solution of what you want to turn into a remedy. Dilute it, one part to ninety-nine parts of water and tap the container thirty times. Take one part of that solution and dilute it with ninety-nine parts of water and again tap it thirty times. You continue this procedure of diluting and tapping as many times as you wish. Each time you do this, you raise the potency by one degree (1c). For example, doing it twelve times creates a 12c potency.

There is a simple method of making these dilutions without any measuring devices. This method makes uses of the fact that a half-ounce bottle, when one-third full, holds about ninety-nine drops of water. When it is emptied quickly (don't let it drain), one drop remains clinging to the sides. Every time you empty it and fill it to one third, you have made another 1:99-part dilution.

The Method

a. Using a clean cup, make a solution of whatever you want to turn into a remedy. If it is a solid, crush it and mix with water. Let it sit a while and pour off (and save) the liquid. Discard the rest.

b. Fill your half-ounce bottle one-third full with the liquid. Put the cap on tight. Tap the bottle firmly against a book about thirty times. Now empty the bottle and quickly set it upright again. Approximately one drop will remain clinging to the sides. Fill it one-third full with water again. Replace the top. Tap the bottle another thirty times. Empty the bottle and fill it one third again. Replace the top and tap thirty times.

Continue this process as many times as you wish. The more times you do it, the stronger the remedy will be. After the last dilution, you have two options, depending on whether you want the remedy to exist as a liquid or as pellets.

Liquid

After the last dilution (you emptied all but one drop), fill the bottle nearly to the top with water and add fifteen drops of pure grain alcohol (drinking alcohol, not rubbing alcohol!) to preserve it. You could also use brandy or vodka. That's it! A dose would be a few drops on your patient's tongue.

Pellets

When you get to the last dilution, empty the bottle and, instead of adding water, add four drops of pure grain alcohol (the drinkable kind—190 proof, available at liquor stores). Twirl the bottle a few times so the alcohol covers the sides. Then fill the bottle three-fourths full with blank pellets and shake well. The pellets will all be coated with the remedy. Leave the bottle open for a few minutes to allow for drying. That's it. A dose is two or three pellets.

Clarifications

a. At each stage of dilution you are discarding all but the one drop that remains clinging to the sides of the half-ounce bottle.

b. Regarding your original solution, you actually use only one drop of it to get the process started. When you empty the bottle, a single drop remains.

c. When making a remedy from a toxic substance, it is recommended that you potentize to at least a 12c (twelve dilutions). That ensures there will be none of the original substance remaining. It's the energy pattern that does the healing.

d. When making a remedy from diseased tissue, let it sit in pure grain alcohol overnight and then use this as the starter solution. Potentize to at least 12c (twelve dilutions).

10
Homeopathy Around the World

Who Uses Homeopathy?

According to the World Health Organization (WHO), over five hundred million people use homeopathy. It is the second most widely practiced form of medicine in the world. The WHO cited homeopathy as a "traditional (holistic) medicine that should be integrated worldwide with conventional medicine in order to provide adequate global health care."

Homeopathy is included in the national health care systems of England, France, and the Netherlands. In 1992 the European Parliament approved guidelines for its use throughout Europe.

In England, homeopathy was recognized as a postgraduate medical speciality by an act of Parliament. Forty-two percent of British doctors refer their patients for homeopathic care. The Royal Family has used homeopathic physicians for three generations. Prince Charles carries a homeopathic kit when he travels.

Homeopathic hospitals in England include the Royal London Homeopathic Hospital, Tunbridge Wells Homeopathic Hospital, Bristol

Homeopathic Hospital, Liverpool Hahnemann Hospital, Liverpool Homeopathic Clinic, Manchester Homeopathic Clinic, and Mossley Hill Hospital.

In Scotland, homeopathy is the fastest-growing alternative therapy. Forty percent of Scots said they would consider a homeopath for medical treatment. The Glasgow Homeopathic Hospital has been in existence for almost a century.

In France, 39% of doctors have prescribed homeopathic remedies, and eight medical schools offer postgraduate degrees in homeopathy (Besançon, Bordeaux, Lille, Limoges, Lyon, Marseilles, Paris-Nord, and Poitiers). French pharmacists are required to learn about homeopathic remedies, which are sold in all twenty-three thousand pharmacies. Forty percent of the French public have used the remedies.

Homeopathy is also practiced in a number of hospitals in France, including the Hôpital Saint-Jacques, the Hahnemann Clinic, Hôtel Dieu, Hôpital Saint-Luc in Lyon, Hôpital Tenon in Paris, and Hôpital Pellegrin in Bordeaux. They offer consultations by homeopathic physicians, including specialists in areas such as gastroenterology, pediatrics, obstetrics, gynecology, and ear, nose, and throat. Four veterinary schools offer training in homeopathy.

In Russia, the "polyclinics" have homeopathic physicians. Patients can be hospitalized and treated by the attending homeopathic physician. The Moscow Homeopathic Center employs 120 homeopathic physicians and celebrated its ninetieth birthday in 2000.

In the Netherlands, 40% of general practitioners dispense homeopathic remedies.

In Germany, 20% of physicians dispense homeopathic remedies. Homeopathic care is provided at Stuggart Homeopathic Hospital and Bosch Homeopathy Hospital, Munchen, Germany.

In India, there are seventy thousand board-certified homeopathic physicians. Homeopathy is practiced in one thousand hospitals. One example is Nehru Homoeopathic Medical College and Hospital. It awards degrees in homeopathy after the completion of five and a half years of training. It has a modern one hundred bed hospital, with departments of X-ray, dentistry, pathology, gynecology, and obstetrics.

In Mexico, approximately 120,000 homeopathic consultations take place each year in official homeopathic hospitals and clinics. There are five homeopathic medical colleges, including the National School of Medicine and Homeopathy at the National Polytechnic Institute of Mexico and the University of La Antiquera in Oaxaca. Three thousand physicians are trained in homeopathy.

In Spain, homeopathic training has been offered for over fifteen years in collaboration with the most prestigious universities (Salamanca, Seville, Valladolid, and Murcia). About four thousand doctors prescribe homeopathic remedies.

In Italy, 7,500 physicians prescribe homeopathic remedies. Training is offered in the major cities, including Bologna, Milan, Rome, Turin, Florence, and Venice.

In Belgium, 40% of the population uses homeopathy and there are about three hundred homeopathic medical doctors. Ten percent of the other doctors prescribe homeopathic medications at least occasionally.

In Eastern and Central Europe, thousands of physicians have been trained in homeopathy (more than eight thousand in Poland, the Czech Republic, and Slovakia). In Romania, the Romanian Institute of Post-University Continuing Education for Medical Personnel offers three-year training courses in homeopathy.

In Poland, homeopathic training is offered to physicians and pharmacists at seven university centers: the Academy of Medicine of Warsaw, the Karol Marcinkowski Academy of Medicine in Poznan, the Collegium Medicum of the Jagellone University in Krakow, the Silesian Academy of Medicine (SAM) in Katowice, the Academy of Medicine in Lublin, the Academy of Medicine in Gdansk, and the Academy of Medicine in Wroclaw.

Homeopathy is also practiced in Vienna, Scotland, New Zealand, Norway, Sweden, Australia, Greece, Belgium, Canada, Brazil, Argentina, Venezuela, and Pakistan.

Well-Known People Who Have Used Homeopathy

The British Royal Family since the 1830s. Queen Elizabeth is patron of the Royal London Homeopathic Hospital.

Pope Pius X consulted homeopaths.

Mother Teresa: Four homeopathic dispensaries are run under the auspices of Mother Teresa's Missionaries of Charity.

Mahatma Gandhi: "Homeopathy cures a larger percentage of cases than any other method, and is beyond all doubt safer, more economical, and the most complete medical science."

Charles Menninger, MD, founder of Menninger Clinic: "Homeopathy is wholly capable of satisfying the therapeutic demands of this age better than any other system or school of medicine."

Mark Twain: "The introduction of homeopathy forced the old school doctor to stir around and learn something of a rational nature about his business. You may feel honestly grateful that homeopathy survived the attempts of the allopaths [orthodox physicians] to destroy it."

Yehudi Menuhin: "Homeopathy is the safest and most reliable approach to ailments and has withstood the assaults of established medical practice for over one hundred years."

Also, **William James**, **Henry Wadsworth Longfellow**, **Daniel Webster**, **Harriet Beecher Stowe**, **Samuel F. Morse**, **John D. Rockefeller**, and **Charles Dickens** have used homeopathy.

A Brief History of Homeopathy in the United States

Homeopathy was first practiced in the United States around 1825. The first homeopathic academy was established at Philadelphia in 1835, by Dr. Constantine Hering.

While studying medicine in Germany, Hering's professor had asked him to write a book disproving homeopathy. In the process of doing that, Hering became convinced that homeopathy was, in fact, the most effective healing art. He went on to become one of the greatest homeopaths of all time and was known as the father of American homeopathy.

The Homeopathic Medical College of Pennsylvania opened in Philadelphia on October 16, 1848. In 1869, it was renamed Hahnemann Medical College. In 1844, the American Institute of Homeopathy was founded.

It was during the 1800s and early part of the 1900s that homeopathy blossomed. By 1900, there were fifteen thousand homeopathic physicians in the United States. That was about 25% of all practicing doctors. There were a hundred homeopathic hospitals. They had all the amenities of the orthodox hospitals, except that homeopathy was practiced. Many cities also had free homeopathic dispensaries for the poor. A thousand homeopathic pharmacies around the country dispensed the remedies.

There were twenty-two homeopathic medical schools, including Boston University, New York Medical College, and Hahnemann Medical College. One of these homeopathic schools, Boston Female Medical College, was the first women's medical school in the world. It was established in 1848. It was another forty years before a conventional medical school in the United States accepted a woman as a student.

The growth and popularity of homeopathy was due to its startling success in treating illness. During the epidemics of the 1800s, survival rates in homeopathic hospitals were often 50% or greater than in conventional hospitals. In the 1849 cholera epidemic in Cincinnati, the death rate in conventional hospitals was 40–70%, but only 3% in homeopathic hospitals.

During the yellow fever epidemic of 1878, survival rates for those under homeopathic care were two-thirds greater than for those treated conventionally.

But it wasn't just in epidemics that homeopathy excelled. Its success in treating common illnesses and in maintaining people's health, led some life insurance companies to offer a 10% discount to homeopathic patients.

With such a record, homeopathy might well have become the prevailing medical practice in the United States. However, it was soon to meet formidable opposition.

Conventional doctors were losing patients to homeopaths and so, in 1847, they formed the American Medical Association (AMA). That organization was founded with the explicit purpose of eliminating homeopathy in the United States. Since homeopaths used minute doses, made their own remedies, or used their own chemists, the pharmaceutical companies also felt threatened by homeopaths. The AMA subsequently formed a coalition with American pharmaceutical companies in 1865, and began a campaign to discredit homeopathy. This campaign included the following measures:

1. The AMA prohibited its members from consulting or even associating with homeopaths on pain of expulsion.
2. The AMA demanded that local and state medical societies purge themselves of homeopathic members.
3. The AMA pressured medical academies to exclude homeopaths from membership.
4. There was a witch-hunting period during which suspected homeopathic sympathizers were removed from the ranks of the AMA.
5. The Flexner Report. In 1910, a commission headed by Abraham Flexner, who was hostile to homeopathy, issued a report on the state of the medical schools. The criteria for rating the schools was purposely biased to reflect poorly on homeopathic schools. Ratings were based on whether the school had a museum with exhibits or elaborate laboratories. They also gave emphasis to courses that were irrelevant or of little importance in homeopathic medicine.

The Flexner Report gave low ratings to the homeopathic schools, in spite of the fact that students from homeopathic schools scored better on licensing exams than students from conventional schools (12% of conventional students failed, but only 3% of homeopathic students did).

State licensing boards started barring homeopathic students from taking the exams. Financial support for homeopathic schools started to dry up. By 1918, only seven schools were left. By 1945, the last one (Hahnemann) dropped its required courses in homeopathy. The last elective course was taught in 1949, and the last degree issued in 1950. (For a more complete account see *Divided Legacy vol. III* by Harris Coulter.)

Another dynamic also led to the end of homeopathic education. Beginning in 1870, commercial medical schools came into existence. They were not associated with a university and had no clinics or hospitals. Homeopaths were hired to teach homeopathy, but conventional doctors taught everything else. Students were given a distorted and negative view of homeopathy. Basic concepts such as the law of similars, the minimum dose, totality of symptoms, and the single remedy were disregarded or ridiculed. The schools graduated many doctors who called themselves homeopaths, but actually practiced conventional medicine.

Homeopathy in the United States Today

Starting around 1970, there was a resurgence of interest in homeopathy in the United States. In the U.S., there are probably less than 1,500 physicians skilled in homeopathy. A few medical schools are starting to offer it as an elective. The Universities of Maryland, Columbia, Arizona, San Francisco, New York, and California, as well as Harvard Medical School have "complementary medicine" centers that offer information on homeopathy. There are also several thousand lay or paraprofessional homeopaths (nurses, chiropractors, naturopaths, physician assistants, etc.). Six or seven insurance companies cover homeopathy, including Blue Cross of Alaska and Blue Cross of Washington State.

Study Groups

In the United States, it is laypeople who have taken the initiative in promoting homeopathy. In every state in the union, laypeople have formed self-teaching groups to learn homeopathy. They meet in churches, community centers, or living rooms. They invite local homeopaths to lecture or they learn from books and tapes. There are now around three hundred such groups. The National Center for Homeopathy (NCH) can help you locate the nearest homeopathic study group, or assist you in starting one in your own community. The NCH can be reached at 877-624-0613 or 703-548-7790, or by e-mail at nchinfo@igc.org. Address: NCH, 801 N. Fairfax St., Suite 306, Alexandria, VA 22314-1757.

II

How to Use a Repertory

A repertory is a book that lists hundreds or thousands of symptoms together with the remedies that cure them. The object of a repertory is to find which remedy covers most of your patient's symptoms. You look up each of your patient's symptoms and write down all the remedies listed there. The remedy that turns up under most of the symptoms will be your first choice. If more than one remedy turns up under most of the symptoms, then you choose the one that received the most emphasis in the repertory. The greatest emphasis is given to remedies listed in **BOLD** print. The next degree is the remedies listed in *italics* The least emphasis is given to the remedies listed in small print. Look for the remedy that appears most often in **BOLD** or *italics*.

The Steps in Using a Repertory

1. Write down your patient's symptoms and whatever you observe about her.

    Does she have fever, nausea, perspiration, diarrhea, vomiting, or pain? Is her face flushed, pale, or blue? Is she bleeding? Is she chilly or warm? Thirsty or thirstless?

What is her mental state? This can be as important as the physical symptoms. Is she anxious, fearful, apathetic, depressed, angry, restless, talkative, delirious, or delusional? Does she want company or prefer to be left alone? What makes her feel better or worse? Is she better or worse from lying down, bending double, moving about, lying still, warmth, cool air, noise, light, motion, or sweating? Is she worse at midnight, 3 a.m., 4 p.m.?

2. Look up each symptom in the repertory and write down the remedies that are listed there. It's a bit tedious, but you can save a life this way. The remedy that turns up in the most number of symptoms will likely cure.

Note: The remedies will be abbreviated (e.g., Bell = Belladonna, Ars = Arsenicum, Pul = Pulsatilla).

Using the Repertory: A Sample Case

You have a patient who is coughing up bright red blood, has intense nausea that is not relieved by vomiting, is frightfully anxious, and is producing lots of saliva.

In the repertory you find the following symptoms and remedies. Notice that "**Ip**" (Ipecacuanha) is found under more symptoms than any other remedy. I've added the parentheses for clarity. Ipecacuanha will probably cure.

1. **Nausea with deathly anxiety:** Ant c, Ant t, Cocl, Crot h, (**Ip**), Lob, Pul, Tab
2. **Nausea, vomiting does not ameliorate:** Dig, (**Ip**), Sang
3. **Saliva—increased:** Am c, Aru t, Bar c, Bor, Dig, Dul, Flu ac, (**Ip**), Iris, Kali c, Lyss, Manc, Merc, Merc c, Nat m, Nit ac, Nux v, Phos, Puls, Ran b, Rhus t, Stram, Ver a
4. **Hemorrhage—bright red blood:** Acon, Arn, Bell, Carbo v, Dul, Erig, Ferr, Hyo, (**Ip**), Led, Meli, Mill, Nit ac, Phos, Plb, Sabi, Dul, Tril

If More Than One Remedy Fits Most of the Symptoms

If more than one remedy fits most of the symptoms, see which one got the most emphasis in the repertory. The greatest emphasis is given to remedies listed in **BOLD** print. The next degree is the remedies listed in *italics*. The least emphasis is given to the remedies listed in small print. Look for the remedy that appeared most often in **BOLD** or *italics*.

Sample Case

Your patient has burning pains in his stomach, an intense fear of death, is restless, wants small but frequent sips of cold water, has painful diarrhea, is worse being alone, and desires company.

A few remedies show up in most of the symptoms, but Arsenicum (ARS) appears most often either in bold (**ARS**) or italics (*Ars*). It has the most emphasis.

Stomach—burning: **ARS**, *Canth*, Caps, Carbo v, *Cic*, Colch, Merc c, Phos, Ran b, Rob, **SEC**, Sep, **SUL**, *Ver a*

Fear of death: **ACO**, Arn, **ARS**, *Calc*, Cimi, *Gels*, Hyd-ac, Kali c, Lac-c, Nit ac, *Phos*, Plat

Restless, with anxiety: **ARS**, *Calc*, Cimi, Iod, Kali ar, Kali c, Merc, Nat c, Phos

Thirst for cold drinks: Acon, **ARS**, Bism, Bry, Valc, Chin, Diph, Merc, **PHOS**, Rhus t, **VER A**

Thirst—little and often: Aco, Ant t, Apis, **ARS**, Bell, Chin, Hyos, *Lyc*, Rhus

Painful diarrhea: Ars, Bry, Cham, Colo, Merc, Merc c, Rhe, Rhus t, Sul

Company, desire for: Arg n, *Ars*, Bism, Bov, Dros, Hep, Hyo, Kali c, Lac c, Lyc, *Pho*, Radm, **STRAM**

The following is a tiny example of the symptoms and remedies you would find in a repertory.

Mini Repertory

Anger: Aconite, Belladonna, Bryonia, Chamomilla, Colocynth, Lycopodium, Ignatia, Nux vomica, Staphisagria.

Biting: Arsenicum, Antimonium tart, Belladonna, Cantharis, Stramonium.

Bones, pain in: Eupatorium, Ruta, Symphytum, Phytolacca, Mezereum, Rhododendron, Silica.

Company, desires: Argentum nitricum, Arsenicum, Phosphorus, Pulsatilla, Stramonium.

Chilly/cold: Aconite, Arsenicum, Carbo veg, Cimicifuga, Caulophyllum, Cinchona, Colocynth, Eupatorium, Ferrum, Gelsemium, Hypericum, Lycopodium, Mercurius, Nux vomica, Phosphorus, Pyrogenium, Rhus tox.

Cold, better from: Antimonium tart, Apis, Argentum nitricum, Bryonia, Chamomilla, Iodum, Ledum, Lycopodium, Pulsatilla, Sulphur.

Cold application/better from applying something cold: Apis, Pulsatilla, Sulphur, Lycopodium, Chamomilla.

Delirium: Arsenicum, Belladonna, Baptisia, Bryonia, Hyoscyamus, Lachesis, Lycopodium, Rhus tox, Stramonium, Veratrum album.

Doubling up, better from: Colocynth, Magnesia phos.

Fear of being alone: Argentum nitricum, Arsenicum, Hyoscyamus, Kali carbonicum, Lycopodium, Phosphorus, Pulsatilla, Sepia, Stramonium.

Fever with chills: Aconite, Arsenicum, Belladonna, Bryonia, Chamomilla, Cocculus, Drosera, Ferrum, Ignatia, Nux vomica, Pulsatilla, Pyrogenium, Rhus tox, Sepia, Stramonium, Sulphur, Veratrum album, Thuja.

Fever without thirst: Gelsemium, Pulsatilla, Apis.

Fever with much thirst: Arsenicum (small frequent sips), Bryonia, Eupatorium, Hepar, Ipecacuanha, Phosphorus, Stramonium, Sulphur, Veratrum.

Fever with vomiting: Arnica, Arsenicum, Crotalus, Ipecacuanha, Nat mur.

Fever with delirium: Anthracinum, Apis, Arsenicum, Belladonna, Bryonia, Chamomilla, Cinchona, Crotalus, Dulcamara, Hepar, Lachesis, Pyrogenium.

Fever without perspiration: Arsenicum, Belladonna, Bryonia, Gelsemium.

Fight, wants to: Belladonna, Lachesis, Mercurius, Nux vomica.

Heat, better from: Arsenicum, Colocynth, Rhus tox, Hepar, Mag phos, Nux vomica, Mercurius (worse either extreme), Lycopodium (can be worse from either hot or cold).

Heat, worse from: Antimonium tart, Apis, Bryonia, Chamomilla, Drosera, Ipecacuanha, Gelsemium, Lachesis, Ledum, Mercurius, Pulsatilla.

Left-sided complaints: Argentum nitricum, Berberis, Capsicum, Lachesis, Phosphorus, Sepia.

Light, worse from: Aconite, Belladonna, Nux vomica, Phosphorus, Stramonium.

Lying down, worse from: Arsenicum, Belladonna, Glonoine, Hyoscyamus, Lachesis, Phosphorus, Pulsatilla, Rhus tox, Rumex.

Lying on the left side, worse from: Cactus, Kali carb, Phosphorus, Pulsatilla, Spigelia.

Lying on right side, worse from: Magnesia muriaticum, Mercurius, Rhus tox.

Lying on the painless side, worse from: Bryonia, Chamomilla, Pulsatilla.

Lying on back, worse from: Nux vomica, Pulsatilla, Rhus tox.

Midnight, worse after: Arsenicum, Drosera, Kali carb, Nux vomica.

Motion, better from: Apis, Chamomilla, Lycopodium, Pulsatilla, Pyrogenium, Rhus tox

Motion, worse from: Bryonia, Belladonna, Colocynth, Hepar, Ipecacuanha, Ledum, Mercurius, Nux vomica, Veratrum album.

Noise, worse from: Belladonna, Coffea, Chamomilla, Cinchona, Colchicum, Ignatia, Nux vomica, Phosphorus, Spigelia, Theridon.

Odors, sensitive to: Colchicum, Causticum, Phosphorus, Nux vomica, Sepia.

Pain—"throbbing": Aconite, Antimonium tart, Belladonna, Hepar, Ledum, Phosphorus, Sepia.

Pain—"burning": Apis, Arsenicum, Cantharis, Carbo veg, Causticum, Euphrasia, Mercurius, Nux, Rhus tox, Sepia, Phosphorus, Silica, Sulphur.

Pain—in small spots: Arnica, Arsenicum, Berberis, Calcarea phos, Colchicum, Conium, Ignatia, Kali Bichromicum, Lachesis, Sabadilla, Sulphur.

Pain—shifts to the part lain on: Bryonia, Graphites, Kali carb, Nux vomica, Phos acid, Pulsatilla.

Pain, which feels like splinters: Hepar, Nitric acid, Agaricus, Argentum nitricum, Silica.

Perspiration, worse after: Cinchona, Mercurius, Phosphoric acid, Phosphorus, Pulsatilla, Sepia, Staphysagria.

Perspiration, better from: Bryonia, Cuprum, Chamomilla, Gelsemium, Hepar, Rhus tox.

Pressure, better from: Bryonia, Cinchona, Colocynth, Conium, Drosera, Mag. Phos, Pulsatilla.

Pressure, worse from: Apis, Lachesis, Cantharis, Hepar, Lycopodium, Mercurius.

Pupils, dilated: Belladonna, Hyoscyamus, Stramonium, Aethusa, Natrum carbonicum, Helleborus, Gelsemium.

Pupils, contracted: Opium, Thuja.

Open air, desires: Pulsatilla, Argentum nitricum, Carbo veg, Lachesis, Sulphur.

Right-sided complaints: Agaricus, Belladonna, Bryonia, Causticum, Chelidonium, Kali carb, Lycopodium, Magnesia phos, Mercurius, Sanguinaria.

Sleep, worse after: Apis, Cocculus, Lachesis, Opium, Spongia.

Slow onset: Ferrum phos, Gelsemium.

Sudden onset: Aconite, Arsenicum, Belladonna, Cantharis, Nux vomica, Pulsatilla.

Sun, worse from: Antimonium crud, Belladonna, Gelsemium, Glonoine, Natrum Carbonicum, Natrum muriaticum, Pulsatilla.

Swallowing, worse from: Apis, Belladonna, Hepar, Lachesis, Mercurius.

Touch/aversion to being touched: Aconite, Arnica, Agaricus, Antimonium tart, Belladonna, Bryonia, Chamomilla, Cinchona, Coffea, Kali carb, Lachesis, Silica, Tarentula, Thuja.

Thirsty (very): Aconite, Arsenicum, Belladonna, Bryonia, Chamomilla, Cinchona (can be thirstless), Eupatorium, Mercurius, Phosphorus, Pyrogenium, Stramonium, Sulphur, Veratrum.

Thirstless: Antimonium tart, Apis, Cinchona, Gelsemium, Ipecacuanha, Pulsatilla.

Vomiting: Arsenicum, Belladonna, Chamomilla, Cinchona, Hepar, Ipecacuanha, Lycopodium, Nux vomica, Phosphorus, Pulsatilla, Rhus tox, Veratrum album.

Warmth, desires: Arsenicum, Hepar, Sabadilla, Causticum, Colchicum, Kali carb, Silica.

12

Remedies for Your Home Kit

Buying a homeopathic kit is the easiest and most economical way to begin. The remedies listed below are the basic ones you should have. If any of these are not in your kit, then purchase them separately.

If you are prone to certain acute ailments, look up the remedies in this book and order any that you don't have. If you get warning of an epidemic, order any special remedies needed for that.

For a description of these remedies see chapter 5, "Remedy Descriptions."

Aconite 30c & 200c, Allium cepa, Antimonium tart, Apis mel, Argentum nit, Arnica 30c & 200c, Arsenicum album, Belladonna 30c & 200c, Bryonia, Calendula, Calcarea carbonica, Calcarea phos, Cantharis, Carbo veg, Causticum, Chamomilla, Cinchona (China), Cocculus ind, Coffea, Colocynthis, Eupatorium per, Euphrasia, Ferrum Phos, Gelsemium, Glonoinum, Hepar sulph, Hypericum, Ignatia, Ipecac, Kali bich, Lachesis, Ledum, Lycopodium, Magnesia phos, Mercurius viv, Natrum mur, Nux vomica, Phosphorus, Phytolacca, Pulsatilla, Pyrogenium, Rhus tox, Ruta grav, Sepia, Silica, Spongia, Staphysagria, Sulphur, Symphytum, Thuja, Veratrum album.

If Not Included in Your Kit, Purchase These Tinctures and Remedies Separately

Urtica urens tincture: Dilute it for topical treatment of minor burns.

Calendula tincture: Dilute it and use it to cleanse wounds. Crucial for preventing infection and speeding healing.

Hypericum tincture: Dilute and bathe wounds that are extremely painful.

Echinacea tincture: Use this full strength internally, in 30- to 40-drop doses, to help fight infections. May be used in addition to selected remedies.

Hepar sulph (6x)**:** This low potency of Hepar sulph is excellent for local infections involving pus. It helps them find a natural drain. The 30c from the kit is too high for this purpose.

Myristica seb (6c)**:** If a local infection does not yield to Hepar (above) then this remedy may prove stronger in getting the wound to drain.

Baptisia (30c)**:** Toxic states due to infections in the blood. Muscular soreness, putrid secretions and breath, indescribable sick feeling, can only swallow liquids.

Pyrogenium (30c)**:** Toxic states due to infections in the blood. Top remedy for childbed fever. High fever and low pulse or vice versa. Great restlessness. Feels bruised and sore and all secretions are putrid (also Baptisia). Tongue dry and cracked. Often follows Baptisia.

Important Nosodes or Unusual Remedies

If epidemics threaten, some of these remedies might become important:

Anthracinum: Anthrax, boils that spread, gangrene, ulcers.

Crotalus horridus: Ailments with hemorrhaging from every orifice, blood poisoning, carbuncles, peritonitis, yellow fever (no prescription needed).

Diphtherinum: Diphtheria, severe sore throat, myelitis.

Influenzinum: Influenza.

Lathyrus: Polio (no prescription needed).

Malaria officinalis: Malaria.

Pertussin: Whooping cough.

Pestinum or **Plaginum** (Yersinia pestis nosode): Bubonic Plague.

Salmonella typhi nosode: Typhoid.

Septiceminum: Septic infections.

Variolinum: Smallpox.

Vibrio cholerae nosode: Cholera.

Yellow fever nosode: Yellow fever.

13
Resources

Looking for a homeopath in the United States? Want to join a homeopathic study group? Contact:

The National Center for Homeopathy
801 North Fairfax Street, Suite 306
Alexandria, VA 22314-1757
tel: 703-548-7790, 877-624-0613
http://www.homeopathic.org
e-mail: info@homeopathic.org

To Read About and Buy Homeopathic Books

Minimum Price Books
P.O. Box 2187
Blaine, WA 98231
tel: 604-597-4757, orders: 800-663-8272
http://www.minimum.com
e-mail: orders@minimum.com

Homeopathic Educational Services
2124B Kittredge St.
Berkeley, CA 94704
tel: 510-649-0294, orders: 800-359-9051
http://www.homeopathic.com
e-mail: mail@homeopathic.com

Recommended Books

Pocket Book of Materia Medica with Repertory by Dr. William Boericke, Indian Edition, in English (Paharganj, New Delhi, India: B. Jain Publishers, Ltd., 1999). To gain more in-depth knowledge, this book would be the next step. It gives detailed descriptions of hundreds of remedies. It also includes a basic mini-repertory with which you can look up hundreds of symptoms and modalities.

Homoeopathic Medicine for Dogs: A Handbook for Vets and Pet Owners by H. G. Wolff (London: C. W. Daniel, 1998). One of my favorites. A clear, concise, easy-to-use work for treating dogs. It has many gems of knowledge not found anywhere else.

Your Healthy Cat by H. G. Wolff (Berkeley, CA: North Atlantic Books, 1991). A little treasure. A user-friendly handbook for treating cats with homeopathy.

The books by H.G. Wolff currently may be out of print or difficult to find, but they are worth tracking down. I would recommend checking with your local library or used bookstore.

Where to Buy Homeopathic Remedies

Remedies and kits are available at many health food stores. Remedies and kits not available locally can be ordered from the pharmacies listed on the next page.

United States

These pharmacies make remedies, sell kits, and will ship anywhere in the world.

Natural Health Supply
6410 Avenida Christina
Sante Fe, NM 87507
tel: 888-689-1608 or 505-474-9175
fax: 505-473-0336
http://www.a2zhomeopathy.com
e-mail: nhs@a2zhomeopathy.com

Hahnemann Laboratories, Inc.
1940 Fourth St.
San Rafael, CA 94901
tel: 888-427-6422, tel: 415-451-6978
fax: 415-451-6981
http://www.hahnemannlabs.com and http://www.Homrem.com
To place orders by e-mail: mqhahnlabs@aol.com

Boiron-Bornemann, Inc.
Box 449
6 Campus Ave. Building A
Newtown Square, PA 19073
tel: 800-258-8823 (professional and wholesale customer service)
http://www.boiron.com
Call for the retail or mail order outlet nearest you: Boiron Information Center: 800-264-7661.

England

Both of these pharmacies will ship worldwide.

Helios Homœopathy, Ltd.
89–97 Camden Rd.
Tunbridge Wells
Kent TN1 2QR
England
tel: 011+44 (0)1892 537254, fax: +44 (0)1892 546850
http://www.helios.co.uk/

Ainsworths
36 New Cavendish St.
London W1G 8UF
tel: 020 7935 5330, fax: 020 7486 4313
http://www.ainsworths.com/site/default.aspx

Websites

These websites (current at the time of publication) will guide you to a myriad of homeopathic resources, including hundreds of other websites on homeopathy. They will help you find a homeopath anywhere, as well as homeopathic veterinarians, nurses, pharmacists, articles, journals and research papers, books to read free online, discussion forums, homeopathic hospitals and clinics, and national and international organizations and schools.

Homeopathy Home
http://www.homeopathyhome.com/index.shtml
Whole Health Now
http://www.wholehealthnow.com/
Hpathy.com
http://hpathy.com/
Homeopathic Medicine for Animals and Humans: Best Links
http://homepage.eircom.net/~progers/homeo.htm

Find a Homeopath Outside the United States

Canada

National United Professional Association of Trained Homeopaths
http://www.nupath.org/
Canada's One-Stop Homeopathy Network
http://www.canadahomeopathy.com/

England

British Homeopathic Association
http://www.trusthomeopathy.org/
England: The Society of Homeopaths
http://www.homeopathy-soh.org/

Australia

Australian Homeopathic Association
http://www.homeopathyoz.org/practitionersHelp.html

New Zealand

New Zealand Council of Homeopaths
http://www.homeopathy.co.nz/

Bibliography

Allen, H. C. *Keynotes.* Paharganj, New Delhi, India: B. Jain Publishers Ltd., 1992.

Bailey, Philip M. *Homeopathic Psychology: Personality Profiles of the Major Constitutional Remedies.* Berkeley, CA: North Atlantic Books, 1995.

Banerjee, D. D. *Textbook of Homeopathic Pharmacy.* Paharganj, New Delhi, India: B. Jain Publishers, Ltd., 1999.

Begley, Sharon. "The End of Antibiotics." *Newsweek*, March 7, 1994.

Blackie, Margery. *Classical Homeopathy.* Beaconsfield, UK: Beaconsfield Publishers, 1986.

Boericke, W. *Homeopathic Materia Medica with Repertory.* Paharganj, New Delhi, India: B. Jain Publishers Ltd., 1999.

———. *The Twelve Tissue Remedies of Schussler.* Paharganj, New Delhi, India: B. Jain Publishers, Ltd., 1998.

Borland, Douglas M. *Homeopathy in Practice.* Beaconsfield, UK: Beaconsfield Publishers, 1998.

———. *Some Emergencies of General Practice.* Paharganj, New Delhi, India: B. Jain Publishers, Ltd., 1991.

Bradford, Thomas L. *The Logic of Figures or Comparative Results of Homeopathic and Other Treatments.* Philadelphia, PA: Boericke and Tafel, 1900.

Castro, D. and G. G. Nogueira. "Use of the Nosode Meningococcinum as a Preventive Against Meningitis." *Journal of the American Institute of Homeopathy* 68 (December 1975): 211–219.

Castro, Miranda. *Homeopathy for Pregnancy, Birth, and Your Baby's First Year.* New York: Saint Martin's Press, 1993.

Centers for Disease Control and Prevention. "Diseases Connected to Antibiotic Resistance." http://www.cdc.gov/drugresistance/diseases.htm.

Chitkara, H. L. *Materia Medica of the Mind.* Paharganj, New Delhi, India: B. Jain Publishers, Ltd., 1994.

Clarke, John H. *Dictionary of Practical Materia Medica.* Paharganj, New Delhi, India: B. Jain Publishers Ltd., 1992.

———. *Diseases of the Heart & Arteries.* Paharganj, New Delhi, India: B. Jain Publishers Ltd., 2001.

———. *The Prescriber.* Essex, England: Health Science Press, 1972.

Coulter, Catherine R. *Portraits of Homeopathic Medicines: Psychophysical Analyses of Selected Constitutional Types, vol. I.* Berkeley, CA: North Atlantic Books, 1986.

———. *Portraits of Homeopathic Medicines: Psychophysical Analyses of Selected Constitutional Types, vol II.* Berkeley, CA: North Atlantic Books, 1988.

Coulter, Harris L. *Divided Legacy: The Conflict Between Homeopathy and the American Medical Association, Volume III: Science and Ethics in American Medicine 1800–1914.* Berkeley, CA: North Atlantic Books, 1982. [An excellent discussion of the history of homeopathy in the United States, including its persecution by the AMA.]

Currim, Ahmed N., ed. *The Collected Works of Arthur Hill Grimmer, MD.* Norwalk, CT, and Greifenberg, Germany: Hahnemann International Institute for Homeopathic Documentation, 1996.

Das, Bishambar. *Select Your Remedy.* Paharganj, New Delhi, India: B. Jain Publishers, Ltd., 1992.

Das, Eswara. *Synopsis of Homeopathic Aetiology.* Paharganj, New Delhi, India: B. Jain Publishers, Ltd., 1988.

de Schepper, Luc. *Hahnemann Revisited: A Textbook of Classical Homeopathy for the Professional.* Sante Fe, NM: Full of Life Publishing, 1999.

Dewey, W. A. "Homeopathy in Influenza: A Chorus of Fifty in Harmony." *Journal of the American Institute of Homeopathy*, May 1921.

Dhawale, M. L. *Principles and Practice of Homeopathy , Vol. 1: Homeopathic Philosophy and Repertorization.* Bombay, India: Institute of Clinical Research, 1985.

Frye, Joyce. "Comprehensive Medical Care for Bioterrorism Exposure: Are We Making Evidence-Based Decisions? What Are the Research Needs?" National Center for Homeopathy. November 14, 2001. http://www.homeopathic.org/crreform.htm.

Gibson, Douglas. *Studies of Homeopathic Remedies.* Beaconsfield, UK: Beaconsfield Publishers, 1994.

Goldberg, Burton, ed. *Alternative Medicine: The Definitive Guide.* Tiburon, CA: Future Medicine Publishing, 1997.

Golden, Isaac. "Homeopathic Disease Prevention." *Homeopathy Online.* http://www.lyghtforce.com/HomeopathyOnline/text/golden.htm.

———. *Homoeoprophylaxis: A Fifteen Year Clinical Study.* Daylesford, Victoria, Australia: Isaac Golden Publications, 2005.

Gray, Bill. *Homeopathy: Science or Myth?* Berkeley, CA: North Atlantic Books, 2000.

Hahnemann, Samuel. *Organon of Medicine.* 6th ed., Kunzli, Jost. trans. Blaine, WA: Cooper Publishing, 1982.

Hoff, Douglas. *Homeo Info.* http://homeoinfo.com/02_history/index.php. [Discusses the use of homeopathy around the world, including its historical development in each country.]

Holvey, D., ed. *Merck Manual of Diagnosis and Therapy*. Rahway, NJ: Merck, Sharp & Dohme, 1972.

Hoover, Todd A. "Homeopathic Prophylaxis: Fact or Fiction." National Center for Homeopathy. http://www.homeopathic.org/crtoddh.htm.

Hubbard, Elizabeth Wright. *Homeopathy as Art and Science*. Beaconsfield, UK: Beaconsfield Publishers, 1990.

Idarius, Betty. *The Homeopathic Childbirth Manual*. Ukiah, CA: Idarius Press, 1996.

Kent, James Tyler. *Lectures on Homeopathic Materia Medica*. Paharganj, New Delhi, India: B. Jain Publishers, Ltd., 1990.

Lazarou, Jason, Bruce H. Pomeranz, and Paul N. Corey. "Incidence of Adverse Drug Reactions in Hospitalized Patients: A Meta-analysis of Prospective Studies," *Journal of the American Medical Association* 279 (April 1998): 1200–1205.

Lessell, Colin B., *The Dental Prescriber*. London: British Homeopathic Association, 1983.

———. *The World Travellers' Manual of Homeopathy*. London: C. W. Daniel, 1993.

Lilienthal, Samuel. *Homeopathic Therapeutics*. Paharganj, New Delhi, India: B. Jain Publishers, Ltd., 1994.

Little, David. "Testimony of Great Homeopaths." National Center for Homeopathy. http://www.homeopathic.org/crhistDL.htm.

Mathur, K. N. *Principles of Prescribing*. New. Paharganj, New Delhi, India: B. Jain Publishers, Ltd., 1994.

Maury, E. A. *Drainage in Homeopathy*. Essex, England: Health Science Press, 1982.

Moffat, John L. *Homeopathic Therapeutics in Ophthalmology*. Paharganj, New Delhi, India: B. Jain Publishers, Ltd., 1995.

Morrison, Roger. *Desktop Guide to Keynotes and Confirmatory Symptoms*. Albany, CA: Hahnemann Clinic Publishing,1993.

Moskowitz, Richard. *Homeopathic Medicines for Pregnancy and Childbirth*. Berkeley, CA: North Atlantic Books, 1992.

Motz, Lloyd, and Jefferson Hane Weaver. *The Story of Physics*. New York: Avon Books, 1989.

Murphy, Robin. *Homeopathic Medical Repertory*. Pagosa Springs, CO: Hahnemann Academy of North America, 1993.

———. *Lotus Materia Medica*. Pagosa Springs, CO: Lotus Star Academy, 1995.

Nash, E. B. *Leaders in Homeopathic Therapeutics*. Paharganj, New Delhi, India: B. Jain Publishers, Ltd., 1993.

National Vaccine Information Center. http://www.909shot.com/. [The NVIC is the oldest and largest parent-led organization advocating reform of the mass vaccination system. Their work includes promoting research, education, evaluation of vaccines, and more.]

Nauman, Eileen. *Poisons That Heal*. Sedona, AZ: Light Technology Publishing, 1995.

Nordenberg, Tamar. "Miracle Drugs vs. Superbugs: Preserving the Usefulness of Antibiotics." *FDA Consumer Magazine* (November–December, 1998). This article can be found online at: http://www.fda.gov/fdac/features/1998/698_bugs.html.

"The Number of Uninsured Americans Continued to Rise in 2004." Center on Budget and Policy Priorities. August 30, 2005. http://www.cbpp.org/8-30-05health.htm.

Perko, Sandra J. *The Homeopathic Treatment of Influenza.* San Antonio, TX: Benchmark Homeopathic Publications, 1999.

Rawat, P. S. *Select Your Dose and Potency*. Paharganj, New Delhi, India: B. Jain Publishers, Ltd., 1992.

Reichenberg-Ullman, Judyth and Robert Ullman. *Homeopathic Self-Care: The Quick & Easy Guide for the Whole Family.* Rocklin, CA: Prima Publishing, 1997.

Roberts, Herbert A. *Sensations As If.* Paharganj, New Delhi, India: B. Jain Publishers Ltd., 1990.

Sankaran, Rajan. *Spirit of Homeopathy.* Paharganj, New Delhi, India: B. Jain Publishers, Ltd., 1991.

Shepherd, Dorothy. *Homoeopathy in Epidemic Diseases.* Essex, England: C. W. Daniel Company, Ltd, 1967.

Smith, Trevor. *Homeopathy for Pregnancy and Nursing Mothers.* Sussex, England: Insight Editions, 1993.

Smits, Tinus. "Homeopathy and Vaccination." http://www.tinussmits.com/english/.

Starre, Jeffrey J. *Vaccine Free: Prevention & Treatment with Homeopathy.* Jewett, OH: Two Hearts Medical Publishing, 1998.

Tobin, Stephen. "Lyme Disease and Homeopathy." Foundation for the Advancement of Innovative Medicine. http://www.faim.org/newslet/95-01/tobin.htm.

Tyler, Margaret L. *Homeopathic Drug Pictures: A Textbook of Classical Homeopathy for the Professional.* Paharganj, New Delhi, India: B. Jain Publishers, Ltd., 1991.

———. *Pointers to the Commmon Remedies: A Textbook of Classical Homeopathy for the Professional.* Paharganj, New Delhi, India: B. Jain Publishers, Ltd., 1991.

Ullman, Dana. *Discovering Homeopathy: Medicine for the 21st Century.* Berkeley, CA: North Atlantic Books, 1991.

———. "Quotes in Support of Homeopathy." Homeopathic Educational Services. http://www.homeopathic.com/articles/media/quotes.php.

U.S. Food and Drug Administration. "FDA Task Force on Antimicrobial Resistance: Key Recommendations and Report." December, 2000. http://www.fda.gov/oc/antimicrobial/taskforce2000.html.

Vermeulen, Frans. *Synoptic Materia Medica.* Haarlem, Netherlands: Merlijn Publishers, 1992.

Vithoulkas, George. *Essence of Materia Medica: A Textbook of Classical Homeopathy for the Professional.* Paharganj, New Delhi, India: B. Jain Publishers, Ltd., 1995.

von Boenninghausen, C. M. F. *Therapeutic Pocket Book.* Paharganj, New Delhi, India: B. Jain Publishers, Ltd., 1990.

Weiner, Michael. *The Complete Book of Homeopathy.* New York: Avery Publishing, 1989.

Whale.to. "VICP & Vaccine Damage Act Payments." http://www.whale.to/v/vicp5.html.

Winston, Julian. *The Faces of Homeopathy: An Illustrated History of the First 200 Years.* Tawa, New Zealand: Great Auk Publishing, 2002.

———. "Influenza 1918: Homeopathy to the Rescue." *The New England Journal of Homeopathy*. 7 no. 1 (Spring/Summer 1998). This article can be found online at http://www.nesh.com/main/nejh/samples/winston.html.

———. "Some History of the Treatment of Epidemics with Homeopathy." National Center for Homeopathy. http://www.homeopathic.org/crhistJW2.htm. [Julian Winston was the most respected contemporary historian of homeopathy.]

Index

Please note: For an alphabetical guide to specific ailments, please see chapter 3, "Ailments A to Z."

BOOKS OF RELATED INTEREST FROM NAB

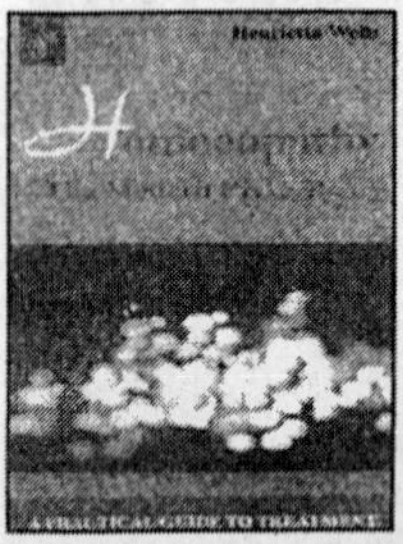

HOMOEOPATHY

The Modern Prescriber

—Henrietta Wells

This book is a very practical approach to using homoeopathic remedies. It gives step-by-step instructions for many first aid situations—from dog bites and wasp stings to tooth abscesses, sunstroke, burns and injuries of all kinds. It explains how to treat everyday coughs, colds, fevers and flu, and gives advice on cures for food poisoning and even hangovers.

ISBN: 81-7822-131-4

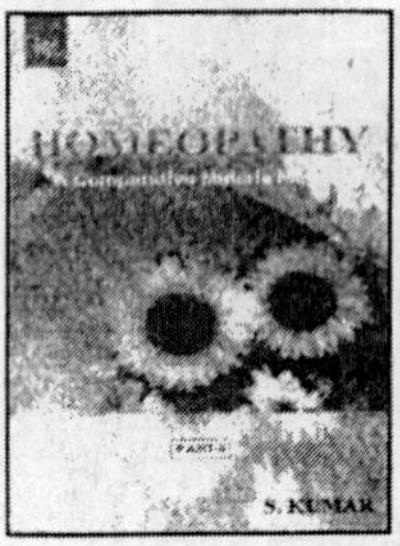

HOMEOPATHY

A Comparative Materia Medica

—S. Kumar

The book, in two parts, has a special feature, "a brief synopsis of the Organon of Medicine" of Hahnemann. All symptoms of a drug included in this book have been taken from leading homeopathic authorities. In this book, a medicine is divided under seven subheadings, all interdependent and interrelated.

ISBN: 81-7822-040-7

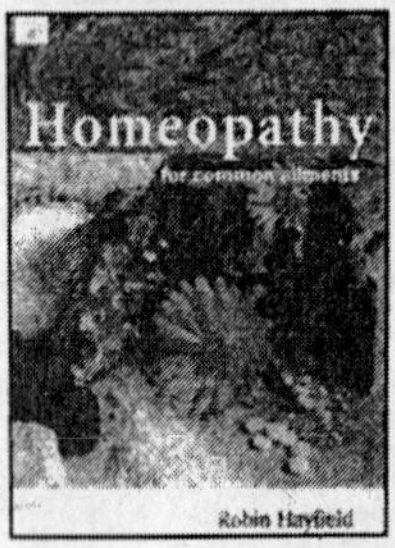

HOMEOPATHY

For Common Ailments

—Robin Hayfield

Homeopathy for Common Ailments is a practical, beautifully illustrated guide that explain and demystifies this safe and simple form of treatment. As well as offering guidance for treating children and using homeopathy for first aid, the book will help you to select and use widely available homeopathic remedies to treat frequently encountered physical and mental health problems.

ISBN: 81-7822-044-x